THE
PALEOLITHIC
PRESCRIPTION

A PROGRAM
OF DIET & EXERCISE
AND A
DESIGN FOR LIVING

**S. Boyd Eaton, M.D., Marjorie Shostak,
and Melvin Konner, M.D., Ph.D.**

Harper & Row, Publishers, New York
Grand Rapids, Philadelphia, St. Louis, San Francisco
London, Singapore, Sydney, Tokyo

*To the memory of our ancestors, whose genes we bear,
and to the small number of remaining hunters and gatherers
who have taught us so much about ourselves*

Ten percent of the authors' earnings from the sales of this book are being divided among the L. S. B. Leakey Foundation (which does research on human evolution), Cultural Survival and the Kalahari People's Fund (which are devoted to the protection of present-day hunters and gatherers and other small-scale societies).

A hardcover edition of this book was published in 1988 by Harper & Row, Publishers.

First PERENNIAL LIBRARY edition published 1989.

Library of Congress Cataloging-in-Publication Data

Eaton, S. Boyd
    The Paleolithic prescription.

    "Perennial Library."
    Includes index.
    1. Health.   2. Nutrition.   3. Exercise.   4. Anxiety—
Prevention   5. Man, Prehistoric.   I. Shostak,
Marjorie, date–.   II. Konner, Melvin.   III. Title.
RA776.E183   1989   613   87–45611
ISBN 0-06-091635-4 (pbk.)

89 90 91 92 93 FG 10 9 8 7 6 5 4 3 2 1

CONTENTS

TABLES

PREFACE

To some people, this book will be worth a lot of laughs.

We know, because when two of us published a technical paper on the same subject in a leading medical journal—*The New England Journal of Medicine*—there were funny cartoons and editorials in many newspapers. The *Washington Post* depicted a future in which a typical suburban man would be seen leaving the house in the morning in an outfit made of skins, carrying a club, and sending every squirrel in the neighborhood running for cover. The *Atlanta Journal-Constitution* ran a cartoon showing a caveman pushing a supermarket cart. Ellen Goodman, the syndicated columnist, made us the butt of her celebrated wit, and an accompanying drawing (it showed old-fashioned savages dancing around a fire) was captioned "Make mine mammoth." We got a kick out of all this too, showed the cartoons around, and even made jokes with waiters in restaurants (one night we ordered saber-toothed tiger with assorted roots and berries).

But officially at least, the medical profession wasn't laughing. We received scores of letters from physicians and medical scientists applauding our analysis and contributing further to our data base. Our article was quoted in many medical journals and at conferences throughout the world. Leaders of preventive medicine as well as anthropology, such as those whose comments appear on the book's jacket, welcomed our perspective as throwing new light on important questions about health and fitness. Alexander Leaf, one of the most distinguished preventive health experts, drew heavily from our article in his keynote address to the International Society of Clinical Nutrition meeting in 1987. And other scientists have begun to reach similar conclusions in their own independent research.

So enjoy the jokes that are sure to be made, but also get the message: In Paleolithic times our ancestors had many health problems, but they didn't have the ones we have. We have conquered many microbes, but we suffer chronically from diseases caused by our life-style—diseases that our ancestors effectively avoided. We need to relearn some important things they knew. The "diseases of civilization" cause untold suffering. We can largely avoid them in our own lives and reduce the colossal burden they impose on our society. Once we overcome our biases about the past, we will realize that the people we see as primitive have a lot to teach us, that looking back can help us to move forward. It's not only good for us—it's philosophically fascinating. And yes, it's even good for a few laughs. Since recent findings suggest that laughter can help fight disease, we're for it as health experts as well as on general principles.

So read, learn, get healthier—and enjoy!

ACKNOWLEDGMENTS

This book has been many years in the making, and many people have helped along the way. For generosity with time and knowledge, we thank the following scientists and physicians: James Anderson, Lawrence Angel, Ronald Barr, Henry Blackburn, Denis Blanton, Barbara Bocek, Jennie Brand, Steven Brandt, Peter Brown, Vicky Burbank, Errett Callahan, William Connor, Patricia Draper, James A. Duke, David Frayer, John Garrow, Antonio M. Gotto, Jr., M.D., Richard Gould, M. R. C. Greenwood, Agnes Estokio-Griffin, P. Bion Griffin, Marvin Harris, Kristen Hawkes, Robert Heaney, Kim Hill, Nancy Howell, Christopher Howson, Magdalena Hurtado, Glynn Isaac, Donald Johanson, Betty Ann Kevles, Daniel Kevles, Laura Klein, Louise Lamphere, Clark Spencer Larsen, Richard Leakey, Anthony Leeds, Roger Lewin, David McCarron, Donald McCormick, Nina Marable, David Martin, Katherine Milton, Harold Newmark, Eileen O'Brien, Kerin O'Dea, Lot Page, Nadine Peacock, Trevor Redgrave, John Rick, William Roberts, John Robson, Otto Schaefer, Margaret Schoeninger, Pat Shipman, Mark Skinner, Fred Smith, D. A. T. Southgate, Geoffrey Sperber, John Speth, Michael Stone, Christy Turner, Peter Van Soest, Alan Walker, Beatrice Whiting, Edwin Wilmsen, Richard Wrangham, D. T. Yen, and especially Denis Burkitt, Irven DeVore, Alexander Leaf, and Richard Lee.

For assistance in library research, we are grateful to Marilyn Littles and Reta Smith. For shepherding our book through the complex process of publication, we thank Lawrence Ashmead, Ann Finlayson, Elaine Markson, Geri Thoma, Margaret Wimberger, and their respective staffs.

Manuscript preparation was expertly done by Angela Bell, Debra Fey, Sharon Minors, and Elaine Warlick.

For crucial institutional support, we thank the administrations and staff of HCA West Paces Ferry Hospital, Altanta; Emory University, especially the Department of Anthropology, Atlanta; the Center for Advanced Study in the Behavioral Sciences, Stanford, California; and the Institute for Research on Women and Gender, Stanford University.

For showing us by their own examples that it is in fact possible to live according to the principles presented here, we thank Fred Allman, David Apple, Peter Berry, Louise Berry, Shirley Brown, George Cahill, John Cantwell, Gerald Domescik, Frank Ferrier, James Funk, John Garrett, John Horney, Robert Lathan, William Whaley, Robert Whipple, Mary Lou Williams, and Tony Williams.

For various kinds of encouragement and support, we thank Farid Ahmed, the Clark A. Baker Memorial Dinner Club, Clifford Barger, Joe and Kay Beck, Michael Cantor, Neal Chandler, William Dismukes, Barbara Erwin, Bradford Fletcher, Gordon Getty, Ellen Goldman, Bill Heidecker, Sarah Hill, Joe Jackson, Laura Smith Kamler, Lois Kasper, Elizabeth Knoll, Lawrence Konner, Ronnie Wenker Konner, William Lang, Arthur Lazik, Bella Linden, Sandra Mackey, Dan Mackey, Richard Matthews, Barbara McKenzie, Kathy Mote, Barbara Newsom, Sandra Nissenberg, Ray Pauley, Lucy Shostak, Sarah Steinhardt, John Stone, Jerome Walker, Melissa Walker, Frank Woods, and Kay Woods; and the technologists and personnel of the West Paces Ferry Radiology Department. Gratitude also goes to our respective parents—Doris and Stanley Eaton, Edna and Jerome Shostak, and Hannah and Irving Konner—and to our children: Catherine, Boyd, and Charles Eaton, and Susanna, Adam, and Sarah (Shostak) Konner; and especially, Daphne Eaton, who has steadfastly and cheerfully endured ten years of this project and whose love and support has made it possible.

The Paleolithic Prescription presents a general plan for recapturing certain features of our ancestors' lives and for integrating these elements with our own life-style. If all Americans and citizens of other industrialized nations adopted these recommendations there is little question that our collective burden of chronic diseases would be greatly reduced. But this is not to say that each individual can, by so living, eliminate all possibility of heart attack, cancer, diabetes, or other diseases. One's previous pattern of health-related practices, one's genetically determined susceptibility, and a certain amount of luck also influence the health of specific individuals.

Exercise programs are not without risk. Previously sedentary readers who wish to begin such a program need to first consult a physician to be sure there is no medical contraindication. For individuals over age forty, the examination should include a stress electrocardiogram (an ECG performed during exercise on a treadmill or bicycle apparatus). Any weight loss program, especially for the obese, should be undertaken with moderation and under appropriate medical supervision.

The concepts presented in *The Paleolithic Prescription* are as up-to-date as possible and, except as noted, consistent with informed scientific opinion at the time the manuscript for this book was completed. Nevertheless, the many scientific disciplines from which the book's material is drawn are fast-moving. Informed opinion or what now seem solidly established facts may be challenged or disproved in the future as our understanding of the past and its application to the present develop and improve.

CHAPTER ONE
THE PALEOLITHIC LEGACY

Who are we? Where do we come from? People have asked these questions for millennia. Their importance is reflected in the myths and religious accounts of human origins common to nearly all the earth's cultures. In our own society, little more than a hundred years ago, existing ideas about human origins were challenged by Charles Darwin, who linked us by blood—or, as we would now put it, by genes—to a long line of apes and other animals.

But we don't say much about that heritage today. The dismay, the outcry that erupted around Darwin's writings jolted polite Victorian society out of its high-minded vision of itself. Yet during the twentieth century, among educated people there has been widespread acceptance of Darwin's ideas; only a handful of scientists and a few religious extremists continue to see issues worthy of debate. The rest of us accept the basic premises of evolution, forget them promptly, and move on with our lives.

How important is evolution, after all? The forces that shaped prehistoric life hardly seem relevant today. Certainly the popular image of our ancient past, evoked by the term "caveman" and exemplified by rude-looking oafs swinging clubs at women and dinosaurs, leaves us feeling more relieved by each day that separates us further from this unappealing alternative to the comforts of modern existence.

A slightly more sophisticated misconception concerns a time when a particularly aggressive prehuman primate ancestor roamed the earth, armed with an insatiable appetite for, and considerable ability to procure, game. We are supposedly unable to shake the genetic legacy of this "killer ape" past, and our human predilection for aggression and violence is thus explained. Our "hunting instinct" has gone awry in

1

"civilized" society, where the thrill of the chase and the kill are no longer part of our experience and there are no clear avenues of expression except, perhaps to our peril, in the streets and subways of today's urban jungles.

Despite these erring views, and whether we like it or not, the ancient past does live in the present—in each and every one of us. We acknowledge, even beam at, the evidence that our children look like us. We know that we ourselves look like our parents and they, in turn, like theirs. We have little trouble accepting the genetic inheritance we are born with and which we pass on.

Yet we rarely look further back; if we did, we would discover the linkage continuing, generation upon generation, back through unimaginable lengths of time, through war and famine, through ice ages and thaws, through geographic and political change, not just to Noah and Adam but to a place and time 40,000 years ago when the most remote ancestors whom we can call fully human spread over the earth, hunting wild animals and gathering wild plant foods. They, too, carried an ancient inheritance in their genes, an unbroken, evolving chain a billion years old. And just as our children reflect our own genetic inheritance, we reflect theirs.

Now that we must own up to these mysterious figures in our family tree, who were they? Even if they were not quite thoroughly brutish cavemen, do we really want to paste their images into our family album?

There is no need for embarrassment. To begin with, people of 40,000 years ago lived in caves only rarely, preferring the open air. They didn't utter grunts and snorts, but expressed themselves in fully human speech. In contrast to our earlier ancestors whose anatomy would have impeded speech as we know it, they had brain structures and throat configurations identical to our own. They didn't live at the same time that dinosaurs lived—that was 70 million years earlier. And they almost certainly didn't drag women around by their hair. In fact, anatomically, physiologically, and psychologically, they were modern human beings, reflecting the same range of variations in human physique and basic biological function as people alive today.

To understand what life was like then, let us suppose for a moment that you and your family and a dozen or more others were living in a reasonably hospitable locale somewhere on the earth 40,000 years ago, long before you or anyone else knew about planting crops or domesticating animals. Despite the untamed environment, the wildlife and physical features of your natural surroundings would be extraordinarily familiar to you. People who live by hunting and gathering, with limited shelter from the elements, are of necessity attuned to natural signs far more subtle than those that trigger the awareness of most people today. And because of the closeness and interdependence of life in small bands you would know the people with whom you lived almost as intimately as you know yourself.

Daily life would abound with the activity of adults and children talking, arguing, laughing, and playing. One young couple enjoying their newborn sit close beside one another, watching with amusement as their four-year-old clumsily struggles to hold the new baby. The young girl's attention suddenly drifts to the sounds of children playing nearby, and she nearly drops the infant in her haste to join the excitement. The mother cradles the startled baby in her arms, and quiets him by putting him to her breast. The couple roasts meat from a recent kill, to be eaten with an abundance of ripe roots that taste like delicious fresh-roasted potatoes, followed by fruit soup and sweet berries.

The woman's younger sister, considered quite beautiful, notices the little feast and sits down to join them. She brings news of the women with whom she has gone gathering earlier that day. On their return from a six- or seven-mile walk, they discovered a large cache of honey in a tree not far from home. A discussion ensues as to the best strategy for obtaining the prize without suffering too many stings. Then talk drifts to a near-mishap that befell one of the men when out hunting.

He had wounded an unusually large antelope and had been tracking it for several hours. Tired, somewhat discouraged, and unaware that the animal was resting nearby, he stumbled into a thorn bush and let out a yelp of pain. The antelope jumped up in fright, practically under his nose, and lumbered off. The surprised hunter frantically and rather comically pulled thorns from his leg and foot as he hopped after it. A fresh animal could have easily escaped such ineffectual pursuit, but because of the spear wound and its sudden burst of effort, the antelope stumbled and fell, allowing the hunter to catch up and kill it. Amid peals of laughter over the hunt's antic conclusion, plans are made for the next day to gather the honey and retrieve the meat—hung safely on tree branches to dry.

The day ends. Firewood is collected for the night as darkness descends. Talk continues long after the children are asleep, but gradually thins even among the late-night stalwarts; at last only the sound of a healer playing a stringed instrument and singing plaintive songs gives voice to the deep quiet of the night. The stars move imperceptibly overhead, but as the hours pass, their motion is so striking that, in the vast silence, they almost seem to make a sound. Figures lie quietly beside the fire, shifting for comfort or companionship, sitting up momentarily to stoke the fire or quiet a child. Hours later, the dark becomes ever-so-slightly lighter, heralding the new day.

This was the Paleolithic period—the Old Stone Age—during which hunting and gathering were the only means of subsistence. People lived in seminomadic bands, dispersed over the various kinds of landscape—savanna, coastal, riverine, and subglacial—that comprised the habitable world. They moved with the seasons, following game, water, and plant foods and aggregated and separated as ecological and interpersonal situations required. They were lean, lithe, and strong—the imprint of the physical activity central to their lives. Although their diet was occasionally insufficient in quantity, and hunger was sometimes part of their world, they usually had enough; and when they did, the food was qualitatively ideal to maintain health. They were often struck down by illness, but it was brought on by microbes—not by deterioration resulting from chronic mistreatment of their bodies. As everyone knows, they had a short life expectancy at birth; but that was mainly because so many died in childhood. Those who survived the assault of accident and infection could look forward to a relatively long, fit life, untroubled by the major diseases *we* bring on *ourselves*.

If, as seems almost certain, they were psychologically similar to hunters and gatherers studied in this century, they were much like us—experiencing most of the same hopes, doubts, desires, pleasures, challenges, disappointments, and conflicts. But they experienced them together. Social isolation, with its now established threat to mental and physical health, was unknown to them. Stresses were numerous, but they arose out of the realities of life, not from clock watching, traffic jams, or class consciousness. Their lives were spent working, playing, eating, sleeping, entertaining, and worshiping—with a close-knit group of people who, as much as they might complain, cared for one another. When tensions arose that couldn't be resolved, they were free to move off and join other friends and relatives in a different band for varying lengths of time. Their children grew up in that same context of closeness, nurturance, and love.

This way of life characterized every generation of human beings on our planet for most of the course of human evolution. But then an event of momentous biological significance occurred: Some of our ancestors abandoned their age-old hunting and gathering way of life for a more settled existence based on agriculture and, eventually, on animal husbandry. Like a genie finally let out of a bottle, powerful and unprecedented forces were unleashed, ones that were unlike those which had controlled the ecology and evolution of plants, animals, and microorganisms during the preceding 3 billion years of life on earth.

This event, known as the Neolithic Revolution, transformed the planet: Whereas 10,000 years ago all people hunted and gathered for a living, fewer than one-thousandth of 1 percent carry on that tradition today. Once introduced, agriculture prevailed as the leading pattern for human subsistence until about two hundred years ago, when another change of immense import—the Industrial Revolution—occurred. With it came a new set of forces that interacted on an ever-increasing scale with the ancient forces of nature, intensifying by a hundredfold an already complex interaction.

Technological progress, aside from its complex influence on the biosphere, has also had a profound effect on human biology. Men and women in modern Western society are exposed to conditions of life that differ radically from those of the pre-Neolithic epoch—those which, through Darwinian natural selection, determined the biological characteristics of the human species as it now exists.

When conditions of life for any animal population deviate from those to which it has genetically adapted, biological maladjustment—discordance—is inevitable. The human species is no exception. For us, discordance between our current life-style and the one in which we evolved has promoted the chronic and deadly "diseases of civilization": the heart attacks, strokes, cancer, diabetes, emphysema, hypertension, cirrhosis, and like illnesses that cause 75 percent of all mortality in the United States and other industrialized nations.

Most of these illnesses simply did not exist, or were very rare, in the society of our Paleolithic ancestors. They, like us, had the genetic potential for these disorders, but it took *our* life-style to bring those genetic susceptibilities to the fore. Of course, our ancestors died earlier than we do on the average, but they died of causes we have now largely controlled, such as deadly infectious diseases, complications of childbirth, and trauma. *We*, in turn, die of illnesses which were uncommon in *their* world—illnesses whose frequency is encouraged by much in our "self-made" environment. With sanitation, pesticides, vaccination, and antibiotics, we hold back what has been called the "restless tide" of microbes. But with comparable technology we have also created other, less beneficial, circumstances and thereby undermined our health in unprecedented ways.

Occasionally one hears the claim that primitive people all died too young to get degenerative diseases. This claim is simply false—many lived well into and through the age of vulnerability for such disorders, yet didn't get them, while in our population even young people often show early signs of them. Sometimes one hears the argument that the few who lived into old age in such societies were exceptionally hardy. But it makes no sense medically to link an ability to fend off microbes in childhood with resistance to heart disease in middle age. Our understanding of the relationships among ancient genes, fast-paced cultural change, evolutionary adaptation, and modern disease has been slow in developing. Its beginnings were intuitive rather than scientific. In 1754, philosopher Jean-Jacques Rousseau wrote that in a "state of nature" men were strong of limb, fleet of foot, and clear of eye. He contrasted this natural condition of health with the proliferating diseases engendered in civilization by wealth and sedentary occupations: "The greater part of our ills are of our own making and we might have avoided them, nearly all, by adhering to that simple . . . manner of life which nature prescribed. When we think of the savages . . . and reflect that they are troubled with hardly any disorders save wounds and old age, we are tempted to believe that in following the history of civil society we shall be telling that of human sickness."

For generations this view was considered no more than naïve speculation, appropriate for the romantic age but without any scientific basis. In fact, it was certainly exaggerated; Rousseau does not even mention infection, and his depiction of the idyllic social life of our ancestors was certainly too good to be true. Although his enthusiasm for the "noble savage" was founded on philosophy rather than on science, some of his views have recently been validated by discoveries in scientific disciplines ranging from anthropology to zoology, from cardiology to preventive medicine. Medical anthropologists, for example, have found that the serum cholesterol levels of foragers (another term for hunters and gatherers) and other traditional peoples are far lower than those of Americans or Europeans, but when the former adopt a more Western life-style their cholesterol values promptly rise.

Such differences have also been observed for blood pressure and diabetes. Before 1940 Native Americans had almost no diabetes mellitus; now its prevalence among tribes such as the Pimas is the highest known. In the same vein, paleontologists have found that the teeth of Cro-Magnons and other late Paleolithic humans were remarkably free of dental caries; these did occur, but were smaller and far less numerous than in the teeth of recent populations.

Current medical research increasingly indicates that by reintroducing essential elements of our forebears' life-style, especially less exposure to alcohol and tobacco, improved nutrition, and more physical activity, we can enrich our own lives while forestalling the development of chronic illness.

Against the background of the life-style of preagricultural humans, cultural changes in the past few centuries have drastically altered our existence. Nutritional practices afford a compelling example. Average daily salt intake—indicted as a cause of hypertension—is five times what it was for hunters and gatherers. In that remote past, the sole "dairy product"—mother's milk—was available only to infants. Older children and adults had none, but despite this their bones and teeth, as shown by fossil study, were stronger than those of people living today. Except for honey, refined carbohydrates were unavailable to Paleolithic men and women, while 20 percent of our calories are derived from sugar (one-third pound per person per day). Instead, our ancestors consumed far more nondigestible fiber and other complex carbohydrates, now considered essential for good health.

Hunting was also a cardinal feature of their lives, so that meat was prominent in their diet. But because the fat content of wild game averages one-seventh that of domesticated beef, their total fat intake was much lower than ours. And what little fat there is in meat from free-ranging game animals has five times the proportion of polyunsaturated fat as is found in the fat of supermarket meat.

The impact of the change has gone far beyond nutrition. Industrial and domestic pollution envelop us. Population pressure is orders of magnitude greater: There are four hundred people alive today for every person living at the end of the Paleolithic period. Natural variations in ambient temperature have been markedly reduced, and incandescent lighting has changed the quality of light while altering the day's natural division into light and darkness. Background levels of ionizing radiation are at least 50 percent higher in Western countries today than they were for our remote ancestors, and noise levels have increased so markedly as to produce widespread late-life hearing loss, a condition almost nonexistent among traditional peoples in rural settings.

Time, as indicated by watches and clocks, exerts a powerful psychic pressure that was not a consideration for men and women who lived before the advent of agriculture. Biologically potent substances including tobacco (a plant foreign to Africa, Asia, and Europe) and alcoholic beverages (whose production by hunters and gatherers has not been observed) constitute health hazards that were much less, if at all, a threat to individuals living under Paleolithic conditions. Effective contraceptive measures have changed the ground rules of reproduction—transforming sexual mores—while other social factors have altered our patterns of child care, changed the structure of our families, and redefined the relations between the sexes.

Not all of these changes are necessarily bad; some are probably trivial, some are of great benefit. But even the beneficial ones can have hidden costs. For example, the Industrial Revolution freed many of us from brutalizing toil, but motor vehicles, spectator sports, supermarkets, electricity, plumbing, central heating, and television have now made it seductively easy for us to live lives in which physical exercise has no place at all. In the long perspective of human existence, we in the advanced nations in the twentieth century have become the soft underbelly of humanity.

In an important sense, of course, there is no going back. We cannot totally recover the Paleolithic way of life, and most of us wouldn't want to. We are too satisfied with our safety and our comfort—and why shouldn't we be? But precisely because of our advantageous position, we should be able to pick and choose among the features of Paleolithic life. We can leave behind what is impractical or unsatisfying while adopting those features that can improve our current health, both physical and mental.

The French poet Apollinaire once described Picasso's strange drawings of animals as natural, saying, "It seems to me that we must return to nature, but not by imitating it like photographs. When man set out to invent a machine that would walk, he invented the wheel, which does not in the least resemble a leg." In this book, to use the same analogy, we intend to "invent a machine that will walk"—a naturally healthy human being whose life-style is consistent with the long, balanced course of evolution. That is, we will show how it is possible to return to the way of life of our Paleolithic ancestors—not by imitating it exactly, but by using its key elements to invent a new pattern. This pattern, designed to work in our supermarkets and kitchens and gymnasiums, will help us match the fitness and strength of our ancestors who lived 40,000 years ago.

First, we show how those ancestors lived and what they have to teach us. Next, we assess the discordance between their lives and ours, and show how the genetic legacy they left us comes into conflict with our present-day habits. Then, we describe and explain the "diseases of civilization," and show how they have been fostered by our new life-style. We also include standards for comparing modern diet, activity patterns, body composition, and blood chemistry to those of our ancestors. We go on to consider child care and development, and also the lives of women, from this same anthropological perspective. Finally, we offer the Paleolithic Prescription: a set of principles for modern-day Paleolithic living that can set us on a new—or, really, an old *and* new—path to health.

Throughout the Paleolithic period, microbial diseases, accidents, complications of childbirth, and infant mortality caused nearly all deaths. Since 1900, however, the incidence of these conditions has been vastly reduced, thanks to safer water supplies, improved sanitary engineering, better housing, widespread immunization, and direct medical intervention. But the Industrial Revolution also brought adverse effects that to some extent counterbalanced its advantages, enabling chronic degenerative diseases—atherosclerosis, diabetes, hypertension, obesity, chronic lung disease, and even cancer—to assume unprecedented significance. For a time these chronic illnesses were viewed by physicians and scientists as natural concomitants of aging, unmasked by the very advances in medicine and public health that have recently lengthened our lives. However, in the past two decades, it has become apparent that they are really "diseases of civilization"—not the inevitable end result of human biology, but the consequences of our particular life-style.

Much of our understanding has resulted from the work of epidemiologists and physicians specializing in preventive medicine. Their studies have shown that "risk factors" (for example high fat, high salt, low fiber diets; inadequate exercise; tobacco abuse) are another way of describing how the lives of contemporary Westerners differ from those of our ancestors. Similarly, both medical anthropologists and pathologists have found that presymptomatic early stages of chronic illnesses (especially atherosclerosis) are common in Western youths, but rare or absent altogether among young foragers and other traditional peoples. Finally, members of technologically simple societies who reach substantial ages (sixty or seventy) are largely spared from the obesity, heart attacks, diabetes, and high blood pressure which plague their "civilized" peers.

Men and women living today enjoy an opportunity for long and healthy life unparalleled in the previous experience of our species. The Industrial Revolution and subsequent public health advances—especially nutrition and sanitation, but also vaccination and medical care—produced a marked increase in life expectancy at birth. This was due largely to improvements in infant survival and reduced mortality from the infectious diseases of youth and young adulthood. But life expectancy at age forty changed much less. In a sense, we exchanged acute medical problems for chronic ones.

However, the last generation has brought a new consciousness into being; we are slowly becoming aware that chronic disease can be forestalled by adopting a new life-style. And, fortunately, this life-style has turned out to be a rewarding one. Thousands of people are jogging, enrolling in health clubs, and eating more intelligently—not only because of some late-life dividend, but largely because it feels right *now*. At some level it must feel right, since it is exactly what we were designed for. And as a result, the last decade has seen substantial increases in life expectancy for older adults.

More exciting still is the fact that older individuals can now expect to maintain a level of physical and mental health that until recently would have been considered exceptional. If physical disability and mental senescence result from the combination of chronic disease and habitual lack of exercise, then it is understandable that Paleolithic-style health should not merely postpone death, but also prolong adult vigor beyond its currently accepted age limits.

In pursuit of these goals it is our unprecedented challenge and opportunity to reinstate essential elements of the Paleolithic life-style into our modern existence. These elements are those for which our genes were selected and without which our bodies and minds suffer. To realize the full human potential for health and longevity, we *do* need twentieth-century technology, including the diagnostic and therapeutic power of modern medicine. But we also need to take a step back in time, if only to have a better understanding of who we really are. If we do, we can restructure our lives so that we measure up not only to conventional modern health standards, but also to an ancient one: the primitive standard of fitness—and protection from key chronic diseases—that is our legacy from the uncounted generations of ancestors whose genes, and whose biology, we bear.

CHAPTER TWO

OUR ANCESTORS, OURSELVES

The theory of evolution—that inherited traits are modified over time—has had a stormy history. The year 1925 marked one of its more sensational moments. John T. Scopes, a high-school teacher in Dayton, Tennessee, was brought up on charges of teaching evolution in his classroom. The trial that followed—dubbed the "Monkey Trial" in the popular press—attracted extraordinary attention. Trial lawyer Clarence Darrow, already famous for handling the sensational Leopold and Loeb murder trial, was Scopes's defender. Pitted against him was none other than religious conservative and three-time presidential candidate William Jennings Bryan, whose famous "cross of gold" speech had established him as one of the era's most powerful orators.

The issue—had humans evolved from a one-cell animal or had they been specially created in seven days as it says in Genesis?—wasn't new; it had been passionately debated since the early nineteenth century. Before that, human beginnings were generally thought to have followed the biblical account of Creation. But as new evidence began to challenge this view, confidence in the literal accuracy of Genesis—and in theological authority generally—began to erode. Most theological scholars today interpret the biblical account allegorically and morally, not as scientifically exact description, but in the late nineteenth century such views were inflammatory. Travelers returned from ever-more-distant lands with tales of great human diversity, much more than had previously been recognized. To reconcile this diversity with Genesis (which describes all people as being created at the same time), theories and speculations flourished: Humans were created a number of different times in a number of different places; only some peoples were descendants of Adam and Eve.

Archaeological findings undermined the Creation account even further. New dating techniques made possible more accurate estimates of past events. These challenged the widely accepted timetable for Creation set forth almost two hundred years earlier by an Irish archbishop, James Ussher. After carefully tabulating all biblical references to the passage of time, he determined the year of Creation to be 4004 B.C. (Another cleric working independently arrived at the same year, but pinpointed the date and time as well: October 23 at 9 A.M.)

Informed opinion in the mid-Victorian era held that all living organisms were created in their ultimate form, with no further modifications necessary. All creatures were rank-ordered from the smallest insect in progression to the most elegantly created one of all: humankind. This ordering was described as the Great Chain of Being, each species a distinct, separate, independent creation, each a separate link in the chain.

Yet newly discovered fossils revealed animals long since extinct—saber-toothed tigers, woolly mammoths, and others—sometimes in conjunction with human remains dating back tens of thousands of years. If all Creation was part of a divine plan, why would some animal species become extinct, others reflect significant changes in body size and attributes, and others remain seemingly unchanged? Perhaps, some argued, God remade the world a number of times, creating it with more sophistication on every try.

One discovery—a human fossil—unearthed in Germany's Neander Valley in 1856, was most puzzling. It wasn't the first example of ancient human remains ever to be found; others had been noted in earlier records. But it was the first to capture the public's interest. It was human, without doubt, yet it also demonstrated a number of significant differences: Its brain capacity was larger, and its body build was stronger than those of contemporary Europeans. Where did it fit in the Chain of Being? The skeleton, called Neanderthal after the site where it was found, was thought by some authorities to date from a period much earlier than Archbishop Ussher's date for Creation.

Geological evidence added fuel to the evolutionary fire by suggesting a much longer developmental history for the earth. Before the nineteenth century, the earth was believed to have remained unchanged since Creation, except for the Flood. Geological findings were initially used as evidence to support theological accounts: The presence of marine remains in mountainous regions "proved" that the Flood had once transformed the earth; fossilized animal remains were interpreted as representing those antiquated, or "lower," species that never reached the ark. But by the early nineteenth century, more sophisticated geological dating proved this thinking implausible. The process of extinction and morphological change occurred so frequently throughout geologic time that a steady progression of adaptation to changing environmental conditions was postulated. Ultimately, that is what nineteenth-century thinkers began to assume: that the same forces observable in the present had always been operating—very slowly and over tremendous lengths of time. This understanding, known as uniformitarianism, continues to provide the basis of our understanding of the history of life.

This was an exciting time intellectually, but most of these ideas seemed ultimately of concern only to scholars. The new thinking, in all probability, would have filtered into the popular press and imagination at a glacial pace if not for a book which so shocked the public that complacency was no longer possible. The bombshell was Charles Darwin's *On the Origin of Species,* which appeared in 1859. An extraordinarily popular book for a work of science, the entire first printing sold out in a single day.

Darwin summarized what other scholars had been saying, added many new insights of his own, and presented an explanation for the evolution of species that was elegant, detailed, far-reaching—and unarguable. Darwin revealed how it worked—a process he called natural selection.

By evolution Darwin meant the variations that occur in living forms and can be passed on from one generation to the next. Central to his argument was the late eighteenth-century idea of Thomas Malthus that more individuals were born within any species than could—or would—reach adulthood. The demise of significant portions of any population was therefore necessary to protect finite resources which would otherwise be outstripped. Population stability had to be ensured from one generation to the next. Life embodied intense competition, all creatures being drawn together in a powerful and brutal "struggle for survival."

Yet not all individuals were equally vulnerable, and mortality was not totally random. Natural forces and environmental factors seemed to favor survival for some individuals and not for others. Those with traits better adapted to a particular environment during a particular time bred more successfully. By analogy with artificial selection—the process used by animal and plant breeders to modify living organisms—Darwin reasoned that if the excess population was culled consistently in a given direction, then new forms would gradually arise in nature. This process could even explain human beginnings as a series of transformations from earlier forms.

The evolutionary principle of natural selection had three essential components. First, within each species "average" traits really reflect considerable underlying variation. Second, some of this variation is heritable from parent to offspring. Third, individuals with characteristics better suited—or adapted—to specific environments will leave more offspring in succeeding generations, a concept currently referred to as differential reproductive success. These more suitable traits—which can be anatomical, physiological, or behavioral—are passed on to the next generation, thus becoming more frequent in a population over time.

"The survival of the fittest," a phrase popularized by writers other than Darwin, referred to individuals who possessed traits that were most adaptive. These did not necessarily involve greater intelligence, strength, aggression, physical beauty, creativity, or even health. Instead, they were qualities best adapted to a specific environment at a specific time—any aspect of the organism that increased the number of surviving offspring an individual left. Theoretically, this could include peculiarities that work *for* the individual in one time period and *against* in another. The concept of natural selection as conceived by Darwin referred to the overall shift in the genetic profile of populations rather than individuals.

Over the last century and a quarter, Darwin's theories have been augmented, modified, and refined. It took about forty years for the mechanism that governs the passing on of traits from one generation to the next to be widely understood. It should have taken only about six years—until 1865, when Gregor Mendel, studying changes in the color of pea flowers over successive generations, conceived the laws of genetic inheritance. He published his findings in an obscure Czech journal, and no one took notice of their implications until nearly forty years later, when his work was finally "discovered."

The resulting science of genetics clarified the mechanisms of heredity and identified genes as the carriers of traits. But it wasn't until 1953 that James Watson and Francis Crick—later to win the Nobel Prize for their work—unlocked the mystery of what genes actually are. They showed that genetic information is carried on chromosomes: long, threadlike molecules composed of desoxyribonucleic acid—or DNA, for short. These strands are made up of links—or genes—each link composed of thousands of bits of genetically coded information. The order in which these bits arrange themselves on the DNA strand is crucial to what makes a person a person or a butterfly a butterfly, just as the arrangement of letters in a sentence is crucial in distinguishing English from French, Shakespeare from first-grade readers, or literature from nonsense. The sequence of these genetic "letters" is the code that directs the expression of all inherited characteristics within an individual.

All the genetic information necessary to make a person or a butterfly is actually contained in every cell of the organism. In order to reproduce, DNA in the sex cells is reduced so that each sperm or egg receives only half the chromosomes present in body cells. When sperm and egg unite, the full complement of chromosomes is reconstituted so that each offspring receives half its genetic inheritance from its mother and half from its father. But what happens if points on the DNA chain break or twist or rearrange somewhat, if the order of the "letters" gets scrambled, or if certain bits are duplicated while others are omitted altogether?

Theoretically, duplication of DNA molecules should proceed with 100 percent accuracy, but it doesn't. Random errors in DNA replication occur naturally in all living forms. Most of these errors are essentially meaningless to the life of the organism. Others are harmful, hampering reproduction or producing less viable offspring. But the most important of these random changes are the "successful" ones that cause the organism and its progeny to thrive, to leave more offspring with the same trait in future generations, and, depending on the trait, even to reorient the species in a new direction.

To contemplate the variations seen among the multitude of living forms on the earth today as the result of DNA duplication errors that have randomly occurred over the past billion years is, to say the least, staggering. Yet, these very errors—or mutations—were responsible for altering, ever so slowly, the characteristics of living forms, generation after generation. By definition, all such changes succeeded in the short run, but not all succeeded equally well over the longer course of time. This is why the process of evolution produces change, but not necessarily "progress." Because, while random errors create variation, only natural selection determines whether or not the variants are viable and for what length of time.

Darwin reasoned that evolution is a cumulative process. It occurs gradually, at a relatively slow rate throughout time, ultimately changing the character of a population. This slow, steady process could account for how modern giraffes grew such long necks and how human brain capacity increased so dramatically over the course of a few million years. The following is an account of another such transformation.

The earliest ancestor of the modern horse was *Eohippus*, the "dawn horse," an animal that lived in the forests of Europe and America over 50 million years ago. It was a small creature, measuring about ten inches at the shoulders and weighing less than ten pounds; a swift runner for its size, it relied on speed for protection. As the vast stretches of subsequent time saw forests dwindle, and in some regions vanish altogether, the descendants of *Eohippus* were thrust onto the open plains.

This new environment favored taller animals that could see predators over the grasses, and swifter runners that could escape a chase.

Random variation in the *Eohippus* population, based ultimately on mutation, produced some animals that were taller or faster than others, or both. (If they were anything like modern horses in their behavior, then increased size and speed may have served the additional function of making certain males more successful in the fierce competition for females.) These were more likely to survive and leave offspring. As a result more of their genes—for size and speed—were passed on to their offspring, who in turn survived to pass them on in succession down the genetic line.

This process, continuing for eons, produced a gradual but consistent trend. By 10 million years ago, *Pliohippus*, an intermediate form closer in size to modern horses than to *Eohippus*, ranged the plains of North America. By 2 million years ago, *Equus*, the modern horse, appeared. When there was no further advantage in gaining yet greater height or speed, horses maintained a fairly constant body form with relatively long necks and long slender legs, serving their original functions in an adequate and stable manner over subsequent evolutionary time.

Although these early members of the genus *Equus* were well suited to their environment, they were still somewhat smaller than most horses are today. They are best represented in this century by Przewalski's horse, which is found naturally only in central Asia, and which is intermediate in size between a Shetland pony and more conventional horses. The horses hunted by late Paleolithic people resembled this somewhat smaller breed. But after domestication, animal breeders exploited random genetic variation to breed selectively for larger and larger animals that could carry a rider or help with heavy farm work, or animals both larger and swifter that could serve in warfare or racing.

This artificial selection by humans is analogous to the natural selection Darwin described, but can be much more rapid. Indeed, Darwin relied on the evidence of artificial-breeding programs to support his initial insights into the process by which the environment shapes the forms of species over time. The horse represents one instance in which the trend begun by natural selection was then extended by artificial selection, underscoring the fundamental similarity between the two processes, just as Darwin suspected.

This gradualist explanation for evolutionary change has faced challenge in recent years. At issue is the paucity of fossils in the archaeological record representing intermediate forms: organisms poised in midstream of an evolutionary process. Theoretically, one might expect to find numerous examples of such fossils, exhibiting both ancestral and contemporary features along one hereditary line. The *Archaeopteryx*, an animal that lived 140 million years ago, part dinosaur and part bird, is just such a case. But additional examples are few and in some cases completely absent.

Paleontologists such as Niles Eldredge and Stephen Jay Gould reconcile these archaeological gaps by theorizing that instead of evolution acting in constant slow gradations, as Darwin postulated, it occurs in occasional bursts. Punctuated equilibrium is their name for the process: Very long periods of evolutionary quiescence during which a species remains basically unchanged (equilibrium) are followed by brief punctuations of rapid genetic change in response to altered environmental conditions.

Other theorists point out, however, that evolutionary change may *appear* to be static when it is, in fact, ongoing. Changes in an organism's "soft" parts—muscle or organ development, for example—are less likely to leave clear evidence in the fossil record than are "hard" skeletal changes. Recent microanalysis of geologic strata also suggests that "spurts" of evolutionary activity in adjacent geologic strata actually represent longer time spans than earlier, less precise analysis suggested, perhaps as long as hundreds of thousands of years—more than enough time for "gradual" (as opposed to "punctuated") evolution to take place.

Evolution, whatever its rate, is an ongoing process, as forceful in the contemporary world as it was in the ancient one. Darwin helped define it and proposed the major mechanisms through which it works. His synthesis sparked a firestorm of controversy that engulfed the popular, religious, and scientific communities of his time and for generations to come.

John Scopes was convicted, but the final court in this case is the court of science. Although the issue still provokes lively debate today, evolution was and is recognized as the only scientifically acceptable account of the history of life.

HUMAN EVOLUTIONARY HISTORY

The story of the discovery of Troy is part of the popular lore of archaeology. Heinrich Schliemann, the son of a poor German pastor, was fascinated in his youth by tales of the Trojan War, considered at that time to be only a myth. He dreamed of one day finding the remains of the city to which Helen was abducted and before which Achilles defeated Hector. As an adult he went into business and amassed a huge fortune, but he never gave up his dream. Leaving the business world behind, he went to Paris to study what was then known of archaeology.

In 1870, at age forty-eight, he was able to begin his quest; with passages from the *Iliad* as his guide, he headed for the Dardanelles. While inspecting possible sites on a promontory jutting out into the Aegean, he noted an imposing mound overlooking a broad plain, which stretched to "the many-mirrored, wine-dark sea," just as described in Homer. He began digging a trench, and almost immediately found the walls of the famed ancient city which had perished in flames perhaps 3,000 years before.

A parallel but less well known story concerns a young high-school student in the Netherlands during the early 1870s—Eugene Dubois—who became intrigued with ideas he had heard in a lecture about Darwin's view of human descent from prehistoric apes. Most people—scientists and the general public alike—rejected Darwin's views not only because they were revolutionary and contradicted the Bible, but also because there was no convincing fossil evidence proving the link between apes and humans. Some of Darwin's supporters confused the debate further by publishing outlandish accounts of the human family tree that were restrained only by the limits of the imagination.

Dubois's fascination with these ideas remained with him through his medical school training in anatomy and six years of teaching in academe. Surmising that our human forebears must have lived in the tropics, Dubois became convinced that caves on the Indonesian islands of Sumatra and Borneo (then under colonial rule and known as the Dutch East Indies) might prove fertile ground for finding what was termed the "missing link"—an intermediate creature between apes and humans. He hoped to provide conclusive proof for Darwin's theories. At age twenty-nine, ridiculed by his peers, denied funding by all those he petitioned, Dubois left his job, home, and security to enlist as a doctor in the Dutch colonial army.

Dubois spent over five years in Indonesia, ultimately focusing his activities on the island of Java, where remains of ancient origin had recently been discovered. By means of extensive, systematic excavation—a technique never before so elaborately employed—at a variety of sites, he discovered a treasure trove of fossils, many of extinct or previously unknown animals: stegodon, ancient hippopotamuses, and primitive forms of deer and antelope. But it wasn't until 1892 that he accomplished his original mission: He found a unique skull in the same geologic layer in which he had already found a thigh bone and several teeth. The pieces were puzzling, seeming to belong to neither ape nor human. They proved to be one of the most important and exciting fossils excavated up to that time.

Pithecanthropus erectus, or Java man, as this discovery was popularly called, caused great excitement throughout Europe. Dubois believed he had indeed solved the mystery of our human past, deducing that the three fossils belonged to one individual. The "missing link," he asserted boldly, had been found. His evidence was the anomalous character of the fossils themselves: a skull that was low, flat, and with a fairly large cranial capacity; a thigh bone that was heavy but designed for upright walking; and teeth that were crinkled, with no clear antecedents.

Dubois exhibited the fossils, gave lectures, wrote treatises, photographed the specimens, sculpted replicas, and defended his views against vehement public opposition. Denounced by the clergy and the scientific community alike (there were at least fifteen different interpretations of the place his fossils had in the evolutionary scheme), he eventually retreated from public view, embittered and reclusive, taking his fossils with him. After thirty years of seclusion, he finally relented, and in 1932 once again allowed the fossils to be viewed.

The controversy sparked by the Java man discovery still smolders. At issue is whether Dubois should have linked the skull, thigh bone, and teeth to the same individual. Opinion today is that the skull belonged to an early human living about 1 million years ago, not a creature half-ape, half-human. The thigh bone is thought likely to have come from a later time, one associated with more modern humans. And the teeth may actually have belonged to a prehistoric, extinct orangutan. Although Dubois may not have discovered *the* "missing link" (we now understand that there are many links, not just one), he did lead the vanguard, setting new standards of scientific rigor in human paleontology while opening the field to others who shared his bent for the excitement of exploration and discovery.

A century has passed since Dubois first set out with a hunch and a great deal of determination. Since then, large numbers of early human fossils have been found throughout the world—in Asia, Africa, and Europe. Within one hundred years of the first Neanderthal find, over six hundred bones of human ancestors had been excavated in East Africa alone. Today that number is several times larger.

With all this evidence at hand, and much more, what picture can we now draw of the past? Starting at our geologic beginnings, our solar system, including the Earth, is thought to have been formed about 4.6 billion years ago. A few hundred million years later, primordial seas formed, and a few hundred million years after that the planet had settled enough for the most spectacular event of all: the beginnings of life—algae and bacteria—around 3.5 billion years ago. Going from nonlife to life, however—from cosmic chaos to genetic order—took much less time than it did to go from simple life forms to more complex ones. At least

2.2 billion years passed before the advent of the first oxygen-breathing organisms about 1.45 billion years ago.

The subsequent events, by comparison, progressed much more rapidly. Around 800 million years ago the first multicellular animals appeared; 400 million years ago witnessed the beginnings of land plants; 300 million years ago insects and amphibians proliferated; 200 million years ago the first mammals appeared; and 100 million years ago birds and flowering plants became widespread even as the large dinosaurs were disappearing.

Primates—the order of mammals that includes ourselves—appeared around 65 million years ago. The early primates proved a very successful adaptation and spread over Africa, Asia, and the Americas. At various junctures in their evolution, these animals generated the forebears of all subsequent primates, including humans. This trail is a convoluted series of branches, splitting here and there into dead ends, continuing elsewhere, creating new paths that never before existed.

Around 45 million years ago, the first major split occurred. Primates in the Old World (Africa and Asia) and those in the New World (North and South America) diverged, as a result of continental drift. Twelve million years later—or 33 million years ago—the Old World became host to the earliest great apes: ancestors of today's chimpanzees, gorillas, and orangutans, as well as of humans. The evolutionary process continued to trace a complex path for millions of years more, splitting repeatedly. The ancestors of gibbons appeared 15 million years ago, orangutans 13 million years ago, and gorillas 9 million years ago. For the next 2 million years, or until about 7 million years ago, the last common ancestor of both apes and humans—which corresponded to the "missing link" as conceived in Dubois's time—existed. From this (still as yet undiscovered) creature, one path led to chimpanzees, the other ultimately to us. Even so, the first creatures with upright posture and bipedal locomotion would not indisputably walk the earth for another 3 million years, or until around 4 million years ago.

Had Eugene Dubois chosen as his excavation site the Rift Valley in East Africa rather than Java, his venture might have been even more successful than it was. Because eroding to the surface of this vast windswept plain, the most spectacular fossils have since been found and excavated. Buried over millions of years, these fossils have helped unravel the mysteries of human evolution, from ancient primates to modern-day people.

One of the most impressive of these fossils was found in 1974 at Hadar in the Afar region of Ethiopia. It was the skeleton of a small female who lived over 3 million years ago. "Lucy," as she was affectionately called by Donald Johanson and the international team of paleontologists who discovered her (at a time when "Lucy in the Sky with Diamonds" was a popular Beatles hit), was ultimately represented by 40 percent of her skeleton. Several hundred additional bones were also found, representing at least thirteen individuals—"the first family"—children, juveniles, and adults, both male and female.

Lucy and her contemporaries, assigned the name *Australopithecus afarensis*, are considered part of the direct human line. Smaller than modern humans and with more marked size differences between adult males (about five feet tall) and females (under four feet tall), their bodies were nevertheless remarkably modern in structure, with hips and legs well adapted to upright walking. Impressions left on a limestone shelf discovered in Tanzania in 1976 by Mary Leakey—"the first footprints"—graphically document their erect posture and bipedal gait.

But smaller stature was not all that separated them from us. Their skulls, including teeth, jaws, and brain capacity, were quite primitive, not having changed much in size for nearly 12 million years. In fact, despite their erect posture, their brains were one-third the size of the brains of modern humans—more like those of contemporary chimpanzees.

Lucy's species was nevertheless quite successful, existing for nearly 1 million years. Then, between 3 and 2.5 million years ago, it apparently diverged into at least three coexisting, independent australopithecine species, also humanlike in body structure but with skulls of fairly small brain capacity. Their speech was therefore probably limited—in all likelihood comparable to the vocal repertoire of contemporary apes. Two of these divergent lines, both robust, large-boned forms, eventually became extinct after existing for at least a million years; the third, more slender and less powerful, ultimately led to us.

How the bipedal but otherwise apelike australopithecines developed into humans is still somewhat in dispute, but all indications point to the presence of the first real humans—in the sense of expanded brain capacity—just over 2 million years ago. Called *Homo habilis*—"capable" or "handy" man—these beings were the first to deserve inclusion in *Homo*, our own genus. Although they were small—a 1986 find, again by Donald Johanson's team, shows they were similar in size to Lucy (*Australopithecus afarensis*)—their brain size and organization had begun to look more like ours. They are the first humans considered to have true culture: learned activities transmitted from one generation to the next. They were also the first to make stone tools. Living by gathering wild plant foods and by both scavenging and hunting, they existed for over half a million years—until about 1.7 million years ago, when they were succeeded by larger and more complex beings: *Homo erectus.* These in turn were the immediate forebears of *Homo sapiens,* our own species.

Although Dubois didn't know it, the remains he identified nearly a century ago were those of *Homo erectus,* not the "missing link" between apes and humans. Since that time, many more fossils of this species have been excavated, but the most spectacular find was made as recently as 1984: the nearly complete skeleton of a twelve-year-old boy whose projected adult height would have exceeded six feet. This find— the work of a team led by Richard Leakey and Alan Walker—led paleontologists to reevaluate many of their ideas about *Homo erectus.* Similar to modern humans in height, *Homo erectus* had a heavier body, but its brain, although larger and more modern in organization than that of *Homo habilis,* was still far smaller than ours. Nevertheless, these early humans were extremely successful and well adapted. They did more hunting, so that meat assumed a more substantial role in their diets, complementing a broad variety of vegetables, fruits, and nuts. They were also the first to control and use fire (as early as 1.4 million years ago), enabling them, about 1 million years ago, to spread from tropical Africa to temperate portions of Asia and Europe—areas never before inhabited by hominids.

Homo erectus thrived for about 1.3 million years—an unusually long period of anatomical and behavioral stability (evidence for the latter comes from their remarkably consistent pattern of stone toolmaking— the hand axe culture). But changes were nevertheless taking place, however slowly, culminating in the appearance around 400,000 years ago of another group called Archaic *Homo sapiens.* These are the first humans to be classified not only in our genus (*Homo*) but also in our species (*sapiens*). Their brains were considerably larger than those of *Homo erectus* and were essentially modern in organization, in all likelihood endowing them with more articulate speech. They gradually supplanted *Homo erectus* throughout the then-inhabited world.

A quarter of a million years later, or about 150,000 years ago, a specialized form of Archaic *Homo sapiens* began to develop in Europe and Western Asia. Eventually this subspecies became classic *Homo sapiens neanderthalensis*—the scientific name for the Neanderthals, who flourished between 90,000 and 30,000 years ago. Despite the negative public image that has been their lot since their initial discovery in 1856, they were actually very similar to people today. They walked fully upright, and although they were massive and muscular, they had, on average, even larger brains than modern humans have. They were also probably very agile, not slow and clumsy as they are often portrayed.

It is now thought that anatomically modern humans—*Homo sapiens sapiens*—may have appeared as early as 90,000 years ago. The location is in dispute (sites from northeast Africa to southeast Asia have been proposed) but the biology is not; these people were physically and physiologically almost indistinguishable from ourselves. At first few in number, by 35,000 years ago they had spread from Europe to Australia. Their exact relationship with preexisting forms of *Homo sapiens* is not clear; in Europe the Neanderthals seem to have been supplanted, while in the Near East they may have intermingled with the advancing modern humans.

Homo sapiens sapiens of 40,000 years ago seem to have had at least the same ingenuity for finding creative solutions to problems posed by their environment as people do today. The longer they inhabited an area, the more sophisticated their cultural adaptation to it became. Stone tool manufacture became increasingly complex, employing such skilled methods as drilling, grinding, and polishing. More varied materials—bone, ivory, and antler—were used. Hunting techniques advanced. Spear throwers greatly extended the striking range. Transportation became more versatile, with boats, sledges, and perhaps snowshoes eventually playing a role. Not surprisingly, these people became increasingly interested in decorating themselves and in creating art.

Whether the process involved replacing earlier peoples or merging with them, *Homo sapiens sapiens*—modern human beings in all respects—had supplanted all other types of humans by around 30,000 years ago. Their dominance and success ultimately enabled them to inhabit all portions of the globe: Australia as long as 40,000 years ago; the Americas at least 12,000 years ago; the extreme Arctic 10,000 years ago, and the Pacific Islands as recently as 2,000 years ago. They are the direct ancestors of all humans living today.

ANATOMICALLY MODERN HUMANS

In the fast-paced mystery novel and film *Gorky Park*, a memorable minor role is played by Andreev, a Russian physical anthropologist. His skills are required for the identification of three victims about whose murder the plot revolves. Their faces and fingerprints have been mutilated to prevent identification, but the anthropologist is able to reconstruct their features on the basis of their facial bones. The character of the anthropologist is actually based on Mikhail Gerasimov, a contemporary Russian archaeologist and artist who has frequently and successfully aided Russian police in identifying the skeletons of missing persons.

Gerasimov has also worked with the skulls of the Cro-Magnons. The faces he re-creates are unequivocally modern, with high foreheads, aquiline noses, wide-set cheekbones, muscular cheeks, large jaws, prominent chins, full lips, and even teeth. They do not exactly resemble any specific national or racial type common today, but their appearance is well within the contemporary range. Clothed in contemporary styles, they would blend quite easily into modern life, attracting little, if any, special notice.

Could these primitive "cavemen" actually have looked so much like us? Yes, according to anthropologist Christy Turner II. By studying the shape of Cro-Magnon teeth—determined by the interaction of about twenty-five separate genes—and comparing them to contemporary humans, Turner found that Cro-Magnon teeth were completely modern. He also found that Cro-Magnon teeth were closer in shape to European teeth than they were to either African or Asian teeth. Analysis of ten-thousand-year-old Paleoindian teeth yields similar results: Paleoindian teeth are more comparable to those of their Amerindian descendants than Amerindian, African, or European teeth are to one another. These findings lend further support to the idea that the human gene pool hasn't changed significantly since anatomically modern humans first became widespread.

The Cro-Magnons, among the first true modern people—*Homo sapiens sapiens*—lived in Europe from around 35,000 years ago until between 15,000 and 10,000 years ago. When this time period—called the Late Paleolithic—ended, a number of radical transformations had taken place. The last of the four great Ice Ages which had visited the planet over the previous 600,000 years was ending and receding glaciers in Europe and North America were precipitating warmer and wetter climates. But from the human viewpoint, the most dramatic development was the debut of an entirely new subsistence pattern: agriculture.

Before about 10,000 years ago there were no farmers. For about 30,000 years, anatomically modern humans had been widespread, yet it had not been necessary for people to alter the natural world around them systematically and deliberately in order to produce abundance. The environment had been sufficiently fruitful and population size still small enough for people to live comfortably from the land most of the time. However, a number of forces—some worldwide, others more localized (population pressure, improving technical skills, and increasingly elaborate social systems) coincided with the transformation in climate to make change not only possible, but ultimately necessary.

Archaeologists have traditionally taught that the first agriculturalists appeared in the Fertile Crescent of the Near East, although very recent investigation suggests that southeast Asia had priority. Either area, however, with its bountiful resources, could have afforded people the leisure necessary to spark such creative innovations. Others reason that agriculture emerged in response to population pressure. As population density slowly rose at the end of the Paleolithic, hunters and gatherers experienced increasing competition for land. Those groups which adopted horticulture enjoyed transient abundance until their own numbers caught up with increased food availability. In the process such groups outbred neighboring hunters and gatherers. Population densities for foragers are rarely greater than one person per ten square miles while, for farmers, the average is one hundred times greater. After the early farmers achieved numerical superiority they were able to displace the remaining foragers from favorable adjacent territory to accommodate their expanding population. In this view the success of the Agricultural Revolution is early evidence that might makes right.

The practicality of agriculture also increased as the Ice Age ended and the climate became warmer and wetter. This change proved a boon to wild grasses—including the ancestors of today's cereal grains—which became abundant, widespread, and ever more attractive as food sources. Modern researchers using the technology of the time—sickles made by placing flint bladelets in a curved antler segment—have shown that a family group harvesting wild wheat at peak season needs only about ten days to harvest a six-month supply of grain.

The step from relying on plants in the wild to "helping them along" a little bit seems a relatively intuitive one, especially when overhunting, displacement by large human settlements, and climatic changes at the end of the Ice Age made wild game less abundant. Cultivation of plants in short supply probably came first, followed by wild grains. As wild grasses were increasingly used for food, they were modified into types more appropriate for farmers. Selective breeding of mutant wheat strains whose seeds didn't detach easily from the stem (as most wild wheat does) resulted in more grain being harvested and less falling to the ground or blowing away in the wind. These developments in the Near East anticipated the later parallel experience of Amerindians who produced what we now know as corn during a few millennia of horticultural experiment and practice, again involving natural mutation.

By about 5,000 years ago agriculture was present on all the inhabited continents except Australia. Cultural diffusion helped it spread, but it probably had independent beginnings in East Asia and the Americas as well as in the Near East. This spontaneous invention in widely separated locations indicates that new forces favorable to agriculture had been broadly unleashed throughout the globe.

The development of farming affected all aspects of human experience. Settled village life became possible, craft specialists became more important, society became more hierarchical, and warfare became possible on an ever grander scale. So unprecedented and radical were the implications of this new subsistence pattern that its beginning has been likened to a revolution.

Called the Neolithic Revolution, the changes wrought by agriculture ultimately eliminated the world of the Cro-Magnons. Again, scientific opinion differs on how this happened. One view is that the surplus populations produced by farming communities, flourishing in the Near East, gradually colonized Europe. As new settlements were founded, lands were appropriated and cultural traditions quite different from those of the original populations were introduced. An opposing view holds that new technology and resources spread, not people; the farming cultures of Europe and of the Near East are archaeologically just too different.

Nevertheless, the Cro-Magnons—whose remains were first discovered in 1868 in a limestone cave (locally called Cro-Magnon) in the Dordogne region of France—seemed to most nineteenth-century Victorians a far more acceptable ancestor than did the Neanderthals discovered a few years earlier. The imagination of the general public was taken by Cro-Magnons then even as it is today. (For example, the heroine of Jean Auel's popular romances about the Stone Age is one of them.) Although they inhabited only a limited portion of Europe and western Asia, the popular image of "caveman," and of preagricultural people in general, derives almost entirely from what is known (and has been imagined) about Cro-Magnon life.

What was the essence of that way of life? The Cro-Magnons lived very much as other people did in the world of that time—by hunting wild animals and gathering wild plant foods. Whether meat was the mainstay of the diet (as with the Cro-Magnons) or vegetable foods dominated (as with many other groups), vastly more generations of humans have depended on hunting and gathering than on any other way of life. It was a more universal and far more long-lasting experience than agriculture, which is only about 10,000 years old, than industrial manufacturing, which is only about 200 years old, or, of course, than computer technology, which is barely a decade old. Put another way, 100,000 generations of humans have been hunters and gatherers; 500 generations have been agriculturalists; ten have lived in the industrial age; and only one has been exposed to the world of computers. Hunting and gathering was the context in which humans evolved, with our impressive intellectual, psychological, and physical endowments—as well as our limitations.

To look at it yet another way, before agriculture actually took hold around 10,000 years ago, 100 percent of the estimated 5 to 10 million people alive were subsisting as hunters and gatherers. By A.D. 1500, the world population had grown to over 350 million and only 1 percent were still maintaining themselves in this mode. Today, with a world population likely to top the 7 billion mark by the year 2000, the few isolated peoples who had been hunting and gathering for a living into the first half of this century will soon completely disappear as independent cultures.

Anthropologists, recognizing the importance of this phase of human experience, have tried to record from among the last remaining traditional hunters and gatherers the essence of their way of life. Although they live in remote areas unattractive or inaccessible to others, recent foragers are fully modern people, no more different from the rest of humanity, biologically, than is any other population around the world. By studying their ancient way of life, and integrating the results with the findings of archaeologists and paleontologists, we open a window on worlds long gone, worlds that helped shape the very essence of our human selves.

Our general ignorance of this way of life was once epitomized by Thomas Hobbes, who characterized living in a state of nature as "solitary, poor, nasty, brutish, and short"—a still widespread but inaccurate view. Contemporary preagricultural people living in areas far less advantaged than those of our distant ancestors seem to manage quite well. In fact, whether living in semidesert conditions (such as the !Kung San in southern Africa and the Aborigines in Australia), in tropical forests (such as the Efe Pygmies in Zaire, the Agta of the Philippines, and the Aché in Paraguay), or on savanna grasslands (such as the Cuiva of Venezuela and the Hadza of East Africa), a modest to moderate amount of work provides a reasonably secure and socially satisfying existence.

Despite their wide geographic distribution, today's hunting and gathering peoples share a surprising number of basic organizational features in common—features probably shared by their Paleolithic counterparts as well. This organization might be called "social simplicity," to contrast with the "social complexity" of most agriculturalists. Recent evidence suggests that just before the invention of agriculture, some foragers with a strong resource base also achieved increasing social complexity. But for most parts of the world for most of the Paleolithic period, the following description probably applies.

Small bands of people—typically between fifteen and fifty individuals—live together, traveling seasonally or more often to maximize resource utilization. The composition and size of these groups vary as members shift from band to band to resolve conflicts or simply to follow personal inclination. Work is usually divided according to sex, with men contributing meat and women plant foods, but crossover is in some cases considerable. Dietary quality is generally excellent, providing a broad base of proteins and complex carbohydrates along with a rich supply of vitamins and other nutrients. Dietary quantity is occasionally marginal or deficient, but this is true of most agricultural cultures as well—probably even more so. Maintenance of the forager diet is accomplished with a moderate work load, leaving ample time for the pursuit of leisure activities.

Territories are maintained, but boundaries are loose and rights of access to resources are liberally interpreted. Sharing of food and material goods is central to the economy. Status hierarchies are usually absent; an egalitarian style delegates comparable rights and privileges to everyone. Although leaders exist, their influence is quite informal, entailing few if any material rewards and no inheritance of titles. Indeed, in some of these societies, those people who are able to distance themselves from selfish, self-aggrandizing, or petty postures are the ones turned to for leadership. Outbreaks of violence certainly exist, as they do in all human societies, and fights may even end in homicide. But when conflict so disturbs a band that resolution is difficult, the essentially fluid nature of group membership allows people to move—temporarily or permanently—to other bands while tempers cool.

The brutish "caveman" with club in hand lording his dominance over women (and anyone else impressed by his strength and ferocity) is an image in opposition to the reality of male-female relationships among recent foragers. Many anthropologists now think that the Agricultural Revolution begun 10,000 years ago was accompanied by a deterioration in the co-existence between the sexes. Although considerable variation in gender relations among contemporary preagricultural people exists, a strong tendency toward equality is also observed in most. Indeed, the extremes of female subordination found in many of today's more "advanced" societies more closely fit the stereotype of "caveman" life than does the more benign alliance generally struck between males and females among the !Kung San and other preagricultural people.

Women in these societies generally exert broad influence over decisions affecting themselves and the group, are quite autonomous, assume roles of major importance within the economy and within the family, and are surrounded by a supportive social network that can be relied on in times of physical or psychological need. Men do maintain a slight edge overall, and exert strong dominance among some hunters and gatherers, but an enviable balance—even cordiality—between the sexes prevails in most of these societies.

The Cro-Magnons living in Ice Age Europe were only one variation on the hunting and gathering theme, but they are the most thoroughly understood of Paleolithic societies. Twenty thousand years ago, thick ice sheets covered northern England, all of Scandinavia, Denmark, northern Germany, Poland, and northern Russia. There was also glacial ice over the Alps, the Pyrenees, and much of northern North America, including the Missouri and Ohio river valleys. Because so much water was trapped as ice, sea levels were about three hundred to three hundred and fifty feet lower than they are now. Ireland and England were joined to Europe; northeast Asia was connected to Alaska by a land bridge—Beringia—nearly eight hundred miles wide; and the sea gaps between Australia and the East Indies were shorter.

No environment in today's world exactly parallels that lived in by the Cro-Magnons. Although sometimes likened to the Arctic, the lands close to the permanent ice wall of the glacier were relatively low in latitude and therefore received considerably more sunlight. The soils were also rich and fertile, and the grasslands with their low-growing shrubs vast, diversified, and flourishing. Wooded river valleys and protected hillsides provided shelter for an additional variety of plant and animal life, and were favored as living sites. The mosaic nature of the landscape—a patchy distribution of diverse microenvironments—attracted Arctic reindeer and alpine antelope, animals found together then but not today. Reindeer, wild horses, antelope, mammoths, and bison roamed in vast numbers. Plant foods were less plentiful, but some, such as berries, were seasonally abundant. The region was a paradise for hunting while allowing more limited but essential gathering.

Of course, most foragers in the world of that time settled far from the glaciers in less extreme environments: on temperate prairies, in woodlands, in river valleys, and on tropical savannas. (They seem to have avoided the deserts and tropical rain forests.) Seasonal variations in temperature and rainfall produced cyclical availability of vegetation and wildlife. Most areas also had a great diversity of large grazing animals, present in almost unimaginable numbers. Early European explorers in the Americas and Australia routinely expressed amazement at the extraordinary abundance of game animals, fish, and birds they encountered. Even today, East African parks support tremendous numbers of wild animals: hippopotamus, elephant, eland, buffalo, gazelle, warthog, zebra, wildebeest, rhinoceros, impala, giraffe, and kudu, among others. This sort of hunters' paradise existed in one form or another throughout much of the inhabited world.

Except near the glaciers, edible plant life—vegetables, nuts, roots, and fruit—was also readily available. Even in the heart of today's Kalahari desert in southern Africa—an environment that early hunters and gatherers would probably have shunned—the /Gwi San (Bushmen) gather around sixty varieties of food plants while their more northern neighbors, the !Kung San, choose from among one hundred five edible species. Before the development of agriculture some regions of the world might have afforded fewer edible plant foods than the Kalahari does now, but in nearly all, plant foods would have made a major contribution to subsistence wherever people lived.

Compared with the devastating environmental consequences of "civilization," humans like the Cro-Magnons lived in relative ecological balance with their surroundings. They did use fire to alter the landscape, to encourage the growth of grass, and to drive prey. And it is even possible that overhunting by humans, combined with the climatic changes that accompanied the end of the last glacial period 10,000 years ago, contributed to the mass extinctions of large animal species—mammoths, mastodons, woolly rhinos, giant sloths, and others—which occurred at that time. Nevertheless, before the development of agriculture the overall impact of humans on the environment was minimal compared to the changes that have occurred since.

HUNTING

A dramatic rock painting in the Transkei of South Africa depicts the death plunge of an eland herd driven over a cliff by Late Stone Age hunters. Another preagricultural rock shelter painting found in Tanzania, East Africa, shows an elephant in a trap. Twenty-thousand-year-old Cro-Magnon cave paintings show bison with spears piercing their chests and flanks.

Although the earliest human hunters were probably limited in their technology and their hunting success, people living between 40,000 and 10,000 years ago were supreme big-game hunters, pursuing a variety of animals in diverse locales. In Europe, mammoths, bison, reindeer, wild cattle, horse, and especially red deer were among their prey. In Argentina 12,000 years ago, llamas, horses, giant sloths, and rheas (birds resembling small ostriches) were hunted. In coastal southern Africa, several antelope species were eaten, as well as Cape and giant buffalo, eland, wildebeest, and hartebeest. In Australia, people feasted on emus, wallabies, kangaroo, and several varieties of now-extinct megamarsupials.

The scope of the hunting carried out by many of these hunters and gatherers was staggering. At an archaeological site near Pavlov, Czechoslovakia, a giant pile of fossilized bones represented the remains of over one hundred mammoths, trapped in pit falls. Near Solutré, France, another heap of tangled bones excavated near the bottom of a high cliff turned out to be the fossilized remains of an astounding number of wild horses—about 10,000—stampeded off the cliff by succeeding generations of hunters.

In America, 10,000-year-old fossil remains of three hundred buffalo were excavated at a site near the Arikaree River in Colorado. The buffalo were efficiently trapped by being driven down sloping banks of ice, packed hard and slick by the hunters, into a streambed filled with drifts of deep snow. There they were slaughtered and their bones arranged in an orderly fashion, suggesting that the Paleoindians may have had an assembly line for butchering.

Our popular image of prehistoric hunters includes the bow and arrow, but this weapon came relatively late in our hunting history, appearing less than 20,000 years ago. The chief weapon throughout the 20,000 or more years before the bow and arrow was the spear—a wooden shaft with a flaked stone, antler, or bone point. (Some of these points are so skillfully executed, with workmanship so far exceeding basic utilitarian need, that they are considered an ancient form of aesthetic expression.)

The spear thrower—a common functional accessory for spear casting—was also used in many areas. This was a simple rod made of wood or antler, about twelve to fifteen inches long, with a hook at one end that could be engaged on the butt of the spear, effectively extending the hunter's arm. It enabled hunters to hurl their spears with increased velocity, providing greater range and penetration. Striking from longer distances in turn made stalking easier and safer; the hunters could stay farther from the animal's sharp hooves, teeth, and horns.

Hunting methods were inventive and varied. Some hunters drove animals, with or without fire, into natural or artificial enclosures. Others drove them over cliffs or into marshes where they were then trapped and slain. Ambushes, pit traps, encirclement, and simple stalking were other common techniques.

Men were most likely the usual hunters, bringing home as much meat as seasonal and regional variation allowed. Hunting was sometimes constrained by long-distance migrations of game animals (for example, bison, mammoths, and reindeer) or by cyclical shifts in game ranges (for example, ibex and chamois summered in inaccessible mountainous terrain but wintered in relatively low lying meadows where they could be more easily approached). In the North African region which has since been replaced by today's Sahara desert, there was a constantly changing succession of wildlife throughout the year. Streams and water holes filling up during the wet season brought wild cattle to graze on the succulent grasses; the dry season, with more savannalike vegetation and drought-resistant grasses, brought gazelles and hartebeests.

Work effort for most groups probably paralleled that of contemporary hunters and gatherers, people whose way of life reflect some of the possibilities of this ancient pattern of subsistence. Some people—such as those living in the Venezuelan Llanos savanna or the Australian out-back where game animals are less abundant than they were for our Paleolithic predecessors—average about twenty hours a week in actual hunting. This translates into a "Paleolithic rhythm" of one or two days of hunting, each lasting around six to eight hours, followed by one or two days of rest. There are other patterns—the Paraguayan Aché hunt nearly every day—but the Paleolithic rhythm probably obtained for most hunters and gatherers in the past since it has been the pattern usually observed among similar groups in the present.

GATHERING

During many periods and at varying locations, game procured by hunt-ing was the dietary mainstay; but in most regions plant foods of great variety were available for much of the year, and gathering was more reliable than hunting. In tropical and semitropical environments (and in some temperate regions as well), gatherers could be virtually certain of returning with a full carrying bag. Hunters—even in the most favor-able areas—could never be quite sure they would not return empty-handed. Among recent hunters, daily success rates vary considerably, from over 75 percent for the Aché of Paraguay to around 25 percent for the !Kung San of Africa's Kalahari.

In contrast, women know that when they leave to gather plant foods for the day they will return with enough to feed themselves, their immediate families, and any other dependents. They can sometimes count on having something left over to share with others in the group as well. In the Kalahari, !Kung women typically spend twelve to twenty hours a week gathering. The resulting pattern of a day spent foraging, followed by one or two days in other activities, is consistent with the "Paleolithic rhythm" of physical activity observed for !Kung hunters.

A core group of staple vegetable foods—usually between ten and twenty—supplemented by sixty or more used less frequently is typical of most recent hunting and gathering diets. Specific resources vary seasonally, and in some instances the same plant provides different portions—leaves, fruit, seeds, stalks, roots—for use at different times of the year. But except in the most extreme environments, edible plants are abundant and available in sufficient variety to allow a wide range of choices. From fruits, nuts, beans, roots, tubers, stalks, bulbs, berries, melons, and gums, leaves, fungi, and flowers a highly diversified, nutritionally rich, and often extremely tasty diet can be obtained.

Gathering requires only light equipment: a digging stick and something to carry the gathered produce in, such as a leather sack or a reed basket. But it also requires great skill, strength, and stamina, as well as knowledge of the distribution of specific foods. Picking wild fruits or vegetables takes less time than extracting bulbs or roots—sometimes buried several feet in the soil—but a day's outing, whatever foods are gathered, requires a significant outlay of energy. In addition to the weight of the day's harvest (which often weighs twenty-five or thirty pounds), women also carry infants and sometimes even older children as well—as much as five miles or more round trip.

SOCIETY AND CULTURE

Most contemporary hunters and gatherers live in small groups called bands. These are typically composed of from five to ten families, related to one another by blood or marriage. The band is the unit that usually travels together, moving from one temporary camp to another every few weeks as the most desirable food resources in an area are used up. The longer a group stays in one place, the farther people have to walk each day to find game or vegetable foods. Bands are loosely organized into larger populations sharing a common dialect and an informally defined geographic range. These units, or tribes, usually consist of about five hundred individuals but range in size from about two hundred to nearly a thousand.

The nature of the camps also varies. Some are hunting camps along expected migration routes. Others are set up at sites of major kills, where many people are needed for butchering. (This also avoids the necessity of carrying heavy loads of meat long distances to a base camp.) Still others are in areas where special plant foods are seasonally available, such as at acorn harvesting sites in northern California. Special-purpose camps are also common—perhaps where good-quality flint is available for tool making, or reeds for basketry, or some other specialized commodity. Most recent forager camps have been out in the open air, and this was also true for Late Paleolithic humans, although in places with severe winters, they sometimes sought the seasonal protection of caves.

People also move to join in social events that bring together as many as several hundred members of the group for specific purposes, such as tribal meetings or ritual ceremonies. On these occasions marriages are arranged, gifts are exchanged, friendships and family ties are renewed, and news of all sorts—stories, gossip, and accounts of outside contacts—is exchanged. When the groups depart, it is often with new arrangements of families or individuals, reflecting the essentially fluid nature of band composition.

Music, art, oral folklore, and ritual are prominent in the lives of today's hunters and gatherers; they reflect great richness of imagination and demonstrate that the human inclination toward aesthetic and religious expression is universal. The evidence for similar human drives in our ancient past is equally clear. Rock shelter and cave wall paintings, small sculptures of game animals, statuettes of pregnant women, and even burials of individuals wearing bone bracelets, shell-, tooth-, or bone-necklaces, and clothing decorated with elaborate beadwork—all attest to the same universal and ancient predisposition. Paleolithic cave paintings of animals and supernatural beings are considered by modern artists and art historians to be among the most impressive images ever drafted by humans, and they may have been at the center of dramatic rituals deep in the torch-lit caves.

FORM AND FUNCTION

By studying skeletal remains of modern humans from the Late Paleolithic period and analyzing the attributes of recent hunters and gatherers, it has been possible to develop a remarkably detailed anatomical and even to some extent a biochemical profile of our preagricultural ancestors. With as little as one limb bone and a formula which relates overall height to limb-bone length, the stature of early humans has been deduced. The height of eastern Mediterranean hunters and gatherers 30,000 years ago, for example, has been estimated as averaging 5 feet 9.75 inches for males and 5 feet 5.5 inches for females—very similar to the stature of present-day Americans. Taken together with the 1984 Leakey-Walker fossil skeleton indicating that *Homo erectus* could reach an adult height of 6 feet 2 inches, these data suggest that for over a million years people have attained heights comparable to or greater than those reached by today's well-nourished industrial populations.

These people were also strong—stronger by all estimates than most agricultural and industrial people (including ourselves) who lived after them. Skeletal remains reflect strength and muscularity; the size of joints and the sites where muscles are inserted into bones indicate both the mass of the muscles and the magnitude of the force they were able to exert. Average Cro-Magnons, for example, were apparently as strong as today's superior male and female athletes. Strange as it may seem, Cro-Magnons and other hunters and gatherers may have worked fewer hours per week than did the agriculturalists who followed, yet they were significantly more robust.

This apparent contradiction is probably related to the pace of work in preagricultural societies: intermittent but demanding of peak effort. Recent studies suggest that brief but strenuous activity occurring at intervals is more effective for the development of muscularity than longer periods of less physically demanding labor.

Because they resist deterioration, teeth are relatively abundant at archaeological sites, and their condition reflects health status and lifestyle just as do bony remains. For example, it is clear that Paleolithic people had limited exposure to sugar. Only about 2 percent of fossil teeth from the Late Paleolithic show evidence of cavities, and even these are shallow and small. In contrast, about 70 percent of the teeth in some recent industrialized populations (for example England in 1900) have had cavities, and these have frequently been very large.

Contemporary hunters and gatherers almost never become obese, yet in most circumstances throughout most of the year, they seem to be adequately fed. A common technique for determining the overall proportion of fat is to measure skinfold thickness at various sites of the body. The back of the upper arm is a favorite place; the skin is gently pinched with a pair of calipers which calibrate the amount of fat underneath. Young men measured in five hunting and gathering societies in Africa, Australia, and North America averaged triceps skinfold thicknesses of 4.6 mm. American and Canadian men of similar age, in contrast, averaged 10 mm of thickness—over twice as much.

Paleolithic hunters and gatherers also seem to have been lean. Stone Age rock wall paintings in Australia, North Africa, Spain, and Tanzania depict slender people. So do many figurines found in Europe and western Asia, which date between 25,000 and 15,000 years ago. Obesity, however, was not unknown. A number of so-called Venus statuettes portray fat Cro-Magnon women. This may have been merely artistic style or convention, but the accuracy of the portrayal indicates that the genetic potential for obesity was present in our earliest ancestors, much as it is in us today. It is quite likely that these statuettes represented an elite group (perhaps priestesses of a fertility or mother-goddess cult) similar to that of the Pacific Polynesians. The Tahitians were thought by eighteenth-century European explorers to be "the comeliest people on earth"; the nobles, however, both men and women, were extremely obese, a tall version of today's Japanese Sumo wrestlers.

Both hunting and gathering require great stamina. Men track, stalk, and pursue game; women walk long distances carrying heavy loads of produce—and children—while gathering. Strenuous dancing is a common recreation. Moving camp every few weeks and extensive visiting among distant relatives demands considerable physical exertion. One of the rewards of this life-style is that it promotes superior fitness, especially for the heart and lungs. Tests of young men from preindustrial societies show that their average maximum oxygen-intake values (the established measure of aerobic fitness) are superior to those of typical American males of similar age.

Endurance activities, in fact, clearly date back as far as the earliest humans (and probably to their australopithecine ancestors as well). Unlike most other animals, humans have two mechanisms which tend to minimize heat buildup during strenuous exercise. First, our bodies have very little hair; exposed skin allows heat to escape easily, especially during running, when air flow over the skin increases. Second, along with a surprisingly small number of other similarly adapted species— such as horses, camels, and cattle—humans release heat by sweating.

These adaptations were favored during our long evolutionary history. Early hominids running on the African savanna during the heat of the day would have had an advantage over animals that were quick to overheat and that had to stop to cool down; both hunters and gatherers had to maintain their arduous activity for long periods of time, sometimes during brutal heat.

Other physiological measures of contemporary hunters and gatherers also reflect their high level of fitness. For example, their blood-pressure and blood-sugar values remain low throughout life; in contrast, in the United States both rise with age. This rise is often so great that levels routinely found in older adults would be considered abnormal in younger people. No such age-related difference occurs among today's preagricultural people.

Serum-cholesterol levels are also typically much lower for foragers than they are for people living in industrial societies. Until very recently, values as high as 300 mg per decaliter were considered "within normal limits" in American laboratories. But around the world hunters and gatherers, small-scale agriculturalists, and pastoralists have much lower levels, generally below 150 mg per decaliter.

This does not mean that hunter and gatherer health is exemplary— people in these societies have high death rates from infectious diseases and trauma, but those who survive the onslaught of microbes do better in many ways than people the same age in our own society. A life-style better suited to our human genetic inheritance help them avoid the degenerative "diseases of civilization."

Such comparisons—Paleolithic and contemporary forager health in relation to ours today—challenges a "pet" idea most of us hold: That with every decade, no less century or millennium, technological advance has been synonymous with progress in human existence on all fronts, a steady climb upward from darkness to light. Indeed, the march of time has been beneficent overall, and our lives *have* steadily improved—at least in many respects. Few would forfeit the advances of modern sanitation and health care, the security of our food sources, the protection from the elements, or the many other comforts of modern life. Admitting this, however, does not necessitate a total rejection of the past. It was, after all, very successful, even with its stresses; this was the context in which our preagricultural ancestors thrived, populating, ultimately, the entire globe. And, as we have seen, in some areas of health and fitness, preagricultural people succeed in ways that we— with all our "advancements"—have failed.

CHAPTER THREE

THE DISCORDANCE HYPOTHESIS

We are the heirs of a process begun over 3 billion years ago with the initial appearance of life on earth. Over the course of that enormous span of time, countless genes have been introduced; some of these have survived over a billion years, while others have come and gone, leaving no trace. Our own current biological makeup reflects this inheritance. It is based on an accumulation of genetic information that originated during a succession of geologic eras. Many more of our patterns are ancient than recent: Fully 99 percent of our genetic heritage dates from the period before our ancestors became human (and of the remainder, 99 percent dates from before the development of agriculture). These biological patterns have been worked out through epochs—proved over and over again in the crucible of natural selection. They are the product of evolution, chosen even as genera and species appeared, evolved, and diverged from one another. Our biology has truly survived the test of time.

It is hard to imagine that only 1 percent of our biological makeup has appeared since 7 million years ago, when the human and great ape lines separated. But it is true. Our most basic biological processes go back much farther than that. The mechanics of cell division, balance of fluids and electrolytes, metabolism, and regulation of energy production are so similar to comparable functions in other living creatures—mammals, vertebrates, and even unicellular organisms—that these essential properties can be dated back 3 billion years, to the very origins of life itself.

But that still leaves us with 1 percent of our genetic makeup having been derived more recently. Considering that this 1 percent has been responsible for distinguishing us from chimpanzees as well as from the earliest humans, it has not been insignificant. Quite a tall order for such a small percentage, but 1 percent of our 50 to 100 thousand functional genes represents a sizable number. These genes have been responsible for our upright posture and bipedal gait, loss of body hair, enlargement of the brain with associated changes in cerebral organization, and modifications of the skull and larynx presumably to facilitate speech, among other traits. We are heirs, of course, to additional and what may seem more recognizable programming, which determines our individual characteristics—the color and texture of our hair and skin, the shape of our eyes, our racial type, some aspects of our personalities and abilities, our likeness to family and kin—in addition to, of course, all our other biologically influenced qualities.

That the vast majority of our genes are ancient in origin means that nearly all our biochemistry and physiology are fine-tuned to conditions of life that existed before 10,000 years ago. In some respects the environment has changed little since then, but in others it is radically different. Consider, for example, current population density and growth rates. When the earliest humans, *Homo habilis*, walked the earth, they numbered only a few hundred thousand. Throughout the subsequent 2 million years, they slowly changed, evolving ultimately into people as we know them today; populations expanded—at an estimated average rate of about one-thousandth of 1 percent per year (as compared with 3 percent in the fastest-growing modern populations).

This rate may seem slow, but human populations expanded more or less steadily throughout the millennia. By 25,000 years ago, about 3.5 million people lived on the earth. By 10,000 years ago—the dawn of agriculture—this same slow rate had produced a world population of between 5 and 10 million.

But then everything changed. Once people started tilling the soil and altering ancient patterns of resource availability and abundance, life became more sedentary, birth spacing became shorter, and annual population growth increased almost a hundredfold, to an estimated .1 percent per year. This rate prevailed for almost 8,000 years. By the birth of Christ, the world population had grown to about 300 million; by 1750, the beginning of the Industrial Revolution, it had reached 700 million.

The effect of the Industrial Revolution during the eighteenth century just about tripled the population growth rate to about .3 percent per year. During the nineteenth century, this doubled again, to .6 percent per year. Today's population is growing at a staggering 2 percent per year—more than 1,000 times faster than it was 10,000 years ago and five times faster than it was at the signing of the Declaration of Independence, a mere two hundred years ago. In preagricultural days, world population doubled (on average) every 15,000 years; after the onset of agriculture, it doubled every 1,000 years. At present, doubling takes only thirty years. The consequence? Our planet is now host to 5 billion people.

When early humans started making and systematically using tools around 2 million years ago, they created a material culture that could be transmitted separately from our genes. Cultural evolution was at first painfully slow. The transition from *Homo habilis* to *Homo erectus* about 1.7 million years ago was apparently marked by significant improvements in hunting technique, so that larger game could be pursued, but thereafter there was little change for over a million years. Archaeologists have been impressed with the almost complete lack of cultural change during the time of *Homo erectus*. Living sites dated hundreds of thousands of years apart show essentially identical tools and subsistence patterns. Even Archaic *Homo sapiens*—the very first members of our species, appearing several hundred thousand years ago—made relatively few improvements.

But after anatomically modern humans became widespread—between 40,000 and 30,000 years ago—the rate of cultural innovation gradually increased. Alterations, embellishments, and even "fads" began to appear in the archaeological record. Each succeeding generation—about 1,500 in all—passed on and often improved existing technology, transforming it into more skillful and sophisticated forms. Complex and beautifully crafted weapons, potent poisons, increased understanding of edible and inedible plants and of medicinal herbs, discriminating insights into animal movements and behavior, skillful extraction of dyes, removal of food toxins, and versatility in various craft media characterized the majority of these societies. The construction of huts, lodges, shelters, and other dwellings, together with better clothing—sewing was introduced during this period—facilitated human penetration into the Arctic and, ultimately, throughout the Americas. Meanwhile, coastal peoples developed oceangoing craft that allowed the settlement of Australia. And true aesthetic expression, ranging from decoration of implements and clothing to the magnificent cave paintings of Lascaux and Altamira, made its first obvious appearance.

These creative and often brilliant innovations arose within the framework of the hunting and gathering life-style. It was in this common and essentially stable context that modern humans evolved biologically and, in some fundamental ways, behaviorally.

In contrast to this slowly measured pace of technological and cultural change, the appearance of agriculture along with the domestication of animals redefined the rules, the game, and the stakes, accelerating the pace and redirecting the process of change in unprecedented ways. The subsequent Industrial Revolution had an even greater impact. More extensive changes in the forms of human existence have taken place within the last two hundred years than within the previous 10,000. So global has this tidal wave been that a Plymouth Rock Pilgrim visiting twentieth-century industrial society—a mere three hundred years in the future—would be more bewildered by life today than an early Archaic *Homo sapiens* transported forward 300,000 years would have been by the life of Cro-Magnon cave dwellers.

Our relationship to the environment—the foods we eat and the types of physical exercise we engage in—are further examples of our changed world. The problem is that our genes don't know it. They are programming us today in much the same way they have been programming humans for at least 40,000 years. Genetically, our bodies now are virtually the same as they were then. Except that "then" was a world we had spent hundreds of thousands of years adapting to, a world we had gradually responded to with subtle alterations in our genetic constitution, a world to which we had slowly molded a reasonably close fit. "Now" is so radically different—its demands so new—that our very old human design has not had time to adapt.

The pace of biological evolution is glacially slow. Unlike the ease and swiftness with which business and industry annually update and unveil their latest models, evolution needs time. It does not "revamp" its human models within, say, hundred-year or even thousand-year intervals. Instead, tens of thousands of years are often necessary for minor changes to occur, hundreds of thousands or even millions for more significant changes. The genetic adaptation of our own ancestors—the hominid line—over the last few million years has actually been exceptionally rapid when compared to that of other mammals.

Nevertheless, there was a certain stability in the human evolutionary line—until 10,000 years ago. At that time, and again 250 years ago, the essence of human experience *was* altered. Agriculture and industrialization each introduced previously unknown components—and pressures—onto the human scene.

In the face of these relatively recent cultural changes, however, few new and successful genetic adaptations have had time to become established; from the perspective of evolutionary change, 10,000 years is just not long enough for major changes. Indeed, the very nature of human existence is now in such constant flux and is being transformed so radically from one generation to the next that even if it were possible for humans to emerge 10,000 years from now with a handful of physiological and psychological mechanisms better adapted to the stresses of our current lives, the circumstances of human life would be so different then that those *new* adaptations would probably be outdated.

There are, however, some simple genetic changes that are known to have taken place within the last 10,000 years, as a response to agriculture. Sickle-cell anemia is one such alteration. Apparently the Neolithic Revolution brought large numbers of people together for the first time in a sedentary context, creating an ideal environment for infectious diseases to breed and spread via people, animals, and insects. The mosquito-borne malaria parasite had been there all along; it had afflicted individual hunters and gatherers much the way it did the agriculturalists who followed. But only after people began living in dense, settled populations, with abundant water sources suitable for mosquito breeding, did it become possible for the malaria parasite to infect and kill in large numbers.

Somewhere, probably in the Arabian Peninsula or along the west coast of India, however, a simple genetic change took place, affording individuals a significant degree of protection. Most people have two genes for normal hemoglobin (hemoglobin A), the oxygen-carrying molecule in red blood cells. This type of hemoglobin, however, is vulnerable to malaria parasites introduced into the bloodstream by the mosquito. But individuals with the genetic mutation had a different pattern: one normal gene for hemoglobin A, and one altered gene for abnormal hemoglobin S, a type less favorable to the parasites. These carriers of hemoglobin S were better able to resist malaria and so left more offspring, passing the altered gene on to subsequent generations. Within a few thousand years—by human evolutionary standards an exceptionally short length of time—this genetic adaptation had spread around the Indian Ocean, across the breadth of Africa, and into the southern Mediterranean.

But this adaptation also contained a major flaw. Through the usual shuffling of Mendelian genetics, some individuals came up with the perfect combination—one gene for hemoglobin A, one for hemoglobin S—and were afforded extra protection. Others inherited two normal hemoglobins and no hemoglobin S—a continuation of the pattern passed on by generations before, which left them still quite vulnerable to the malaria parasite.

But for those who inherited two hemoglobin S genes and no normal hemoglobin, the genetic change meant disaster: the double hemoglobin S genes afflicted them with sickle-cell anemia, a disease that nearly always produced death in childhood. The majority, however, were more fortunate. With one hemoglobin S gene, they "carried" the disease but did not actually get sick from it, contracting neither sickle-cell anemia nor malaria. This clearly was a beneficial evolutionary novelty.

Another simple genetic change that seems to have occurred during the last 10,000 years is the persistence into adulthood of lactase, an enzyme found in the intestinal wall of almost all infant mammals, including humans. When this enzyme is present, the major sugar found in milk—lactose—can be absorbed. Since all mammals nurse their young, it follows that the enzyme must be found in the young. However, lactase disappears in late childhood because there is no need for it after weaning. That is, for all mammals except humans who, by domesticating animals, devised a way to make milk products available throughout life. How, then, did humans handle the lack of lactase?

One solution was cultural: they converted fresh milk into yogurt, rennet, buttermilk, and a wide variety of cheeses, in such a way that its undigestible sugar was almost completely broken down by bacterial action before eating. Another solution was genetic and arose through natural selection in populations with long traditions of herding cattle, goats, yaks, camels, or horses. A simple genetic change allowed these people to continue production of lactase not only into late childhood, but throughout adulthood, affording them maximum benefit from the nutrients in fresh milk and its various products.

These two changes—sickle-cell hemoglobin and the persistence of intestinal lactase—are examples of relatively recent genetic evolution. A limited number of other single-gene changes (for example, such hemoglobin variations as thallassemia, which also protects against malaria, and possibly the capacity to tolerate gluten, the major wheat protein) are generally recognized by geneticists and anthropologists. Even certain relatively recent adaptations to extreme environments, such as high altitudes, may have a partial genetic basis.

But apart from these examples, most recent trends—such as changes in jaw and tooth size and decreased skeletal robustness—are considered nongenetic in nature. Comparable to the increasing height of Japanese people raised in America as opposed to those raised in Japan, these variations demonstrate the broad range of physical plasticity that is triggered by the complex interaction of our environments, our cultures, and our genetic constitutions.

So, here we are in the late twentieth century, with a 40,000-year-old model body, trying quite nobly to understand what it means to be human, adjusting as best we can to the complex demands of our lives. Yet with genetic makeups essentially out of synch with our life-styles, an inevitable discordance exists between the world we live in today and the world our genes "think" we live in still. This mismatch—referred to here as the discordance hypothesis—can account for many of our ills, especially the chronic "diseases of civilization" that cause 75 percent of the deaths in industrial societies.

And the diseases of "noncivilization"? People certainly get sick and die in technologically simple societies and do so at younger ages and in larger numbers than we do. But how people live and what makes them die are connected. The health—and causes of death—of people living as did our hunting and gathering ancestors provides a stunning contrast to our own pattern.

It has only been about thirty years since scientists turned their attention to the quality of life among preagricultural peoples; their approach has been to look at the health of contemporary hunters and gatherers along with estimating the health parameters of individuals in the fossil record. Their findings have confirmed a limited but important part of what philosopher Jean-Jacques Rousseau—one of the first to recognize the healthy bearing of people living in a "state of nature"— had conjectured. To be sure, Rousseau underestimated the disorders of such people; they suffer not only from wounds, but from a variety of deadly infectious diseases for which we have cures. But today's preagricultural people are in some other ways surprisingly fit, and their counterparts of the past show evidence in their fossil remains of having been similarly strong and robust.

The world's few remaining hunters and gatherers inhabit jungle, desert, and Arctic environments far more extreme than those of our remote ancestors. This may help explain why skeletal remains of early humans show they were larger, more muscular (and probably healthier) than are today's hunters and gatherers. Nevertheless, the Australian Aborigines, the North American Eskimos, the Tanzanian Hadza, and the San (Bushmen) of Africa's Kalahari desert have much to offer us. All are people who have lived by hunting and gathering into modern times and all have had, until recently, viable traditional cultures.

Perhaps the most intriguing discovery emerging from these studies is that the diseases which cause most deaths in our society are infrequent among hunters and gatherers. Even pastoralists, rudimentary horticulturists, and simple agriculturalists avoid many of these diseases. Although their adaptations are relatively recent, people living in these kinds of societies still resemble Paleolithic peoples in certain fundamental ways. Given the paucity of data on "pure" hunters and gatherers—those most analogous to Paleolithic humans—we can broaden our data base and sharpen our analysis by amalgamating certain carefully selected findings on nutrition, exercise, and disease prevalence among these other preindustrial peoples with what is known about recent hunters and gatherers.

For example, autopsies conducted in the early part of this century showed no significant coronary atherosclerosis among a traditional group of 1,000 Kenyan Kikuyu. Diabetes is unknown, even today, among Broaya pastoralists who maintain a traditional nomadic life in the Sahara. Examination of a number of preindustrial societies in Africa, Australia, and South America show the virtual absence of hypertension (high blood pressure) and obesity. As long as these societies maintain their age-old life-styles, they seem to be protected; but as soon as they move to urban centers and adopt a more Western life-style, they experience hypertension, diabetes, coronary atherosclerosis, and other urban diseases. In the past fifty years of rapid cultural change, this has proved true for people as diverse as Africans, Eskimos, Polynesians, and Amerindians.

One common suggestion is that traditional people do not contract these diseases simply because they do not live long enough to get them. Reasonable though this argument may seem, recent studies have refuted it. Young men in industrialized societies show early signs of many of these illnesses—atherosclerosis, hypertension, and obesity, for example—while young men from more technologically simple societies do not. In addition, even people aged sixty and above in traditional groups continue to avoid these diseases. This is not true for their Western counterparts who—even if they have no symptoms—still show silent but ominous evidence of the key disease processes. If, as we suggest, it is the life-style of preindustrial people that protects them from these dreaded diseases, what factors are involved? Or, rather, what have we abandoned, and how have we changed, to have rendered ourselves so vulnerable to them?

To begin with, hunters and gatherers of both the past and the present obtained all their food from wild game and uncultivated plants. Although the types and proportions of foods consumed varied widely from one group to another, a generalized profile of their diet (as compared to ours) can nevertheless be drawn. It was low in saturated fat and salt. Water was the major, and usually only, beverage. Refined sugar—mainly honey—was available only seasonally. And roughage, or dietary fiber, was consumed in large quantities from wild, noncultivated plant foods—a major component of this diet. Although meat was prominent, wild game contains so much less fat—about one-seventh as much as domesticated meat—that their total intake of fat, especially saturated fat, was much lower than ours. As for alcohol, most contemporary hunters and gatherers began consuming it only *after* being introduced to it by technologically more advanced people. This, along with limited and unsuitable storage capability, makes it unlikely that alcohol consumption among preagricultural people was common or frequent.

Even routine use of wild tobacco is likely to be recent in origin because of its seasonal availability. Except for the Aborigines, who chew tobacco indigenous to parts of Australia, no hunters and gatherers are known to have used the uncultivated plant. As an agricultural crop, tobacco was first grown in the Americas around 5,000 years ago. Europeans, Africans, and Asians had no access to it until after the voyages of Columbus. Cigarettes—the historic key to the widespread use and abuse of smoking—were not manufactured until the late nineteenth century.

The patterns of activity among hunters and gatherers generate high levels of physical fitness. Men and women are strong and muscular, with impressive endurance capabilities. Their strength is consistent with the skeletal remains of Late Paleolithic people, which generally show them to have been more robust than their agricultural descendants, including ourselves. Even comparing our own fitness with that of traditional preindustrial people is unflattering to us in many ways, suggesting that certain aspects of human health and fitness declined not only across the boundary from the Neolithic, but additionally with the advent of industrial life.

This should not suggest that all twentieth-century affluence has been bad for human health. Indeed, improved nutrition (in a quantitative sense), housing, sanitation, preventive measures, and medical care have all but eliminated the ancient impact of infection and greatly reduced the toll from trauma, the chief causes of mortality from the Paleolithic until 1900. As a result, the average life expectancy of industrial populations is double that of preindustrial ones. Nevertheless, because we have so little routine exercise in our daily activities, consume foods so different from those available to preindustrial and earlier populations, and are exposed to the deleterious effects of alcohol and tobacco, we have finally estranged ourselves from the broad continuum of general mammalian experience. And with this estrangement has come an unprecedented rate of chronic illness; a new prevalence of conditions rare among recent hunters and gatherers.

THE DISEASES OF CIVILIZATION

Having defined the differences in our life-styles, it becomes possible to explore their impact on our patterns of health and illness. Contemporary hunters and gatherers are not models of perfect health, but the diseases they contract are ones we can largely avoid or control through sanitation, safety precautions, vaccination, and medical care. Chronic diseases we cannot yet control or treat—the major killers of people in modern times—are ones that barely afflict them at all. These are the diseases fostered by technologically complex societies, or civilizations: atherosclerosis, hypertension, diabetes, chronic obstructive lung disease, and several common cancers, as well as less deadly disease processes such as osteoporosis, hearing loss, dental caries, alcohol-related diseases, diverticulosis, and obesity. A discussion of these diseases and their causes will lay the foundation for an understanding of how we can use lessons from the hunting and gathering life-style to avoid and control such problems.

Atherosclerosis

Atherosclerosis is by far the most important deadly disease in the United States at the present time. It is the pathologic process underlying most heart attacks and strokes, which together far outweigh cancer as the leading cause of death. The process consists of the gradual deposit of fat and cellular debris in the walls of the arteries to form plaques. These plaques slowly but surely thicken the walls of the arteries, making them less supple and restricting the channel through which the blood must flow as it carries oxygen to the tissue.

This condition poses grave risks. In the arteries of the heart, reduction in blood flow may have serious consequences when the person is at rest. But physical exertion or even psychological stress causes the heart to pump faster, increasing its demand for oxygen. When the channel has been tightly restricted, the pumping heart muscle may become starved for oxygen, and severe chest pain—known as angina pectoris—may result. If the blood vessel is contracted still further by a spasm of the diseased artery—or by a blood clot at the same site—a section of that muscle may die for lack of oxygen. This is the irreversible damage known as a myocardial infarction, or heart attack.

In the brain, exertion does not increase the demand for blood flow the way it does in the heart. But narrowing of the arteries to the brain can produce a result comparable in some ways to a heart attack. This is one major form of stroke, which results in destruction of a part of the brain and frequently in devastating losses of physical and mental function—or even in death. Another kind of stroke depends on atherosclerosis more indirectly: A small clot, formed on an atherosclerotic plaque in the carotid artery, may subsequently break off and travel to the brain.

Although heart attacks and especially strokes most often occur late in life, the process that underlies them—atherosclerosis—begins during childhood. Studies of young men killed in action in World War II, Korea, and Vietnam, as well as studies of young people of both sexes killed in automobile accidents, show that healthy people in their late teens or early twenties have already begun the lifelong process of laying down the atherosclerotic plaques that, over a period of years, will narrow their arteries and make them vulnerable to heart attack and stroke.

Autopsies of young or even middle-aged men in preindustrial societies, however, fail to show a similar process. The absence of atherosclerosis in these postmortem studies (one of which included 1,000 consecutive autopsies) is consistent with the absence of clinical signs of atherosclerotic heart disease among people in these groups. Arctic Eskimos, Kenyan Kikuyu and Masai, Solomon Islanders, Navajo Indians, Australian Aborigines, Kalahari San (Bushmen), New Guinea Highlanders, and Zairian Pygmies are among the peoples shown to be protected from the signs and symptoms of atherosclerosis.

A large number of experimental and clinical studies on industrial populations can be correlated with these anthropological data to throw new light on the nature of atherosclerosis. The process begins with a microscopic injury to the wall of the artery—the sort of injury that is natural, unavoidable, and occurs regardless of genetic or cultural background. But the events set in motion by the tiny injury differ greatly from one society to another. Among hunters and gatherers and other preindustrial peoples, the injury is repaired and leaves no significant damage. But in societies such as ours, the same injury becomes a focus for the development of a plaque.

The difference lies in part in the level of cholesterol in the blood. Although genetic predisposition can play a critical role in determining blood-cholesterol levels, for most people environmental—especially dietary—causes are more important. Habitually high levels of fat intake, especially when saturated fat is a prominent dietary constituent, can chronically elevate blood cholesterol concentration. As we have seen, in our society cholesterol levels of about 200 have until very recently been considered safe by most physicians, but the same levels would be very high among preindustrial groups, where values over 150 are unusual.

A likely explanation for these contrasting cholesterol levels lies in differences in diet and, to a lesser extent, activity patterns. Studies of traditional people who become Westernized or migrate to industrialized countries show that dietary changes can elevate blood cholesterol within a relatively short time span and, over a longer period, can produce clinical signs and symptoms of atherosclerosis.

Several recent studies have demonstrated that aggressive therapeutic and dietary intervention can actually reverse the atherosclerotic process in both coronary and peripheral arteries. Merely slowing the rate of plaque formation may be sufficient to forestall the disease's clinical manifestations. By recreating the pertinent life-style features of Paleolithic existence, we may thus be able to reduce the incidence of heart attack and stroke, and to ward off other consequences of atherosclerosis.

Hypertension

Hypertension, or high blood pressure, is a disorder with few direct manifestations of its own, but it becomes a major contributor to other ailments—heart attack, kidney failure, and especially stroke. It appears to exert its effect primarily by accelerating the process of atherosclerosis, but the way this works is not well understood. (It is also associated with hemorrhagic strokes—those that result from bleeding into the brain tissue—in addition to its association with ischemic strokes—those that result from arterial narrowing and oxygen starvation.) What is clear is that hypertension is widespread in industrial societies such as ours, and rare in technologically simple ones. Furthermore, blood pressure commonly increases with age, in our society, from a baseline normal pressure of 120/80. (The higher number represents the pressure in the arteries when the heart muscle has contracted, the latter when it has relaxed.) Among people such as the San (Bushmen), the Eskimo, the Australian Aborigines, the Zairian Pygmies, the Tanzanian Hadza, and many other preindustrial groups, blood pressure remains low throughout life.

The translation of elevated blood pressure into stroke and heart disease can be expressed numerically. For each increase of 10 points in the higher figure (known as the systolic pressure), the risk of stroke increases by about 30 percent. In the well-known Framingham study, 5,000 men were followed for a period of eighteen years. During this time, 105 strokes occurred—95 in men with high blood pressure, and only 10 in men with normal pressure. The impact on heart disease is also impressive. Someone with a systolic pressure of 180 runs twice the risk of developing clinically evident coronary artery disease as someone with a systolic pressure of 120. In recent years, the control of high blood pressure with drugs has been one of the key factors in reducing the risk of stroke and heart attack. Ideally it should be possible to achieve this same effect or an even greater reduction without drugs, by identifying and removing nongenetic causes of hypertension.

A number of epidemiological studies have linked hypertension to diet and other life-style factors. The blood pressure of populations has been related to their salt intake, specifically to the amount of sodium consumed. Populations consuming little sodium—amounts comparable to those our ancestors likely obtained—have no hypertension and no age-related increase in blood pressure. Obesity is another contributing factor. Still other studies suggest that diets high in potassium and calcium may have a protective effect. Finally, populations that avoid hypertension tend to be those with high levels of exercise and aerobic fitness, and this may exert an independent effect against blood-pressure elevation.

Diabetes

Diabetes (or, strictly speaking, diabetes mellitus) is a common disorder of blood-sugar metabolism that has many serious physical consequences. It causes the body either to produce insufficient insulin or to respond insufficiently to the insulin it does produce. The function of insulin, a hormone, is to remove sugar from the blood so that it can be used by the cells, and thus elevated blood sugar is the hallmark of the disease. Diabetes can cause blindness, kidney disease, nerve degeneration, lowered resistance to infection, and atherosclerosis, with its resulting risk of heart attack and stroke (and, for diabetics, additional risk for blockage of the arteries of the legs and penis).

There are two major types of diabetes. Type I (insulin-dependent), which typically begins in childhood and is more severe, depends little on life-style factors. It may be viral in origin, and it results in lifelong dependency on insulin. It probably exists among preindustrial peoples, but has not been studied among them, presumably because it is rapidly fatal when untreated. Type II (noninsulin-dependent) diabetes usually begins in adulthood. It is much more common in our society than is Type I (about 90 percent of American diabetics are in this category) and is less serious—at least at first. Its occurrence is closely related to the patient's dietary habits. Over 80 percent of adult-onset diabetics are obese, and one of the best predictors of the disease is the degree and duration of obesity.

In a Scandinavian study, moderate obesity increased the risk of diabetes tenfold, while still greater degrees of obesity (45 percent above normal body weight) increased it thirtyfold. In experiments with laboratory animals, overfeeding sufficient to produce obesity predisposes to diabetes, while caloric restriction prevents the disease. And in one similar experiment with eight human volunteers, a 25 percent weight gain produced abnormal glucose utilization patterns in every case.

Apparently obesity either reduces the number of insulin receptors on body cells, or disperses these receptors, and thus produces resistance to insulin. This insulin-resistance mechanism eventually allows abnormally high levels of glucose to build up in the blood, and this in turn results in unfortunate effects on various body tissues. Interestingly, athletic training and other physical conditioning have the reverse effect; that is, activity enhances insulin sensitivity, thus protecting against abnormalities of glucose metabolism. Yet another protection against this form of diabetes is eating a diet high in nonnutrient fiber and complex carbohydrates.

These facts help to explain historical and cross-cultural trends in its incidence. In New York City, for example, between the years 1866 and 1923 there was a tenfold increase in deaths from diabetes in the over–forty-five age group, this against the background of a steady fall in the overall death rate from all causes during the same time period. This trend is most likely attributable to dietary alterations (for example, fiber intake declined after roller-milled flour became widely available in the 1880s and 1890s), changes in exercise patterns (as industrial mechanization and increasing general affluence decreased the need for physical exertion), and an increase in the prevalence of obesity (between 1863 and 1963 the average weight of men similar in age and height increased by 22 pounds).

Unfortunately, the same phenomenon has repeated itself many times in the nonindustrial world. Studies of Native Americans, Alaskan Eskimos, Australian Aborigines, Pacific Islanders, and Yememite Jews show that abandonment of traditional dietary and exercise patterns increased the prevalence of obesity and diabetes. While it is difficult to separate the effects of dietary changes from those of a more sedentary life-style, it is likely that both factors contribute to the problem. Current estimates are that from 3 to 10 percent of people over age twenty in industrialized nations have diabetes. In twelve traditional societies the comparable prevalence rate was in all cases under 2 percent and averaged only 1.1 percent.

Chronic Obstructive Lung Disease

This term includes emphysema and chronic bronchitis, two degenerative lung conditions that often occur together, and that frequently result from breathing impurities and toxins. Chronic obstructive lung disease (sometimes abbreviated to COLD) entails progressive deterioration of respiratory function culminating in death, usually from a superimposed case of pneumonia. But before this release there are often years of chronic air hunger, a particularly painful form of suffering: a sense of smothering, of suffocation, of being unable to "get a good breath." Death is preceded, literally, by years of starving for air.

Occupational and general urban air pollution play roles in these and other lung conditions, but the overwhelmingly dominant cause in the United States today is inhaled cigarette smoke. Ninety-five percent of patients with chronic obstructive lung disease either are or have been regular cigarette smokers. In one series of 1,400 autopsies, 90 percent of the nonsmokers had no evidence of emphysema, and none had advanced emphysema. Of people who smoked less than a pack a day, 75 percent had some evidence, and 12 percent had advanced disease. Of those who smoked more than a pack a day, all had some emphysema, and 20 percent had advanced disease.

Chronic bronchitis is often the first step on the road to emphysema. Defined simply as the daily coughing up of phlegm for at least three months in each of two consecutive years, chronic bronchitis predisposes the patient to repeated infections of the respiratory tract. Persistent inflammation of the bronchial tree due to irritation by microbes and by smoke and other pollutants partially obstructs the flow of air.

Of patients with chronic bronchitis, 25 percent—probably a group with some underlying genetic vulnerability—go on to develop emphysema. This occurs when the obstructed flow of air causes breakage of the alveoli, or air sacs, in which the exchange of oxygen and carbon dioxide takes place. This irreversible deterioration continues as long as the irritation (usually cigarette smoking) does. Chronic obstructive lung disease, or COLD, lacks the dramatic effect of "cancer" or "heart disease," but the condition kills 60,000 people annually in the United States alone.

Cigarette smoking is the prime villain in this destructive process. In addition there are minor contributions from general urban pollution and, for some individuals in selected occupations, industrial pollution. All three factors were absent from the lives of our late Paleolithic ancestors; indeed, even in this century hunters and gatherers such as the San (Bushmen) and the Hadza of Africa, and the Aché and Mashco-Piro of South America had no tobacco until it was introduced by outside contacts. Although the Mayans used pipes and cigars over 2,000 years ago, no people in the Old World had tobacco until after the initial exploration of the Americas. Even then, pipes, cigars, chewing tobacco, and snuff were all that were available until the Crimean War of the mid-1850s, when French and English officers learned of cigarettes from their Turkish allies. Automated manufacture of these inhalable-smoke producers began a few decades later, with three major consequences: Tobacco use by men increased tenfold; smoking by women became socially acceptable, especially after 1920; and inhalation of smoke became the rule rather than the exception.

While general atmospheric and workplace pollution are only minor contributors to emphysema and chronic bronchitis, it is a different matter with certain other lung conditions. Occupational exposure to dusts of various types plays a primary role in producing asbestosis, silicosis, black lung disease, and other chronic lung diseases. Typically these conditions involve inflammation and hardening of the lung tissue itself rather than airway obstruction. Even collectively, they are less common than COLD (chronic obstructive lung disease), but to the same extent they are caused by civilization.

Cancer

Although atherosclerosis—the root cause of most heart attacks and many strokes—is numerically the most prevalent modern killer, the specter of cancer takes hold more firmly on the minds of most of us. Because of the (sometimes irrational) fear of cancer, it is particularly important not to slip into easy explanations. There are many different malignancies, and they result from different processes—some genetic, some viral, some chemical, and some unknown—or in many cases from a combination of processes. However, in recent years it has become clear that several of the most widespread cancers in our society are either primarily caused or heavily contributed to by environmental factors—specifically, by cigarette smoke, dietary fat, and alcohol. The removal or reduction of these agents would prevent more cancers than have been cured by all known treatment methods, and far more than have been detected by all known screening methods.

The single most common cause of cancer death—now true for women as well as for men—is lung cancer. Once a relative rarity, it is now responsible for about 100,000 deaths a year in the United States. There is no longer serious debate about the reason for this enormous increase: the rise in cigarette smoking. Women provide an instructive lesson; they lagged behind men in lung-cancer rates to the same extent as they lagged behind men in smoking (about one generation), and now they have caught up in both. The average smoker's risk of lung cancer is about ten times greater than that of a nonsmoker, and the risk increases with the duration and amount of smoking. As every medical student learns, the number of "pack-years" a patient has logged—packs per day times number of years smoked—is one of the most important facts to be determined during the initial interview.

The mechanism is relatively straightforward. Normal bronchi (the tubes that carry air from the trachea, or windpipe, to and from the lungs) are lined with special protective cells. On the surface of these cells are thousands of tiny, fingerlike projections called cilia. Cilia ordinarily sweep away microscopic debris, but cigarette smoke immobilizes them and ultimately destroys the lining of the airway.

Once this protective, ciliated layer is gone, there is nothing to prevent inhaled particles—including the irritants in tobacco smoke (some of which are radioactive)—from collecting at strategic sites within the branching airway, usually at points where a larger passage divides into two or more smaller ones. In turn, unprotected cells from the deeper layers of the airway wall are stimulated to grow in an abnormal, uncontrolled fashion that can eventually become malignant, or cancerous. Cancers of the mouth, throat, and larynx—stimulated by similar mechanisms—are also much more likely in smokers than in nonsmokers.

Cancers of the colon, or large bowel, and rectum are about as common as lung cancers, although only about half as deadly. Their causes are not as clear, but there are now many strong clues. One striking feature of the geographical distribution of large-bowel cancer is its constant relationship to the modern industrial life-style. Its prevalence is invariably lowest in rural areas where a traditional life has been maintained. For example, the rate of colon cancer in black Americans far exceeds that in rural black Africans.

The experience of Japanese-Americans is also instructive. The Japanese in Japan have a rate of colon cancer less than one-fifth that in the United States; but when their descendants move to the United States and adopt American dietary habits, they approach American whites in their rate of this disease. A similar trend has occurred in Yemenite Jews moving to Israel and adopting the Western life-style of the dominant population.

Detailed epidemiological studies, backed by experiments with laboratory animals, have produced insights into the mechanism of these differences. Three main dietary factors appear to be important: fat, nondigestible fiber, and calcium. Although it is difficult to separate the three influences, evidence suggests that fat has a carcinogenic effect on the colon, while fiber and calcium are relatively protective. One mechanism may involve transit time through the colon, which is speeded up by fiber. The faster material passes through, the less time cancer-causing agents spend in contact with the colon wall. Even the sheer bulk provided by fiber dilutes such agents so that their concentration at the colon wall is reduced.

Fat, whose cancer-promoting effects on the colon are even better documented than are the protective effects of fiber, may act through another intriguing, indirect mechanism. When the body has a large fat intake, some of it is eliminated by the liver through its secretion of bile. This inevitably results in higher levels of bile acids and cholesterol-breakdown products in the intestine—the route through which bile is excreted. Colon bacteria break them down even further into substances that have been shown in animal experiments to cause cancer. Dietary calcium acts by combining with bile acids to produce insoluble substances that have no (or at least less) cancer-causing potential.

Breast cancer, only recently edged out by lung cancer as the biggest cancer-killer of women, is probably the most dreaded of all diseases affecting women specifically. Mutilating surgery looms almost as large as death in the fears of some women, and in a large number of cases a breast-cancer patient ends by having to face both. Although many advances in treatment have been made, no development of recent years could be called a breakthrough.

Breast cancer appears internationally in almost the same distribution pattern as does bowel cancer. In Europe and North America—until 1985, when lung cancer surpassed it—breast cancer killed more women than any other malignancy. But it is relatively uncommon in less-affluent, developing countries. As with colon cancer, immigrants coming from Taiwan, where breast cancer incidence is low, to the United States, where it is high, acquire the American rate in the second generation—underscoring the power of our environment in promoting the disorder. In epidemiological studies, fat consumption and breast tumors are correlated. In laboratory-animal studies, diets high in fat enhance the development of both spontaneous and chemically induced breast cancer.

The mechanism by which high-fat diets induce these cancers is unknown, but informed speculation centers on hormones as mediating the effect indirectly. The female reproductive hormones—estrogens—help promote breast malignancy, and fat cells have the capacity to convert noncancer-causing adrenal hormones into estrogens. It is reasonable to conjecture that excess fatty tissue promotes breast cancer by means of this hormonal conversion. (Some studies indicate that women in underdeveloped countries have lower estrogen levels than do women in industrialized nations—possibly in part a result of lower fat levels.) Whatever the mechanism, the relationship between dietary fat and breast cancer has appeared in many studies.

Other environmental influences on cancer have been frequently documented. Smoking has been implicated not only in lung cancer, but also in cancers of all surfaces contacted by the smoke, in bladder cancer, and to a lesser extent in cancers of the pancreas and cervix. Dietary fat has been implicated in prostate cancer, possibly caused by a mechanism similar to that of fat in breast cancer. (For example, African blacks have lower androgen levels, and less prostatic cancer, than do American blacks.) Excessive alcohol consumption has been strongly implicated in cancer of the esophagus and larynx (the "voice box"), which has been increasing in prevalence in the United States. Even moderate consumption of alcoholic beverages—three drinks a week—has been shown to increase breast cancer risk by 60 percent. And, of course, specific environmental agents such as asbestos and radiation are well known to cause certain cancers. In each of these cases, as in the more common lung, colon, and breast cancers, both the causative environmental agents—usually elements of our life-style—and the prevalence of the disease increases with the advent of Western industrial civilization.

Osteoporosis

Osteoporosis means a weakening of the bones, resulting from a loss of bony material at a rate in excess of the rate at which it is replaced. It becomes more frequent with age, is most common in postmenopausal women, and can be indirectly life-threatening. Osteoporosis increases the likelihood of breaking a bone. Injuries, such as falls, that might have only trivial effects in people with healthy skeletons, can begin a vicious cycle in osteoporotic individuals. Hip fractures, common in people with osteoporosis, are notoriously slow to heal and a long period of inactivity often follows such injury. In turn muscle weakness, bed sores, and pulmonary embolism may develop. The latter is potentially fatal: a blood clot forms in the leg or pelvis, passes through the veins and heart until it lodges in the lungs where, in severe cases, it may block all blood flow to the lungs and thus cause death. Not infrequently, a broken hip in an osteoporotic older person is the initiator of final deterioration and death.

Two factors important in preventing osteoporosis are sufficient amounts of calcium in the diet and muscle-building exercise—features more consistent with the hunter and gatherer's life than with our own. Their calcium intake was great, partly because they ate large amounts of fresh plant foods (often three pounds a day), and partly because wild fruits, vegetables, and roots usually contain more calcium than do our cultivated varieties—typically 50 percent more for a given weight of vegetables.

In addition, hunters and gatherers exercise much more than most people do in modern Western societies. Recent studies have shown that exercise, especially resistance exercise (the kind used in muscle building), strengthens bones as it increases musculature. This helps explain the impressive skeletal mass accumulated during youth and young adulthood by Paleolithic hunters and gatherers, as seen in their skeletal remains. A low "initial bone density" has come to be recognized as a prime risk factor for osteoporosis; it was rare among our remote ancestors, but is common in modern populations.

Hearing Loss

Life in Western nations is an assault on the ears. Industrial noise—at foundries, quarries, and manufacturing plants—has long been recognized as an important cause of hearing loss. But in recent years the impact of recreational noise has assumed equal status: Rock concerts, auto races, firearms, video arcades, motorcycles and dirt bikes, home power tools, and audio headphones are in this category. Of course, a further cacophony is neither recreational nor industrial: traffic noise, household appliances, building construction, farm machinery, subways, lawn mowers, sirens, chain saws, and airport noises.

Most people consider such high noise levels just one more annoying element of twentieth-century life, like smog or traffic congestion. But ear specialists regard the noise in our environment with more concern. Their experience indicates that noise levels common in Western society are a major threat to hearing. About 25 million Americans have enough hearing impairment to qualify for workmen's compensation. And these are not just old people; many are in their teens and twenties. The U.S. military services reject thousands of applicants each year because of hearing loss, and a study at the University of Tennessee showed that 60 percent of entering freshmen had measurable hearing loss. Ear specialists believe that the decline in auditory function is occurring at ever-earlier ages and that more and more Americans will enter their "golden years" with severely impaired hearing.

The ear is an organ of dazzling efficiency and sensitivity. Many components are necessary to achieve its unparalleled ability to detect, process, and retransmit the information it receives. Sound waves produce eardrum motion which, in turn, is transmitted by the tiny bones of the middle ear to create oscillation of fluid within the cochlea of the inner ear. This fluid motion is sensed by hair cells located on the cochlear lining; they respond by sending electrical signals via the acoustic nerves to the brain. The cochlear hair cells are readily damaged by exposure to loud noises, a form of injury termed "acoustic trauma." Just one extremely loud burst of noise may be sufficient to destroy enough hair cells to produce sudden, permanent hearing impairment.

However, the more common pattern is an ongoing, repetitive exposure to sounds of lesser but still harmful intensity. Thirty years may be required for this gradual process to become noticeable, but the hair cells are irreplaceable. Each of us is born with about 16,000, and as they are destroyed, one by one, hearing is gradually and permanently erased. The cumulative effects of chronic noise-induced acoustic trauma are irreversible: They produce sensory-neural hearing loss, which cannot be helped by hearing aids.

We are all familiar with older people whose hearing interferes with their ability to participate in conversation. If the predictions of ear specialists come true, such impairment will become common among ever-younger Americans. It is clear that the ear was not designed to withstand the kind of noise to which it is now subjected.

The acoustic environment of our ancestors was relatively noise free. Otologists (ear specialists) have studied the hearing of Maaban agriculturalists living in the southern Sudan and of San (Bushmen) in the Kalahari—people whose lives are spent amid noise levels similar to those encountered by Paleolithic humans. When the hearing of these people is contrasted with that of Westerners, marked differences in the patterns of age-related hearing loss become evident. Average seventy-year-old Maaban men have a 15 decibel (dB) hearing loss (at a standard frequency of 4,000 cycles per second) when compared with fifteen-year-old Maaban boys. But, among American males, seventy-year-olds have a 65 dB loss when compared with fifteen-year-old American youths— five times as much hearing impairment! The difference between Maaban and American women is slightly less pronounced, but still dramatic: a 20 dB loss for Maabans, as opposed to a 50 dB loss for Americans!

None of the Maabans or the San have presbycusis (hearing loss with age) sufficient to produce functional impairment. Before these studies were conducted, presbycusis severe enough to interfere with conversation had been considered a "normal" concomitant of aging, but the absence of significant hearing impairment among people who, like our ancestors, live in an environment where there is little exposure to noise suggests that what we have accepted as the normal accompaniment of advancing years is just another indication of the abnormally traumatic nature of our "civilized" environment.

Dental Caries

Dental caries, or "cavities," is caused by the bacterium *Streptococcus mutans*, which colonizes the surface of the teeth in susceptible individuals exposed to ample presence of simple, refined carbohydrates, especially sugars. Dental caries, although scarcely a major threat to health, is a source of annoyance, pain, expense, and eventual loss of teeth.

Caries is rare among nonindustrial peoples unaffected by modernizing influences. These peoples may show severe tooth wear over time, but such wear patterns result from grinding teeth on food particles harder than those we are accustomed to, or from the use of teeth as implements. They do not affect the basic structure of the teeth. The absence of tooth decay in these populations is well documented, as is its dramatic rise following the introduction of widespread sugar consumption. Unlike most of the diseases of civilization, the absence of caries has been documented directly in populations of our ancestors. The best preserved of human remains, teeth have been shown over and over again to be relatively little affected by decay in a variety of archaeological and paleontological populations.

The rise of sugar consumption during the recent past makes a story as dramatic as that of smoking. Developers of sugar beet and sugarcane plantations, together with industrialists, food technologists, and advertisers, have encouraged the sweet tooth of the civilized world. Dental caries—many times more common now, especially in areas without fluoridated water, than it was in the preindustrial era—has been repeatedly related to increasing sugar consumption. For example, the English experienced a stepwise increase in dental caries, as first honey (from domesticated bees) and then sugar became commonly available. By 1900, caries was thirty-five times as frequent as it had been in prehistoric Britain.

Alcohol-related Diseases

Research suggesting that moderate alcohol ingestion protects against coronary heart disease and reduces cardiac mortality has received considerable media exposure and popular attention. Investigators concur that heavy alcohol use markedly increases overall mortality, but light to moderate drinking (two to three drinks per day) has been shown to raise levels of HDL-cholesterol—the "good" cholesterol which protects against atherosclerosis—and this effect was proposed as the mechanism whereby light to moderate drinkers were protected from heart disease.

Subsequent articles which cast doubt on alcohol's benefits have been less publicized. These show that the HDL subfraction affected by alcohol is HDL_2 and that this factor has neutral, not beneficial effects on coronary disease. (HDL_3, elevated by exercise, is the subfraction which protects.) Why then have light drinkers had the lowest cardiac mortality—lower than that of nondrinkers—in several studies? Researchers have been unable to establish a physiological basis for this pattern and it is now thought likely that methodological and psychological factors may explain the association. From the standpoint of the study design, most investigators grouped lifelong teetotalers together with reformed drinkers, some of whom had previously imbibed to a considerable extent, in the "nondrinker" category. And from the psychological point of view, light drinkers tend to be better educated than either teetotalers or heavy drinkers. Such individuals are generally more conscious of diet, weight, exercise, and other health factors. Accordingly they constitute a low-risk group for heart disease. The increasingly widespread view of health professionals is that alcohol's potential as a protective influence against atherosclerosis is highly questionable.

In contrast to the dubious evidence suggesting a beneficial role for alcohol, the diseases it can promote are numerous, well-documented, and often devastating. Alcohol has a direct toxic effect on liver cells, the result depending on the extent and duration of alcohol abuse as well as on individual susceptibility. Large daily doses of alcohol can produce liver damage—fatty infiltration—within two weeks. In chronic alcoholics liver fat content can rise to eight times normal levels (40 percent of total liver weight), but fatty infiltration itself does not actually destroy liver cells. Alcoholic hepatitis does. This condition, which usually develops only after five to ten years of heavy drinking, is more serious and often produces jaundice. Furthermore, about a third of these patients go on to develop cirrhosis. Cirrhosis, the eighth leading cause of death in the United States, consists of extensive liver destruction, severe scarring, and markedly impaired function—often progressing to hepatic failure and death.

Other major diseases resulting from alcohol abuse include cancers of the esophagus, larynx, oral cavity, and breast. Even modest social drinking (two to three drinks a *week*) increases a woman's risk of breast cancer by approximately 60 percent. Alcoholic cardiomyopathy (a deterioration of the heart muscle), pancreatitis, alcoholic psychosis (hallucinations), and two other brain disorders, one affecting movement and one affecting memory, are further alcohol-related disease conditions. Withdrawal symptoms, including the DT's (delirium tremens), are often incapacitating. Babies carried by mothers who drink heavily often have abnormalities of facial and brain structure with associated mental impairment—the Fetal Alcohol Syndrome. Even moderate drinking by pregnant women can produce lesser fetal alcohol effects. Finally, intoxication itself, because it impairs normal functioning, increases the risk of accidents, homicide, suicide, unwanted pregnancy, wife beating, and child abuse.

Exposure to alcohol must have been rare if it occurred at all during the Paleolithic. Honey and many fruits can undergo spontaneous fermentation, so it is likely that at least some preagricultural peoples occasionally consumed alcoholic beverages. In the present century nearly half of all preliterate societies studied by anthropologists have made use of beverage alcohol; yet *none* of the groups actually producing it were hunters and gatherers.

When farming first began, the concurrent development of agriculture and ceramics (for storage) led quickly to regular manufacture and widespread consumption of alcoholic beverages. Barley beer was brewed in the Near East 7,500 years ago and, 3,000 years later, 40 percent of the grain crop in ancient Sumer was used for beer production. The Egyptians appear to have been the first wine makers. They used grapes, but later the Babylonians used dates and the Chinese used rice, for the same purpose—both long before the Christian era. Distilled spirits date only from the current millennium—a by-product of the alchemists' search for gold.

The easy availability of alcohol has rarely abated since. At present two thirds of all American adults drink alcoholic beverages more or less regularly and 7 to 10 percent of the average adult's energy intake is derived from this source.

About 10 million adults can be considered either alcoholics or at least problem drinkers. These unfortunates cause problems for themselves and for everyone with whom they come in contact. Alcoholism shortens life expectancy by ten to fifteen years and increases mortality rates to two or three times those of otherwise similar nondrinkers. It has been estimated that fully 10 percent of all deaths in the United States—as many as 200,000 a year—are alcohol related.

Population groups such as practicing Mormons who reject alcohol are spared this needless tragedy. Indeed, whole nations have experienced a significant reduction in alcohol-related deaths, especially cirrhosis, during periods of reduced alcohol availability as in continental Europe during the latter stages of World War II.

Preindustrial societies that did not have alcohol were also free from these illnesses. Unfortunately, when alcohol was introduced these societies were often violently disrupted. In several tragic cases alcoholism became almost universal, its related disease conditions widespread, and its resulting mood of dejection, paralyzing.

Diverticular Disease

Colonic diverticula are small saclike protrusions of the colonic lining, which project through weak spots in the bowel's muscular coat. There may be only one or there may be large numbers of them, but, taking all into account, the condition—diverticulosis—is the most common bowel disorder; it affects nearly half of all Americans over age fifty.

By themselves colonic diverticula are relatively innocuous, but occasionally a diverticulum ruptures so that intestinal content escapes into or through the bowel wall, resulting in infection, fever, and lower abdominal pain. Termed diverticulitis (as opposed to diverticulosis), surgery is sometimes required; very rarely, it even proves fatal. Under other circumstances a diverticulum may erode into one of the small arteries of the colon wall, producing massive lower-intestinal bleeding. While less common than diverticulitis, diverticular bleeding is the most frequent cause of extensive colonic hemorrhage; it, too, can end in death.

While colonic diverticula are extremely common in today's older Americans, they were regarded as rare curiosities by nineteenth-century pathologists. It was not until 1920 that descriptions of diverticulitis began to appear in medical and surgical textbooks, and as recently as 1930 diverticula were found in only about 5 percent of patients over age forty.

The English physician Denis Burkitt clarified the pathophysiology of colonic diverticular disease even as he offered an explanation for why the condition "emerged" as a major medical problem only in this century. Burkitt noted that rural blacks in Africa, whose diets contain ample nonnutrient fiber, have almost no diverticulosis. This resistance to the condition is not racial, because the prevalence of diverticular disease in American blacks equals that in American whites.

For millions of years, our ancestors consumed large amounts of crude dietary fiber as an integral component of the fruits, roots, seeds, and other vegetable foods that made up a major portion of their diet. As a result the large bowel became genetically adapted to function properly only in the presence of such bulky residue. It is designed to operate on a relatively large volume of waste material, moving it through the bowel by waves of muscular contraction.

Toward the end of the nineteenth century, the fiber content of diets in western Europe and the United States declined precipitously as finely milled flours and refined sugars became the chief carbohydrate staples, replacing whole-grain porridges and breads which had previously been dietary mainstays. Then and now, people who eat these largely fiber-depleted foods make trouble for their large intestines because there is not enough waste bulk for effective bowel function. Consequently, intestinal muscles contract with greater force, creating higher pressures within the bowel in order to move along the small volume of waste. This higher pressure can produce herniation of the bowel lining at weak points in the muscular wall, forming diverticula.

Burkitt and other researchers have found that reintroduction of insoluble fiber (usually in the form of wheat bran) into the diet markedly alleviates the symptoms associated with diverticular disease, and most investigators believe that a lifetime high-fiber diet—like that of our ancestors—can prevent formation of diverticula altogether.

Obesity

For over one hundred years, Americans have been getting fatter. A comparison of American Civil War draftees with those of the Korean and Vietnam conflicts shows that men's body mass index, a measure of obesity, has increased about 16 percent over the past century. In 1979 women were determined to be three to seven pounds heavier, at the same age and height, than their mothers had been only twenty years earlier. A more graphic example involves New York's Yankee Stadium. Originally built in 1922, it was renovated in 1978. However, in order to accommodate the expanding American posterior, the seats had to be widened from 19 to 22 inches, resulting in a decrease of 8,000 in "seating" capacity.

Obesity can be defined arbitrarily as weight 20 percent or more above that actuarially "desirable" from the insurance standpoint. By this standard about 30 percent of American men and 20 percent of American women between the ages of thirty and sixty are obese. But a more meaningful definition of obesity relies on *body composition*. When body weight alone is the criterion many athletes might be considered "overweight" because of their well-developed musculature; conversely, individuals in the "normal" category may have achieved their "desirable" weight by balancing an excessive amount of fat against a deficit of bone and muscle. In contrast, an evaluation of body composition (which can be accomplished by underwater weighing, skin-fold measurements, or by determining a series of body girths) establishes the proportions of fat and lean tissue in the individual being examined.

The desirable ranges of body fat content in healthy young Americans are commonly accepted as 13 to 18 percent for men and 20 to 30 percent for women; however, among hunters and gatherers body fat content is appreciably less. Considering these differences, "compromise" ranges of 10 to 15 percent for men and 20 to 25 percent for women may more nearly represent what human evolution has designed us to carry in the way of adipose tissue. (For women, the lower adaptive limit of body fat is easier to establish. There is some evidence that when fat constitutes less than 20 percent of a woman's weight, reproductive function may be disrupted in minor ways; further below this level menstrual cycling may stop.) Finally, in economically developed Western countries people tend to gain fat and lose lean body mass as they grow older. However, individuals in preagricultural societies do not gain fat and lose only a minimal amount of lean body mass as they age. Accordingly, a desirable goal would be to maintain the body composition appropriate for young adults throughout our lives.

None of the other diseases of civilization has such a straightforward mechanism as does obesity. Since the ability to store fat during times of plenty has had such strong survival value, it is no wonder that genetic adaptation for efficient conversion of food energy into fat has been selected during human evolution. But this genetic heritage leads to trouble when an affluent environment offers abundant food and leisure.

There are two main elements in the development of obesity: *energy intake*—the number of calories consumed as food and drink—and *energy expenditure*—the calories required for work, exercise, play, and the maintenance of ongoing bodily functions, or basal metabolic rate. Formerly, appreciable caloric expenditure was needed to generate or dissipate heat as required by the ambient conditions. However, central heating and air-conditioning have largely insulated us from our primal need to regulate body temperature.

These key elements—intake, activity, and heat production—are related in the energy balance equation, which states simply that for body weight to remain constant, the number of calories consumed in the diet must balance those expended. Since 3,500 calories can be equated with one pound of stored body fat, it follows that an excess of 100 calories a day on either side of the equation, over the course of a year, will amount to a ten-pound weight gain or loss. An eight-ounce nondiet soft drink, four ounces of cole slaw, or a single fried chicken leg each provide more than 100 calories. Conversely, a 1.5-mile jog, forty-five minutes of not-too-strenuous canoeing, or twenty minutes of disco dancing each require more than 100 calories.

Most foods available to affluent industrial peoples are calorically concentrated compared to the wild game and uncultivated fruits and vegetables that constituted the Paleolithic diet. So many calories are packed into such small quantities that an unsatisfyingly small volume now provides all the calories our low level of physical activity expends. To obtain 3,000 calories, hunters and gatherers had to eat five pounds of food, which kept their stomachs full. If we ate five pounds a day of typical supermarket or fast-food fare, we would all shortly resemble blimps.

Over the last hundred years, while the prevalence of obesity has risen alarmingly, the incidence of atherosclerosis, heart attack, adult-onset diabetes, hypertension, and cancer has also increased. The relationship between excess body weight and these chronic illnesses is a complex one, but in underdeveloped areas of the world where obesity is uncommon these diseases are rare. Also, when people move from such underdeveloped areas to the Western world (for example, when Yemenite Jews move to Israel or Greenland Eskimos to Denmark), the incidences of both obesity and these particular chronic illnesses increase in parallel.

Elevations of body weight up to 15 to 20 percent above the "ideal" level produce little or no impairment of health. Above that proportion, however, further increases cause a steady rise in morbidity (illness) and mortality (death). People 50 percent overweight have up to 100 percent excess mortality. This excess mortality, and an additional burden of excess morbidity, is caused by obesity-related increases in the above diseases plus gallbladder disease, disorders of pregnancy, musculoskeletal problems, and psychosocial disability.

Obesity increases the risk of developing atherosclerosis, especially in the arteries supplying the heart and brain. Its influence seems to be mediated indirectly through other risk factors, chiefly diabetes, hypertension, and elevated blood-cholesterol levels. Even if the relationship between atherosclerosis and obesity is an indirect one, it is powerful. One report of autopsy studies on 1,250 subjects showed that severe atherosclerosis was 2.5 times more common among obese than nonobese individuals. This increased risk is especially notable in people between ages twenty and forty; after age forty the influence of obesity has a lesser, though still important, effect.

Obesity's influence on blood pressure is also marked; for every 10 percent increment in body weight, there is a 6.5 mmHg rise in systolic blood pressure. The highly regarded Framingham study has shown that high blood pressure develops ten times more often in people 20 percent overweight than in people who maintain a "desirable" weight.

The theoretical explanation of the relationship between obesity and adult-onset diabetes has already been considered: Excessive fatness causes a diminished sensitivity to the action of insulin, setting up a vicious cycle of overproduction and underresponsiveness. One medical study showed that normal people produced 31 units of insulin over a twenty-four–hour period while obese subjects produced 114 units. Eventually, in genetically susceptible individuals, the stress of excess insulin secretion leads to relative insulin deficiency and, accordingly, to a pattern of abnormal glucose utilization.

Adult-onset diabetics, on the average, produce 46 units of insulin in twenty-four hours. This amount is 50 percent above the level produced by normal people, but in the obese, it is insufficient to regulate the uptake of glucose by the body tissues. Moderate obesity increases the risk of developing adult-onset diabetes about ten times. People whose weight is 45 percent above desired levels have a thirtyfold increased risk of diabetes.

As already shown, the frequency of several important malignancies is correlated with dietary practices, especially the proportion and amount of animal fat consumed. Since obesity is also correlated with these factors, it is not surprising that obesity and, for example, colon cancer are related, at least statistically. A more direct relationship between obesity and cancer of the endometrium (cancer of the uterus in one of its two main forms) has been shown to result from abnormal levels of estrogenic sex hormones—especially in postmenopausal women. Fat cells biochemically convert inactive forms of these hormones—made by the adrenal glands—into active and potentially carcinogenic forms. A similar effect of obesity on cancer of the breast, again as a result of relatively high estrogen levels in obese postmenopausal women, has also been suggested.

Other diseases are precipitated by obesity as well. Medical students learn to suspect gallstones in patients who are "fat, fair, and forty." This homily merely recognizes that gallstones are more common in women than in men, and that their frequency increases with age and weight. The obese tend to form bile that is supersaturated with cholesterol; such bile has an increased tendency to form gallstones. Degenerative arthritis—that is, arthritic changes occurring as a result of wear and tear on the weight-bearing joints, especially the knees and hips—is a greater cause of disability among obese individuals than among people of normal weight. Arthritic involvement of the spine is increased in obese women though not, for unknown reasons, in comparably overweight men.

Certain obstetrical complications are also influenced by obesity. The clearest relationship is between body weight and toxemia—a serious complication of pregnancy, which consists of fluid retention, rising blood pressure, and failing kidney function. It can progress to convulsions, coma, and death. If an overweight woman gets pregnant, and her weight places her in the highest 10 percent of pregnant women, she has twenty-five times more risk of toxemia than do women whose prepregnancy weight is in the lowest 10 percent.

Psychosocial disability is the ultimate insult and final cost of the syndrome. As Jean Mayer, prominent nutritional scientist and president of Tufts University, points out, the obese have become a new minority against whom strong prejudice is expressed in every way possible. The stigma of being overweight includes rejection and disgrace; the condition is viewed as both physical deformity and behavioral aberration. Unlike most handicaps, obesity becomes a moral issue; fat people are chastised for their lack of self-control and are held responsible for what is seen by some as a voluntary, self-inflicted disability.

There are six times as many obese women in the lowermost social classes as in the uppermost. Also, there is much less obesity among those moving up the social ladder than among those who stay in the social class into which they were born. Obese high-school students are less likely to be accepted by top-ranking colleges than are their non-obese peers who have similar academic grades and test scores. In the working world, obese people are discriminated against in hiring, pay raises, and promotions.

Because they deviate from prevailing esthetic standards, fat people suffer from social as well as economic discrimination, tending to be excluded from peer-group interactions. Surveys of groups ranging from schoolchildren to doctors show that the obese are consistently characterized in negative terms: unlikable, weak-willed, awkward, less attractive, and less desirable as friends.

These societal prejudices have important psychological and psychiatric consequences. Many fat people feel mortified and ashamed, full of self-disparagement and self-hatred. In terms of psychosocial disability they have a triple disadvantage: They are discriminated against; they are made to feel that they deserve that discrimination; and they come to accept their treatment as just.

Never before have so many members of a mammalian species eaten so much, burned away so little of their food, and accumulated so much surplus fat. As Jean Mayer says, *Homo sapiens sapiens* is evolving into *Homo sedentarius obesus*. The cause of this unique development is a deceptively simple imbalance in the energy equation; its cure is an alteration of life-style away from the deleterious elements of the affluent twentieth century and toward a way of life based on the pattern for which humans have been genetically adapted through eons of evolution.

CONCLUSION

This dismal yet incomplete catalog of the diseases of civilization (see Table I) illustrates and substantiates the discordance hypothesis. In each case, our genes are adapted to the circumstances in which we evolved, but in which we no longer live. Our industrial present includes increased levels of saturated fat and salt, decreased levels of fiber and exercise, the widespread use of alcohol and tobacco, a state of continual abundance, and universal caloric concentration. These factors, rare in the past, together result in a mismatch, or discordance, between the genes carried forward from our environment of evolutionary adaptedness and the new environment we have "suddenly" created. This mismatch, in turn, promotes, accelerates, and fosters the diseases associated with affluent civilization. And, together, these afflictions account for three-fourths of all deaths in the modern industrial state.

TABLE I.

Leading Causes of Death in the United States—1985

Cause of Death	Percent of Total Deaths
Heart Disease (chiefly coronary atherosclerosis)	37.0%
Cancer (Lung, colon, and rectum; breast; and prostate together cause 54% of all cancer deaths)	22.1%
Stroke	7.3%
Accidents	4.5%
Chronic Obstructive Lung Disease	3.4%
Pneumonia	3.2%
Diabetes Mellitus	1.8%
Atherosclerosis (not including heart or brain, but including aortic aneurysm)	1.8%
Suicide	1.4%
Cirrhosis	1.3%
	83.8%

Source: *Vital Statistics of the United States*, 1985.

CHAPTER FOUR
THE STONE AGE DIET

Well over 200 million years ago a successful and fairly large group of mammal-like reptiles, the therapsids, walked the earth. Ironically, they resembled us more than they did their successors, the dinosaurs. The early dinosaurs began their 150-million-year reign only after mass extinction nearly exterminated their mammal-like predecessors; but those therapsids who survived—small, quick, and carnivorous—eventually outlasted the giants, giving rise to the mammals and, ultimately, to us.

If the Victorians were nonplussed at the thought of descent from monkeys or even Neanderthals, imagine how they would have reacted to the idea that their earliest mammalian ancestors bore an unflattering resemblance to today's rats. These creatures were primarily insect-eaters, and they remained so throughout the reign of the dinosaurs, which ended around 70 million years ago. This (for us) fortuitous occurrence opened the floodgates for mammalian evolution, and a prompt flowering of species—called an adaptive radiation—produced forms from sloths and shrews to bats and whales.

The mammals in our ancestral line during this period (from 70 to 50 million years ago) had the basic features of today's mouse lemurs, bushbabies, and tarsiers: small, active, and much more primitive than monkeys. These early primates were also largely insectivorous. Without suggesting that katydids, fire ants, and dragonflies should be among our dietary staples, consideration of the nutritional properties of insects—eaten by our ancestors for 150 million years or so—is illuminating. And, since evolution is basically a conservative biological process, it is not too farfetched to suggest that our genes partially reflect that very long-standing adaptation. Indeed one might think of these creatures as extremely early "hunters." With the exception that they contain much more calcium, the insects they preyed on are nutritionally remarkably similar to wild game. In both cases protein far exceeds fat, sodium is low, and potassium is high. (See Table II.)

TABLE II.

Nutrients in Insects and Wild Game
Components of a 100-Gram Portion

Nutrient	Insects	Wild Game
Fat	4.30 gm	3.91 gm
Protein	21.90 gm	24.30 gm
Energy	118.00 kcal	141.00 kcal
Calcium	82.90 mg	10.00 mg
Sodium	96.90 mg	68.75 mg
Potassium	212.00 mg	387.50 mg

From L. B. Page, J. G. Rhoads, J. S. Friedlander, J. R. Page, S. Curtis, "Diet and Nutrition," in J. S. Friedlander, ed. *The Solomon Islands Project.* Oxford: Clarendon Press. 1987: 55-88.

In fact, in certain vital ways (for example, low fat, low sodium, and high potassium) this nutrient spectrum continued to characterize the diet of our intermediate ancestors as well—between 50 and 10 million years ago—even though the specific foods they consumed were different. Because over the course of millions of years of evolution, as primates became larger and more varied, their diet slowly shifted toward plant foods. The first hominoids—the great apes—living 30 million years ago subsisted largely on fruit, although fossil remains show that their teeth were also suitable for processing other vegetable foods and meat. This pattern—fruits primary, with other vegetable foods and meat a distant second and third—seems to have prevailed for about 20 million years.

Around 7 million years ago—when the protohuman line diverged into two paths, one leading to chimpanzees, the other to humans—meat began to assume greater importance, although whether it was obtained by hunting, scavenging, or both is not clear. What *is* clear is that meat was included as regular fare in the early human diet soon after the first stone tools were manufactured around 2 million years ago, and that the proportion of meat increased with the later appearance of *Homo erectus*. Wherever they lived and whatever their physical form, ancestral humans made tools designed for processing game, and their living sites were near the grazing grounds or migratory routes of large herd animals. Animal remains from this period bear clear marks of having been butchered with stone tools, and in one or two cases it is evident that the animals were killed by humans; spear points are embedded in the bones.

The role of vegetable foods has been harder to assess, since plant remains and even gathering tools—most are made of wood or plant fiber—are poorly preserved. But, in most cases, these foods are likely to have been the mainstay of the hunting and gathering diet, then as now. A probable major exception was a relatively short period beginning about 35,000 years ago in Europe, not long after truly modern humans appeared. With well-developed equipment, sophisticated hunting techniques, and human population densities low in relation to numbers of game animals, people such as the Cro-Magnons concentrated on big-game hunting. In some areas during this time meat probably provided over 50 percent of the diet. But this didn't last very long in evolutionary terms; even before agriculture appeared 10,000 years ago, overhunting, climatic changes, and population growth had caused a shift from big-game hunting toward a broader spectrum of subsistence activities.

This subsistence pattern included fishing and shellfish collection along with gathering plant foods and hunting wild animals. Although shells and fish bones first appear in the archaeological record 130,000 years ago (during the time of Archaic *Homo sapiens*), it is only in sites dating from 20,000 years ago or more recent periods that these remains show up frequently, suggesting that widespread use of aquatic foods is relatively new. (Whether this was true along the seacoast as well is not known since those regions were permanently submerged when the glaciers melted.) Remains of small game animals and tools for processing plant foods—such as grindstones and mortar-and-pestles—also date from this period, which is known as the Mesolithic, a period between the Paleolithic and the Neolithic, or from around 20,000 to around 10,000 years ago.

This shift—from greater to lesser meat consumption—is evident from chemical analysis of strontium and calcium in fossil bones: the ratio of these atoms reflects the relative proportions of animal and vegetable foods consumed during life. Since strontium reaches bone mainly when plant foods are consumed, the bones of herbivores have a higher strontium-calcium ratio than do those of carnivores. When fossil remains of people living in the Middle East, prior to and after the advent of agriculture, are subjected to this analysis, it is clear that the latter were eating more vegetable foods and less meat. This pattern has characterized the transition from hunting and gathering to agriculture whenever it has occurred.

The effect of slowly evolving changes over millions of years pales compared to the immediate impact agriculture (and more recently, industrialization) has had on the human diet. Within a few thousand years of agricultural life, vegetable foods came to make up as much as 90 percent of the diet. At the same time, the broad range of wild plant foods typical of hunting and gathering diets was replaced by a narrow range of cultivated crops. The result? People living after the advent of agriculture were four inches shorter, on average, than early European *Homo sapiens sapiens* living 30,000 years ago. Even *Homo erectus* of 1.6 million years ago was tall; a remarkably complete fossil skeleton recently found in Kenya by Richard Leakey and Alan Walker suggests that these remote humans were as tall or taller than we are today.

A similar trend was observed in the fossil remains of Central American Indians. Those living as hunters and gatherers 11,000 years ago—the Paleoindians—were big-game hunters. Their agricultural descendants, just before European contact, ate little meat. Eventually their diets became so deficient in protein that clinical malnutrition occurred, as is evident in their fossil remains. In addition, in some regions their intake of calcium and tryptophan (an essential amino acid) probably declined as corn became the staple. Together, these nutritional deficiencies increased the population's susceptibility to infectious diseases, which became widespread. The toll? People were considerably shorter than their ancestors, and their bone structure reflected less than ideal nutrition.

Since the Industrial Revolution, the animal-protein content of Western diets has once again increased. This may help explain the increase in the average height of Americans and Europeans observed within the last 150 years. We are now nearly as tall as were the first biologically modern humans. Even so, our diets still differ dramatically from those of hunters and gatherers in many fundamental—and detrimental—ways.

RECENT HUNTER AND GATHERER NUTRITION

Although few have survived late enough into the twentieth century for their diets to be analyzed with scientific rigor, over fifty hunting and gathering societies have been sufficiently well-studied that some generalizations about their nutritional status can be made. The spectrum of foods they consume—wild game and uncultivated vegetable foods—

is similar to the spectrum consumed by our ancestors throughout 4 million years of human and prehuman existence.

Nevertheless, hunters and gatherers of today are different from their Paleolithic counterparts in significant ways. Contemporary preagricultural people live in marginal environments—the desert, the tropical forest, or Arctic regions. The food quest in such settings is more difficult than it would have been 25,000 years ago, when the most fertile and productive areas were available and game was more abundant.

Even in the recent past, we can see examples of such environmental largesse. Explorers in North America and Africa recorded staggering numbers of animals. In the nineteenth century, American bison herds stretched from horizon to horizon, sometimes requiring two days to pass by. Flocks of passenger pigeons literally darkened the sky and were easily killed when they landed because their numbers were so great. Similar sights were common in Africa within the last few decades. But human population expansion and settlement, with consequent logging, farming, fencing, and construction—as well as our penchant for hunting, often only for trophies—has drastically decreased the quantity of game, especially big game animals.

Modern hunters and gatherers are also more technologically advanced than their Paleolithic forebears. The bow and arrow, for example, are only about 15,000 to 20,000 years old. And virtually all known groups have had considerable contact with the outside world, which has influenced to different degrees their economies, technologies, and social organizations. Even with these differences, contemporary hunting and gathering life still operates under constraints sufficiently similar to those that shaped the life-style and the diet of their (and our) forebears that these data can be systematically enlightening. This is, therefore, a good place to begin our exploration of what humans are genetically "programmed" to eat, digest, and metabolize.

An overview of contemporary preagricultural diets shows great variation—from the Aborigines of central Australia, who obtain only 10 to 20 percent of their food from meat, to the Arctic Eskimos, for whom animal foods provide 90 to 95 percent of the subsistence—and suggests an average pattern of 35 percent meat and 65 percent plant foods. (See Table III.)

While each of these examples provides no more than a dim and skewed reflection of a vast, long past, together they form a helpful, if clouded, mirror. The similarities between them, despite their diversity, form a rational basis for important generalizations about the hunting and gathering life-style, both recently and in the remote past.

But first, a look at some terms. *Meat* and *plant foods*—words quite

TABLE III.

Subsistence Patterns of Contemporary Hunters and Gatherers

People	Environment	Subsistence Pattern (Plant : animal)
Hadza	Tanzania: inland, semitropical	80:20
!Kung San	Botswana: desert	65:35
Aborigines	Australia: variable from extreme desert to swampy to seacoast	90:10 (desert) 25:75 (coastal)
Aché	Paraguay: forest	50:50
Agta	Philippines: tropical mountainous forest	40:60
Eskimos	North American Arctic	10:90

familiar to us—often require modification when discussed in the hunting and gathering context. Wild plants breed to maximize their own reproductive advantage, not for the taste or convenience of humans. Never having been cultivated, these plant foods are often found thinly spread over wide areas. Berries are usually more pit than flesh; pods may have hard, starchy seeds; fruits are often sour, with tough inedible skins; and nuts and beans have thick shells difficult or impossible to crack without special tools. The negatives are not universal, however. Many wild plants are delicacies of the first order; consider truffles, wild strawberries and blueberries, various nuts, and numerous tropical fruits. Most wild plants have more protein and calcium than do their domestic cousins, and unadulterated wild plant foods are fiber-rich.

Whatever their virtues and drawbacks, plant foods have been a dietary mainstay of preagricultural people living at all but the highest latitudes. And these plants are not limited to a meager few. Hunters and gatherers typically consume a wider range of vegetables and fruits than do agriculturalists, who concentrate on a smaller number of planted crops. Cereal grains—an agricultural staple for the past 10,000 years—play only a minor part in the diet of recent hunters and gatherers. (The almost total absence of grindstones and mortars-and-pestles in archaeological material dating from before 20,000 years ago suggests that this was true in the Late Paleolithic as well.) Roots, beans, nuts, tubers, fruits, flowers, and gums provide hunters and gatherers with a greater quantity and wider variety of vitamins and minerals than farming did for agriculturalists.

Similarly, wild meat also differs from that of domesticated animals, which have always been fatter than their wild counterparts because of steady food and reduced physical activity. During the past century, breeding and feeding practices increased the proportion of fat still further in response to consumer demand for ever-more-tender meat. The marbling of muscle and thick layers of insulating fat found in supermarket meat shows the results of these efforts. Indeed, the carcasses of today's domesticated animals are 25 to 30 percent fat, while a survey of forty-three different species of wild game animals from three continents has revealed an average fat content of only 4.3 percent.

Not only the quantity, but the quality of fat differs. Fat from wild game contains a much higher proportion of polyunsaturated fatty acids—five times as much per gram—as does fat from domestic animals. It also contains about 2.5 percent of an essential fatty acid—eicosapentaenoic acid, or EPA—currently thought to offer protection against atherosclerosis. Domestic beef, in contrast, contains so little EPA it is hard to detect.

Because it is lean, meat from wild animals has fewer calories and more protein than comparable portions of domestic meat. (The amino acid spectrum is the same in both.) Many drawbacks attributed to red meat in general should actually be attributed only to modern fatty meat; game meat is leaner and its fat less saturated. One might guess that it would be lower in cholesterol as well, but because the cholesterol content of lean tissue is roughly equivalent to that of fat, this is not the case.

The change to agriculture had less impact on the fiber content of diets than on protein intake. Paleolithic methods of food processing—ranging from none (eating fruits and vegetables raw) to pounding, scraping, roasting, or baking—meant that most nonnutrient fiber remained. The processing techniques of early agriculturalists were scarcely more transforming, although when grains assumed new dietary significance, insoluble fiber became relatively more prominent than soluble fiber in the diet (at least in Europe and Asia). However, with the development of roller mills in the nineteenth century, finely ground flours replaced the coarse, fiber-rich flours that had been in use for the previous 10,000 years. Thereafter, the decline in total fiber intake was dramatic. A study of the Welsh diet, to take only one example, shows that starchy foods have decreased by 50 percent in this century, with dietary-fiber intake only a third of what it was a hundred years ago.

Sugar consumption has also changed over the centuries. After three generations of steady increase, the American diet now boasts a yearly consumption of over one hundred pounds of sugar per person per year—about four to five ounces per day. (The actual range varies greatly—some individuals eat over two hundred pounds a year!) In contrast, hunters and gatherers consume sugar only as it occurs naturally in plant foods and in the honey of wild bees. Paintings found in Spain dated between 10,000 and 12,000 years ago show a woman climbing to obtain honey from a tree. She is surrounded by bees, a testimony to both the strength of the human sweet tooth and the difficulty of satisfying it. Recent observations of !Kung San and Pygmy hunters and gatherers have revealed similar scenes.

Our human predilection, even craving, for sugar is as powerful as it is ancient. But in the wild that craving is hard to indulge; honey is available only seasonally, and even then, it requires considerable effort to extract: chopping and climbing trees, and smoking bees out while enduring painful stings. For hunters and gatherers, sugar was a highly prized commodity—all the more so for being available only irregularly.

With the domestication of sugarcane, however, all that changed. Sugarcane, apparently, was first cultivated in New Guinea around 8,000 years ago. (The domestication of honeybees took much longer, and is first recorded in Egypt a mere 4,500 years ago.) Cane sugar production spread far and wide, reaching Southeast Asia and India by 500 B.C. and the Mediterranean regions, including North Africa and Spain, around A.D. 700. Even so, by the late fourteenth century—Chaucer's time—cookbooks still specified honey in recipes; sugar was never even mentioned. By the seventeenth century, it had become much more common, although very expensive. It remained a luxury for the wealthy until the nineteenth century. From then on, the story is simple and familiar. By 1900, sugar provided one-fifth of all calories in the English diet—about the level we maintain in the United States today.

Vegetable foods, meat, sugar—even what we drink differs from what hunters and gatherers ate and drank. A 1985 American trade publication *Impact Beverage Trends in America: Review and Forecast* revealed some pretty sobering sales statistics. Soda is the most common beverage consumed in the United States—more common than water, milk, alcoholic drinks, coffee, or tea. Not only are most soft drinks heavily laden with sugar, but they also pack a wallop of concentrated calories. For hunters and gatherers, water—the ultimate low-calorie drink—was the primary thirst quencher. Of course, seasonal tea-like beverages, soups, and fruit juices were alternatives. (Milk was not; only those not yet weaned were so privileged.) Much the same could be said of alcoholic beverages. No hunters and gatherers studied in this century independently developed their own brew; in all instances, these were introduced by outsiders. Because of seasonal fluctuations, geographic constraints, and limited storage capacity, it seems unlikely that such drinks—for example, mead or fruit wine—were regular fare for our Paleolithic ancestors.

Diseases of nutritional deficiency, such as scurvy, pellagra, and beriberi, were probably less common among hunters and gatherers (with their varied fruit- and vegetable-based diets) than among agriculturalists. The same is true for widespread famine; when climatic aberrations produce crop failure and starvation for farmers, nearby hunters and gatherers often remain relatively unscathed. Given their wide choice of wild vegetable plants—plants proved capable of surviving climatic change over time—this is not surprising. Because, while hybridized plants imported from distant regions may succumb to unseasonable cold, drought, or flooding, indigenous wild plants continue to survive, ensuring that hunters and gatherers will as well. Indeed, during one year when extreme drought killed crops and decimated cattle herds in Botswana, technicologically "advanced" Bantu-speaking people were able to survive only by adopting the foraging techniques of the "primitive" !Kung San, their hunting and gathering neighbors.

PROBABLE DAILY NUTRITION OF OUR PALEOLITHIC ANCESTORS

By compiling studies which detail the diets of recent hunters and gatherers, it is possible to reconstruct a prototype of what was probably the nutrient content of our ancestral diet. Since the estimates average the diets of many groups, they should be considered ballpark figures, encompassing local variations in climate, season, terrain, and other environmental conditions, as well as differences in the specific plants and animals available. The nutrient content for Paleolithic foods is reconstructed by averaging the composition of meat from current free-living game animals and contemporary wild plant foods. These values have been determined for forty-three different game animals—including such diverse creatures as wild boar, bison, eland, kangaroo, oryx, and deer—and for over one hundred species of plants consumed by modern-day hunters and gatherers. (See Tables IV, V, and VI.)

TABLE IV.

Nutritional Properties of Wild Game and Domestic Meat

| | Average Content per 100 g | |
Constituent	Wild Game*	Domestic Meat**
Energy, kcal	133.1	385.5
Protein, g	21.9	15.8
Fat, g	4.3	29.0
Cholesterol, mg	67.0	75.0

*43 species
**4 varieties

TABLE V.

Nutrient Properties of Wild Plant Foods*

Constituent	Average Content per 100 g	Number of Species with Data Available
Dietary Fiber	12.6 g	109
Calcium	131.0 mg	119
Vitamin C	30.6 mg	64
Iron	6.4 mg	101
Sodium	26.9 mg	102
Potassium	424.6 mg	112

*Total number of species = 153

Energy Sources

As our ancestors sat around the fire savoring the aroma of a roasting venison haunch, the meat they were eating gave them about 133 calories for every four-ounce chunk. (In contrast, when we wolf down a quarter-pounder at the local burger joint, we're getting about 319 calories from the meat alone, even in the unlikely event that it's ground from four

TABLE VI.

Wild Game—Lipid Characteristics

Constituent	Average Content per 100 g	Number of Species with Data Available
Total Fat, g	4.3	43
Cholesterol, mg	67	8
Polyunsaturated Fat, % of all Fat	32	17
EPA (C 20:5), % of all Fat	2.5	7

TABLE VII.

Proposed Average Daily Macronutrient Intake for Late Paleolithic Humans Consuming 3000 kcal (35% Meat and 65% Plant Foods)

	Grams	Percent Total Energy
Protein	250	33
Animal	190	
Vegetable	60	
Fat	70	21
Animal	30	
Vegetable	40	
Carbohydrate	340	46
Total Fiber	150	—

Updated from S. B. Eaton, and M. Konner. "Paleolithic Nutrition: A Consideration of Its Nature and Correct Implications." *New England Journal of Medicine* 312 (1985): 283-89.

ounces of pure sirloin.) The fresh roots and other plant foods that completed our predecessors' meal would have provided an additional 129 calories per 100 g portion.

Their daily energy requirements can also be estimated and related to the caloric content of their food. Preagricultural people were quite tall and considerably more muscular than we are today; they also led lives that required much more physical exertion. A reasonable estimate of their average daily energy need would therefore be around 3,000 calories.

If we assume that they were eating about 35 percent meat and 65 percent vegetable foods—the most common pattern among recent hunters and gatherers—then they must have been eating about 2,250 g (nearly five pounds) of food every day and, of this, meat would have been 790 g and plant foods about 1,460 g. If the proportions were reversed (65 percent meat, 35 percent plant foods), total energy intake (calories) would be relatively unaffected because of the close caloric similarity between game meat and plant foods. (With our concentrated diets we get the same number of calories from only three pounds of food—less bulky and thus less satisfying.) After eliminating water content (almost two-thirds of the total weight), the daily diet, broken down even further, would probably have looked something like what is shown in Table VII.

Fat and Fatty Acids

Wild game animals have less total fat than domesticated animals (just over 4 g fat per 100 g wild meat, as compared to 29 g fat per 100 g domestic meat), and the fat in game is much less saturated. For example, the fat from a Cape buffalo is 30 percent polyunsaturated, 32 percent monounsaturated, and 38 percent saturated. This finding is typical of other wild animals as well. Of seventeen wild animals analyzed—Cape buffalo, eland, kangaroo, caribou, seal, giraffe, grouse, warthog, and nine others—the proportion of polyunsaturated fat averaged 32 percent. (Domestic meat—beef, pork, lamb, veal, and chicken—in contrast is only about 7 percent polyunsaturated, one-fifth that of wild animals.) Assuming a similar ratio for most wild animals, our reconstructed Paleolithic diet would have provided 8.9 g polyunsaturated fat, 9.5 g monounsaturated fat, and 11.3 g saturated fat from animal sources.

Most vegetable foods contain little fat, and this fat usually has a high proportion of polyunsaturates. When the fat content of thirty-six wild foods eaten by the Hadza, the San (Bushmen), and other African tribal groups was analyzed, polyunsaturates averaged 39 percent of total fat.

Cholesterol

The cholesterol intake of Paleolithic people was probably a little higher than ours. Meat from modern domesticated animals averages 75 mg (1/1,000 of a gram = 1 mg) of cholesterol for each 100-g portion. Since the proportion of cholesterol in meat is surprisingly little affected by its fat content, the amount of cholesterol in meat from wild game is only slightly less—67 mg/100 g. Our ancestors consuming a theoretical 790 g of meat daily would therefore have ingested about 520 mg of cholesterol. This is slightly more than our consumption today—most recently estimated at 300-500 mg/day.

Sodium and Potassium

All mammals except humans normally consume more potassium than sodium, and until salt became an inexpensive commodity (sometime after A.D. 1000) this was true for our ancestors as well. However, because sodium (as common table salt, or sodium chloride) is added to food today at almost every step in preservation, processing, preparation, and consumption, and because potassium is consistently leached out during these same procedures, people in affluent countries now consume about one and a half times as much sodium as potassium. Total sodium intake commonly ranges from 2,300 to 6,900 mg a day, but in some areas (such as northern Japan) it can exceed 20 g (20,000 mg!) a day. An analysis of vegetable foods and meat consumed by traditional hunters and gatherers indicates that they averaged a sodium intake of about 700 mg daily and that potassium far exceeded sodium in their diet—by tenfold or more.

Calcium

At present there is considerable controversy among nutritionists and physicians about the proper amount of calcium recommended for daily human consumption. An analysis of over one hundred plant foods used by recent hunters and gatherers supports the notion that high levels of calcium intake are desirable. Wild vegetable foods average about 130 mg of calcium per 100 g portion; since Late Paleolithic people were eating about 1,460 g of such food each day, plant foods would have provided over 1,800 mg of calcium while the meat they ate would have given another 100 mg. Chewing bones from fowl or small mammals might have substantially increased this last value.

Even if plant foods made up only 30 percent of their estimated daily diet, calcium levels would still be high by American standards. The more typical Paleolithic calcium intake of about 1,900 mg per day would bring us closer to (though still below) what is known about calcium requirements in other mammalian species. Lower requirement estimates (figures as low as 400 mg per day have been suggested by some nutritionists) are far below the proportional estimates for other mammals.

Ascorbic Acid

Wild plant foods can be excellent sources of vitamin C. The Australian green plum, favored by Aborigines, contains over 3 g (3,000 mg) of vitamin C per 100 g portion. Not including it, the mean ascorbic acid content of sixty-four vegetables eaten by recent hunters and gatherers is about 30 mg per 100 g, so 440 mg of vitamin C would have been a typical daily intake in the Paleolithic period. This is five times what Americans normally consume, and over seven times the current authoritative recommendation.

Other Nutrients

Even at the lowest levels of meat consumption (as little as 10 to 15 percent meat), the intake of animal protein, iron, vitamin B_{12}, and folic acid would have been adequate, by modern standards, in the Paleolithic diet. By contrast, widespread deficiencies in these nutrients are evident in many agricultural populations of today's less developed countries.

Great diversity of plant foods—with a correspondingly wide spectrum of nutrients—is typical of hunting and gathering diets, but not of agricultural ones. This made available most of the essential trace elements, although limited geographic distribution of iodine may have meant deficiencies for some groups. Even today, people in inland mountainous regions are frequently iodine deficient.

Fiber

Since hunters and gatherers consumed large quantities of vegetable foods and had relatively crude techniques for processing them, they obtained substantial dietary fiber. The average total fiber content of one hundred and nine plants eaten by modern hunters and gatherers is 12.6 g per 100 g eaten. Calculated according to our model diet with 1,460 g of vegetable foods, the estimated daily fiber intake of Paleolithic peoples would have been on the order of 150 g as opposed to less than 20 g for ourselves. This, to us, seemingly high estimate for fiber intake is supported by independent research involving human coprolites (fossilized fecal remains). Analysis of this material suggests that Archaic Amerindian hunters and gatherers were consuming about 130 g of fiber each day.

Furthermore, the proportion of soluble fiber (a major fiber component in most fruits and vegetables) in their diets would have exceeded that in ours because wheat and rice (major components of the modern diet) have predominantly insoluble fiber. While both types of fiber have important physiological benefits, soluble fiber has been shown to lower serum cholesterol levels.

Shortages

All people before the Industrial Revolution, whether they were hunters and gatherers or agriculturalists, experienced occasional nutritional stress due to seasonal or local variations in climate. More extreme periods of food shortage also occurred, but were less frequent. Although Paleolithic hunters and gatherers often lived in areas teeming with game and wild plant foods (in contrast to recent hunters and gatherers who have lived in marginal areas), it is likely that they also faced periodic shortages great enough to produce weight loss. Since food was rarely stored, a severe depletion of the environment's natural storehouse could have precipitated perilous deprivation. For individuals with little or no body fat, starvation and death may have resulted.

The way this problem was solved—a solution apparently favored by natural selection—was for people to be "programmed" to eat more than was necessary during times of abundance to ensure against times of scarcity. This pattern has been observed among modern hunters and gatherers even as it has among ourselves. But for those of us living in affluent countries our seemingly insatiable appetites produce fat stores we no longer need. Unless we create a deliberate personal shortage known as dieting, we never use them up. Because of this literal and figurative "cushion," our survival (as individuals) is now threatened by plenty instead of by dearth.

THE PALEOLITHIC DIET IN MODERN PERSPECTIVE

Whether based on as much as 80 percent or as little as 20 percent meat, the spectrum of nutrients eaten by Paleolithic hunters and gatherers differs dramatically from that consumed by most Americans today. In some ways, it is even at odds with what many established nutritionists are advocating, including those working with the American Heart Association and the United States Senate Select Committee on Nutrition and Health. (See Table VIII.) For example, we traditionally divide our foods into four basic groups: (1) meat and fish, (2) vegetables and fruit, (3) milk and milk products, and (4) breads and cereals. Two or more servings from each group are considered necessary for a balanced diet. Yet before agriculture, people derived their nutrients from just the first two groups.

TABLE VIII.

Late Paleolithic, Contemporary American, and Recently Recommended Dietary Composition

	Late Paleolithic Diet	Contemporary American Diet	Recent Recommendations
Total Dietary Energy (%)			
Protein	33	12	12
Carbohydrate	46	46	58
Fat	21	42	30
Alcohol	~0	(7–10)*	—
P:S Ratio	1.41	0.44	1
Cholesterol (mg)	520	300–500	300
Fiber (gm)	100–150	19.7	30–60
Sodium (mg)	690	2,300–6,900	1,000–3,300
Calcium (mg)	1500–2000	740	800–1,500
Ascorbic Acid (mg)	440	90	60

Updated from S. B. Eaton and M. Konner, "Paleolithic Nutrition: A Consideration of Its Nature and Current Implications," *New England Journal of Medicine* 312 (1985): 283–89.

*Inclusion of calories from alcohol would require concomitant reduction in calories from other nutrients, mainly carbohydrate and fat.

"Give us this day our daily bread," says the ancient prayer, and 2,000 years ago foods derived from cereal grains were the staples of most people's diets. But in relation to our long human existence, dependence on bread is a very late phenomenon. Artifacts related to the harvesting, processing, and storage of grain (such as wood or bone sickles set with multiple microlithic flint blades, and tools such as grindstones, mortars-and-pestles, and storage pits) are rarely found in archaeological material dating from before 20,000 years ago, but they become relatively common thereafter.

Earlier humans knew of grains, but in order to be utilized, they had to be collected, winnowed, processed, and stored. Other plant foods were usually preferred even in areas where wild grain was abundant; that is, until toward the end of the Paleolithic, when population growth and climatic changes increased the pressure on available wild food resources and it became expedient to include grain in the diet. Only then could the prayer for daily bread become one in which people around the world found meaning.

Since they had no domesticated animals, Late Paleolithic hunters and gatherers had no dairy products after weaning. Even so, in most areas, their calcium intake would have exceeded that of most people today. Wild fruits and vegetables contained more calcium than do today's cultivated hybrids (grains are an especially poor source), and the great quantities they consumed provided abundant amounts. Even the Neanderthals of 50,000 years ago and the Cro-Magnons of 35,000 years ago—who both lived near the glacial edge and consumed an exceptionally high proportion of meat—had massive bones, demonstrating sufficient calcium intake. Current calcium recommendations range from 400 to 1,500 mg per day, while the average American consumes an estimated 740 mg. This amount is less than half the average for Late Paleolithic people who probably consumed from 1,500 to 2,000 mg per day.

As ever-more-sophisticated processing transforms our basic foods into canned, frozen, reconstituted, and "fast" forms, their natural fiber content is being reduced or completely lost. With (at most) mortars-and-pestles and minimal cooking, and with preference for raw fruits and vegetables, preagricultural peoples consumed much more dietary fiber—in both soluble and insoluble forms—than most of us do. Even when we do increase our fiber intake, we tend to get it mostly from grains, while fiber in Paleolithic diets came mainly from fruits and vegetables. The importance of such differences in fiber type is still controversial, but initial research suggests they may be significant.

Hunters and gatherers consumed only one-sixth the sodium that typical Americans do—about a third the amount considered acceptable by the United States Department of Agriculture. Even Paleolithic people who consumed more sodium—those on 80 percent meat diets—would still have had an intake of less than half of ours. Their high potassium intake would also have contrasted with our low levels; like all mammals except for present-day humans, they would have consumed more potassium than sodium.

The wide range of vegetable foods eaten by hunters and gatherers normally ensured adequate vitamin and trace element intake. But meat—with its high levels of iron and folic acid—also represented a larger proportion of Paleolithic diets than of most modern Western diets. For those who believe that as we go back in time, life (and diet) become steadily less attractive, it may come as a surprise that present-day levels of meat (and, by extension, of protein) consumption are only about one-third that of people living 35,000 years ago.

But high meat consumption also meant high cholesterol intake. Indeed, Paleolithic hunters and gatherers probably consumed more cholesterol than most Americans do—far more, in fact, than is currently recommended by nearly all health authorities. That today's hunters and gatherers seem to escape cardiovascular complications may be due to their different pattern of fat intake; they eat much less of it, and the fats they do eat—derived from wild game and vegetable foods—have a higher ratio of polyunsaturated to saturated fats.

A bottom-line comparison between the million-year-old diet of our ancestors and the mere decades-old diet of today's Americans reveals stark differences, all of which are likely to promote the chronic disorders that lead to so much illness—and early death—in the United States:

- They ate only half the fat we do, but about three times the protein.
- The fat they ate was more polyunsaturated than saturated, the reverse of our proportion, although their cholesterol intake equaled or exceeded ours.
- They had very little refined carbohydrate—far less sugar than we do, and no finely ground flour.
- Their sodium intake averaged one-fourth of ours, and they consumed much more potassium than sodium.
- Their calcium intake was roughly twice ours.
- Their diet provided an abundance of essential micronutrients, particularly iron, folate, ascorbic acid, vitamin B_{12}, and essential fatty acids.
- They had five to ten times our level of nonnutrient fiber, most of it from fruits and vegetables rather than from grains.
- Their foods were bulky and filling, while ours are calorically dense, due to higher levels of fat and refined carbohydrates and lower levels of fiber.
- They probably had little or no alcohol, and in any case could never have consistently obtained 7 to 10 percent of their calories in this form, as average adult Americans now do.

Health advisory bodies around the world see the need for industrialized Westerners to alter their diets—to correct what has been appropriately called affluent malnutrition. However, the dietary recommendations frequently differ in details and change as new data become available. It would be helpful to have some general guidelines that might serve as an external standard against which to consider and evaluate the various changing recommendations.

Without arguing that it is a perfect solution, we consider the Paleolithic diet such a standard. Recent clinical, experimental, and epidemiological evidence, summarized in the next two chapters, supports many but not yet all of the nutritional principles suggested by the diet of hunters and gatherers. Only this kind of evidence can provide absolute verification, but anthropological data can provide a series of anchor points while also defining promising avenues for research.

Our genes were selected to operate within the most ancient human spectrum of experience. They provide us with enormous versatility, but the largely new dietary pattern adopted since the invention of agriculture, and especially within the past one hundred years, appears to go beyond what our genes can tolerate. Anthropologically derived principles can serve as a guide to planning and interpreting new research, and can offer a yardstick against which we can measure the conflicting advice and exotic fads that continually bombard us. Following a diet comparable to the one that humans were genetically adapted to should postpone, mitigate, and in many cases prevent altogether, a host of diseases that debilitate us—diseases almost unknown among recent hunters and gatherers.

CHAPTER FIVE
OUR DAILY BREAD

Is it possible to eat as our ancestors did 25,000 years ago? Mammoths, aurochs, and mastodons are long since extinct, and wild game in any form is in limited supply. Most of our vegetables and fruits are botanically new; the wheat and corn we eat today were unknown 10,000 years ago. Potatoes, squash, and pumpkins are also relatively recent New World additions to human consumption; people living in Asia, Africa, and Europe before A.D. 1500 had no exposure to them. Dairy products, now an essential part of our diet, were not available (except as mother's milk) before the domestication of animals. And "bread for the morrow," which is a better translation of the New Testament Greek than is "our daily bread," didn't become the staff of life until about 8,000 years ago at the earliest.

Fortunately, our bodies do not know (or care) whether the building blocks necessary for proper metabolism and biochemical function enter in the form of mammoth or as boiled shrimp. Our nutritional needs can just as easily be met by California grapefruit as by the baobab fruit of the Tanzanian Hadza. What is important is that the foods we eat provide the same spectrum and proportion of nutrients—protein, carbohydrate, fiber, fat, cholesterol, vitamins, and minerals—as were eaten by our hunting and gathering ancestors, the nutrient pattern for which our genes were originally selected. If it had not been so overworked and misused, the word *natural* would most accurately describe the dietary principles outlined in this book. But *natural* has been applied to so wide a range of commercially prepared fare and has been used so often as an advertising ploy that it has lost much of its original import. It really should mean "in accord with our genetically determined biochemistry and physiology." That *is* the sense in which it is used here.

88

After all, these nutritional principles are derived from a perspective accommodating a million years of human evolutionary experience, enriched by data accumulated in numerous anthropological field studies and refined by the findings of modern nutritional and medical science.

To develop a practical "soup to nuts" approach to Stone Age eating in today's world, then, we must reassess our basic nutritional requirements from this complex perspective. This chapter and the next provide such a reassessment and translate it into daily life, offering guidelines for the re-creation of an ancestral diet with twentieth-century foods.

CARBOHYDRATES

Carbohydrates are made up of carbon, hydrogen, and oxygen. Their basic structural unit is the simple sugar or monosaccharide; the most common are glucose, fructose, and galactose. Glucose (also called dextrose) is the main sugar in our blood and can be found in fruit, flowers, and the sap of trees and plants; fructose also comes from fruits, as well as from honey; and galactose can be found in milk. Double sugars, or disaccharides, are formed when two simple sugars link together. Common examples are maltose (found in grain), formed from two glucose units; sucrose, or common table sugar, formed from one glucose unit and one fructose unit; and lactose, or milk sugar, from the combination of glucose and galactose.

When more than two simple-sugar units link together, chains of varying lengths are formed, creating complex carbohydrates, or polysaccharides. Some polysaccharides, such as pectin and cellulose, are nondigestible (by humans) and provide, respectively, soluble and insoluble dietary fiber. Others, such as starches, are digestible; once in the digestive tract they are broken down into simple sugars and absorbed. Through the intestinal lining, they enter the bloodstream and travel to the liver, where they are converted into glucose for use as energy. Any excess is stored, first as glycogen (a polysaccharide unique to animals) in the liver and skeletal muscles, then as fat. The list on the following page shows the relationship among these carbohydrates.

Carbohydrates are the main energy source for the body. Each gram provides about 4 kilocalories (the more scientifically precise term for "calories"). Protein can also be used for energy, but only after it has been converted to glucose and/or fatty acids. While the body can generally use fatty acids to produce energy directly, the brain can use only glucose.

Carbohydrates		
Simple Carbohydrates		
Monosaccharides (simple sugars)	glucose	
	fructose	
	galactose	
Disaccharides (double sugars)	maltose (glucose-glucose)	
	sucrose (glucose-fructose)	
	lactose (glucose-galactose)	
Complex Carbohydrates		
Polysaccharides (multiple sugars)	starch	
	cellulose	
	guar	
	pectin	
	glycogen (animal starch)	

Dietary fiber is found almost exclusively in plant foods. Also called nonnutritive fiber, nondigestible carbohydrate, roughage, and bulk, it is not absolutely essential; Eskimos eat very little, and breast-fed infants consume almost none. Because a deficiency of dietary fiber doesn't produce immediate symptoms, its impact on health has been ignored until recently. Nevertheless, it *is* a basic component of the human diet; our hunting and gathering ancestors consumed large quantities, as did most agriculturalists who followed. Its functions vary from regulating muscular activity in the intestinal tract to affecting the absorption of cholesterol, sugar, and minerals. (For example, in diabetics, regular consumption of high-fiber meals results in lower blood-sugar levels.) Our intestines evolved in response to a diet rich in fiber and, by design, operate most effectively when fiber is present in significant quantity.

Dietary fiber can be defined as plant food material, resistant to human digestion, which passes through the small intestine without being absorbed. It comes in two basic forms: water insoluble and water soluble. Most plants provide both types. The actual proportions and amount depend not only on the specific plant, but also on how it has been stored, processed, and cooked.

Insoluble fiber comes from the structural components of plant cell walls, where it helps maintain the plant's shape and texture. It is made up of complex carbohydrates, but has no caloric value for humans; unlike ruminants (such as cattle, camels, sheep, giraffes, and deer), we are unable to digest it. The most common types of insoluble fiber—cellulose and lignin—are found in fruit and vegetable skins, whole-grain products including bran (especially wheat bran), and some seeds.

Soluble fiber, on the other hand, comes from the pulp of fruits, vegetables, and beans as well as from some cereal products such as oat bran. The most common types of soluble fiber are pectin, pentose polymers, some hemicellulose (found widely in plants and vegetables), and gums (found in the seeds and stems of various plants).

Our bodies recognize and respond differently to each of the two main kinds of fiber. Insoluble fiber—a major component of most cereal brans—absorbs water as it moves through the small and large intestines. This tends to increase stool bulk, reducing the time it takes for material to pass through the intestinal tract (the "transit time"). By helping to normalize gut function and dilute intestinal content, disorders resulting from abnormal muscular activity in the large bowel wall may be prevented: irritable bowel syndrome (spastic colon), diverticulosis, and diverticulitis. The prevalence of hiatus hernia and hemorrhoids may also be reduced. Diluted intestinal content and faster transit time may even minimize the effects of ingested carcinogens and thus reduce the risk of colon cancer.

Soluble fiber—such as that found in oat bran and beans—also increases stool bulk, but less dramatically and by a different process. It supports the growth of normal intestinal bacteria which, by their very presence, increase the bulk of colonic waste material. This effect, however, is limited and has less impact on transit time than does insoluble fiber. Soluble fiber nevertheless has other beneficial functions. Most importantly, it modifies cholesterol metabolism in ways that can lower serum cholesterol levels.

Carbohydrates eaten by Late Paleolithic hunters and gatherers came from wild tubers, berries, roots, shoots, edible leaves and flowers, seeds, fruits, gums, fungi, nuts, and honey. Except for the simple sugars found in fruits, honey, and tree sap, most of these carbohydrates were complex. Honey is exceedingly popular with recent hunting and gathering peoples and presumably Paleolithic humans held it in equally high regard; they made rock wall paintings which show how they robbed bees' nests. For today's foragers, honey is abundant for only a few months a year (for example, during July and August for the Efe Pygmies of Zaire's Ituri forest). In good years and in season, honey supplies from 5 to 35 percent of the band's total caloric intake. However, during the remainder of the year there is essentially no honey available, and in bad years foragers may be unable to obtain any even during the usual honey season. For average Americans the pattern is quite different. Refined sugar (14 percent) and other sweeteners—molasses, honey, and syrup (4 percent)—provide a constant 18 percent of calories year-round.

The first major shift away from the long-standing Paleolithic pattern of carbohydrate consumption came with agriculture, which limited the variety and range of plants consumed. Only a handful of plants were chosen for cultivation; many more were abandoned. Slowly, those that were cultivated became physically different from their wild forms, and as they gradually changed, their nutritional properties were altered as well.

Cultivation of wheat, for example, began in the Near East around 10,000 years ago, then spread to places where wheat had never previously grown. Within a few thousand years, a new kind of wheat had evolved, a spontaneous hybrid form: a cross between wild emmer wheat and goat-faced grass. The resulting "bread" wheat withstood cold better, had more gluten, and had kernels that held fast, so that fewer were lost during harvesting. Corn went through a similar transformation. Wild corn had tiny ears, typically less than an inch long. About 4,000 years ago in Mexico, it spontaneously crossed with a closely related wild grass, perennial teosinte. The resulting hybrid had longer, more numerous ears and strong husks, triggering corn's explosive spread as a cultivated plant; succeeding generations of farmers gradually adapted it into the forms we know today. Beans and tomatoes were also transformed, becoming larger and hardier after centuries of cultivation and selection.

But these changes came at a cost. Cultivation did provide abundant food for rapidly expanding human populations, but as the wild strains were repeatedly and selectively bred, many foods declined in nutritional quality. Wild einkorn wheat, for example, has 50 percent more protein than does hard red winter wheat (the most common type grown in North America), and many wild plant foods contain more calcium than do their cultivated forms.

While the dietary and societal revolution heralded by the Neolithic change to agriculture was ubiquitous, certain beneficial elements of the hunting and gathering diet continued, especially the consumption of complex carbohydrates, which even increased. In fact, high intake of complex carbohydrates persisted until the Industrial Revolution, but since then there have been dramatic changes.

Sugar consumption, for example, was quite modest until recently. As late as 1800, the annual per capita consumption of refined sugar was only four pounds. Increasingly efficient methods of harvesting and greater ease of transportation, however, quickly changed that. Today, the average American consumes those same four pounds in just two weeks. We are now eating roughly a third of a pound of sugar per person per day—or close to one hundred pounds per year—so that nearly 20 percent of our average daily caloric intake is sugar. To make matters worse, sugar consumption skyrocketed as dietary fiber intake plummeted; modern food processing techniques—especially modern roller milling—greatly reduced nonnutrient fiber in carbohydrate foods. For most Americans and Europeans today, cereal fiber intake is a small fraction of what it was in the mid-1800s.

Today's carbohydrate foods are "energy-dense"—concentrated in calories—rather than "nutrient-dense"—bulky, high in essential nutrients, and low in calories. Their energy:satiety ratios are therefore high, which means they provide plenty of calories but fail to "fill us up." This affects the rates of obesity as surely as low levels of dietary fiber predispose us to a variety of diseases ranging from diverticulosis to colon cancer. The unprecedented prevalence of these conditions today is clearly related to our having veered from the path of carbohydrate consumption known to our ancestors.

PROTEIN

Like complex carbohydrates, proteins are large molecules made up of many smaller units: the amino acids. These contain carbon, hydrogen, and oxygen as well as nitrogen and sometimes sulfur. By altering the sequence of twenty-two amino acids many thousands of different proteins are formed by our bodies. Of the twenty-two, we can synthesize all but nine "essential" amino acids, which must be obtained from our food.

Dietary protein, to be of use, must be broken down in the digestive tract into its constituent amino acids. These are absorbed through the intestinal wall into the bloodstream and distributed throughout the body, to be formed into new proteins as needed. Babies are able to absorb some proteins directly, such as antibodies from mother's milk, but this capacity is lost after infancy.

Proteins function in many ways and, excluding water, they comprise 50 percent of our body's weight. They form tissues such as muscles, tendons, ligaments, and blood vessel walls. All growth—from conception to adulthood, including repair from bodily insults such as burns, surgery, or infections—is dependent on proteins. Certain intracellular enzyme and carrier proteins are vital to cell function, being formed, used up, and formed again and again in a cyclical pattern and in large volume. Other proteins function extracellularly as digestive enzymes, hormones, antibodies, and as carriers of cholesterol and fatty acids in the bloodstream. Still others—such as those found in protective structures like nails, hair, and skin—are dense and tough for protection.

Proteins differ from fats and carbohydrates in two important ways: (1) they cannot be stored in the body and any excess is converted into fat; and (2) because the "essential" amino acids cannot be made by the body, we must always consume new protein to meet our daily needs. Only in times of stress are some of the body's proteins, especially those in the muscles and the liver, broken down and used for energy: during intense endurance-type exercise, during starvation, and while on reducing diets. This protein loss can be minimized by carbohydrates in the diet—carbohydrates are used preferentially for energy and thus have a protein-sparing effect. Resistance exercise, such as weight training, also minimizes structural protein loss.

Animal and vegetable proteins differ in value. Protein derived from animals and fish more closely resembles that found in our bodies. Since all nine essential amino acids are present in these sources, they are called *complete* protein. Most vegetables and plant foods, in contrast, provide *incomplete* protein, which lacks one or more of the essential amino acids. However, the presence of essential amino acids is not the whole story; the proportion in which they are consumed is also crucial. Just as letters in the alphabet are used with different frequency, the need for each amino acid varies. Foods containing optimal proportions of amino acids, such as those derived from animal sources, are rated high-quality protein. Foods are also assigned biological values—a numerical expression indicating the quality of their protein. In these terms, human milk is rated as the most perfect protein source for humans, with a value of 100. Other commonly consumed foods have decreasing biological values, as shown in Table IX.

Paleolithic hunters and gatherers obtained an abundance of complete protein, mostly from wild game; their vegetable foods were an ancillary protein source. This pattern prevailed until agriculture transformed it, shifting the human diet away from meat and toward plant food. Cultures around the world soon learned how to "create" complete, high-quality protein from vegetable sources; when they mixed a variety of plant foods in the same meal, an amino acid missing in one food could be balanced by its presence in another. As long as all nine essential amino acids were present in suitable proportions, it did not matter whether they came from one source or many. Corn or wheat with beans, for example, or rice with peas are combinations that provide adequate protein. A small amount of meat or milk could also play a balancing role. These and various other combinations are prepared and consumed throughout the world.

This process, called complementary protein balancing, can be very effective. However, because protein synthesis is fairly rapid, the balancing must be accomplished at the same meal or soon after. If an amino acid is absent or if the proportions are inadequate, the remaining amino

TABLE IX.

Biological Values of Common Foods

Food	Complete	Biological Value
Human milk	yes	100
Egg	yes	94
Cow's milk	yes	84
Fish	yes	83
Meat	yes	74
Soybeans	yes	73
Brown rice	no	73
Whole wheat	no	65
Green leafy vegetables	no	64
White rice	no	63
Potato	no	60
Corn	no	60
Kidney beans	no	58
White bread	no	52

acids will not form protein, but will be converted into fat. Persistent, inadequate protein balancing can ultimately result in protein deficiency, a condition rarely found among Americans or, for that matter, among recent hunters and gatherers. People in developing countries, however, with economies based on limited agricultural produce and little meat, are more vulnerable. Children are the primary victims; for them, advanced cases of protein malnutrition often lead to death.

There is some evidence that protein intake affects height. First-generation Americans are taller, on average, than their immigrant parents. Their children, second-generation Americans, are taller yet. The trend continues into the next generation as well, as evidenced by third-generation Japanese-Americans who average almost five inches taller than their immigrant grandparents. Eventually, these growth increases level out. A variety of factors seem implicated: (1) increased overall caloric intake, (2) improved general health during childhood, and (3) increased protein intake. This helps explain why the average height of *all* Americans increased several inches between the mid-1800s and the present.

Nevertheless, we have not quite reached the height of Cro-Magnon hunters and gatherers living 25,000 years ago, when males averaged nearly 5'10" and females nearly 5'6". These heights made them generally taller than most later people, including ourselves, although we are coming close. It was once thought that, except for the Cro-Magnons, our remote ancestors were short, much shorter than we are today. However, the 1984 discovery of a nearly complete *Homo erectus* skeleton 1.5 million years old caused this view to be revised. The skeleton, found in Kenya by a team led by Richard Leakey and Alan Walker, was that of a twelve-year-old boy whose projected adult height would have been 6'2". Intrigued, human paleontologists began to reexamine existing fragmentary remains of other early humans and found, much to their surprise, that their heights had been systematically underestimated.

The evidence now suggests that preagricultural humans were essentially similar to us in height, or even slightly taller, for well over a million years, but that after the appearance of agriculture inadequate, limited protein intake "dwarfed" most succeeding human populations until this century. Of course the time frame for the changeover from foraging to agriculture varied with specific geographic locations, but in nearly all cases the shift was accompanied by a decrease in body size. This suggests that agriculture could not consistently provide the abundance of calories, vitamins, minerals (particularly calcium), and especially proteins that were available to Paleolithic hunters and gatherers and, more recently, to ourselves. As nutrition gets better, it seems, human height attains levels near the peak of our genetic potential.

This may come as a surprise to people who have, for the sake of health, cut back on the one protein source most readily consumed by hunters and gatherers: red meat. Yet the "bad press" red meat has received in recent years has not been undeserved. The meat available to us—beef, lamb, pork, veal, mutton, and ham—is simply less healthful than the meat our ancestors ate; it has more fat and higher proportions of saturated fat. Today, fish, shellfish, and poultry more closely match the nutritional properties of the meat our ancestors ate. So, too, do the very lean cuts of red meat becoming available in select markets as producers attempt to recreate, often with considerable success, the low-fat beef of the past. If the burgeoning growth of commercial game farms stocked with exotic wild species are any indication, this trend is likely to continue.

The human diet and that of our prehuman ancestors has included meat for millions of years. Yet meat is not an absolute necessity. Strict vegetarians eating a vegan diet (which, except for breast milk, avoids all animal products including eggs and dairy foods) can be basically healthy, although there is some evidence that children raised exclusively on such diets have slowed growth and development. To propose humans as basically vegetarian in nature, however, is clearly unjustified. Meat is, and has always been, a major constituent of the human diet.

Current estimates as to how much protein is necessary for optimal growth during childhood range from 6.5 to 15 percent of each day's total caloric intake. Protein quality influences the amount required; generally, about one-third more protein is necessary when it is obtained from vegetable sources than when it is derived from animal sources.

What about athletes—do they need extra protein? For years dietitians and nutritionists have argued this point with coaches and trainers, the former saying no, the latter saying yes. The correct answer depends on which exercise is involved. Athletes wishing to increase muscularity and lean body mass through strength training and young athletes still growing need extra dietary protein; athletes engaged in endurance or pure skill-type activities (for example, diving) do not. To increase lean body mass (muscles, tendons, ligaments, and bones) through strength training, dietary protein should approximate 20 percent of daily calories. The results of programs combining strength training with extra dietary protein can be seen in the bodies of high-school, college, and professional athletes.

For adults, current health authorities recommend that between 10 and 20 percent of total caloric intake come from protein. Paleontological findings, together with anthropological data from contemporary hunters and gatherers, suggest that late Paleolithic humans obtained 20 to 60 percent of their calories from protein, with most groups typically between 30 and 35 percent. Our bodies therefore seem genetically constituted to accept a fairly high protein load.

Nevertheless, recent studies provide evidence that very high levels of dietary protein can promote renal degeneration and accelerate aging of the kidneys. Our protein intake, therefore, should be aimed at the lower end of the Paleolithic range, at about 20 percent—the point at which current recommendations overlap with the Paleolithic experience and below the level at which protein intake is likely to damage otherwise healthy kidneys. Today's Eskimos continue to consume a high-protein diet (25 to 35 percent of total calories), but autopsy studies reveal no more renal degeneration than would be found in an age-matched series of Americans. This 20 percent level will very adequately supply the amino acids necessary for health, even for the most exuberant growth of lean body mass. Less than 20 percent is inconsistent with our evolutionary past and much more would be unnecessarily costly and possibly harmful. Further research is needed to establish both the lower and upper limits of safe protein intake.

FATS

Fats, like carbohydrates, are made up of carbon, hydrogen, and oxygen. (The term *oil* is used for fats that remain liquid at room temperature.) Fats found in food consist primarily of triglycerides: three (*tri*) long chains of carbon and hydrogen atoms (called fatty acids) attached to a glycerol (*glyceride*) molecule backbone:

```
          H
          |
   H— C —fatty acid
          |
   H— C —fatty acid        Triglyceride
          |
   H— C —fatty acid
          |
          H
```

glycerol + 3 fatty acids

Cholesterol, frequently considered together with fats, is a complicated substance, more like a wax than a true fat. Chemically, its structure is based on four interconnected rings, so that it does not look like a fat and, technically, it is classified as an alcohol. It enters our diet only from animal sources: meat, fish, shellfish, and dairy products. It does not occur in plants. Together, fats and cholesterol are referred to as *lipids*, a term commonly used by physicians and nutritionists in discussing the relationship between diet and heart disease.

In the intestines, dietary fat is efficiently digested; less than 5 percent passes through without being absorbed. (This was fortunate for our ancestors, who needed efficient conversion of food into energy, but not for most of us who consume more fat calories than we need.) Cholesterol absorption is less complete, being influenced by a number of factors including the level of nonnutrient fiber in the diet. Together, triglycerides and dietary cholesterol are absorbed into the lymph system, where they form relatively large saclike particles, or chylomicrons. These eventually enter the bloodstream, destined ultimately for the liver and other body tissues. There they are disassembled and used for energy, for structural purposes, for storage, or to manufacture other kinds of molecules.

Lipoproteins

Unlike simple sugars and amino acids, neither triglycerides nor cholesterol dissolve in blood; they must be transported by special protein carriers called lipoproteins. These are assembled in the liver, which produces different types, two of which are central to human health: low-density lipoproteins (LDL) and high-density lipoproteins (HDL).

HDL, with less fat and cholesterol—less fatty but with a greater specific qravity—is considered "good" cholesterol. Its levels are determined by genetic makeup and by life-style. Regular physical exertion, especially endurance exercise, can increase it, while sedentary living, obesity, and tobacco use can decrease it. Fat and cholesterol consumption also affect HDL levels, but less directly than they do LDL concentration, for example, which is mainly determined by diet; LDL rises when total dietary fat (and, to a lesser extent, dietary cholesterol) content is high and when the proportion of saturated fats exceeds that of polyunsaturated fats.

In contrast to HDL, LDL has been called "bad" cholesterol. It appears to carry cholesterol *to* the body tissues, including the blood vessel walls, where it is then deposited. These deposits, or plaques, slowly accumulate, causing the vessels to narrow; atherosclerosis, or hardening of the arteries, is the result. HDL does the opposite. It carries cholesterol *away* from the tissues (including the blood vessel walls) and ferries it to the liver, where it is removed from the body. High blood levels of HDL are therefore considered protective against atherosclerosis, while high levels of LDL indicate additional risk.

Fatty Acids

There are a large number of different fatty acids in our bodies and in our foods. Butter alone contains more than twenty-nine kinds. Fatty acids consist of long chains of carbon and hydrogen molecules with a simple organic acid group at one end (shown at the right-hand end in the diagram). This group is similar in all fatty acids; the length of the chains and the kinds of bonds between the carbon atoms determine the differences. Single bonds are present when all the carbon atoms are filled—or "saturated"—with hydrogen atoms.

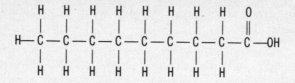

Saturated fatty acids are found most typically in the fat of domesticated animal meat (beef, pork, lamb, poultry), in their by-products (lard, butter, cream, eggs, cheese), and in certain vegetable oils such as palm and coconut oil.

Other fats, mainly vegetable in origin, contain one or more "double" bonds between carbon atoms:

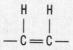

The double bond signifies a pair of carbon atoms with one less hydrogen affixed to each. No longer filled or "saturated" with hydrogen atoms, these fatty acids are called "unsaturated fats." Two different types exist. The first, *mono*unsaturated fat (prominent in peanuts and olives), has one double bond in the carbon chain:

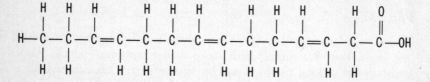

The second, *poly*unsaturated fat (prominent in walnuts, corn, and safflower and sunflower seeds, as well as in the fat of wild game), has two or more double bonds in the carbon chain:

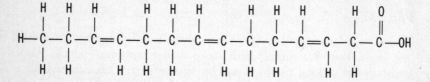

The most recent research has shown that the precise location of double bonds in the chain can also have significance for health. Specifically, those with the double bond three carbons from the left-hand end— known as omega-3 fatty acids—are especially protective.

Hydrogenation

Fats that occur naturally in plants and meats are a mixture of saturated and unsaturated fatty acids. Many of the fats found in processed foods, however, have been altered; the open carbon slots in the unsaturated fats have been artificially filled with hydrogen. This process—called, logically enough, hydrogenation—eliminates some or all of the double bonds in the carbon chain:

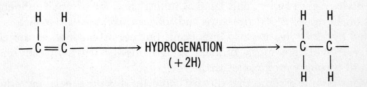

Hydrogenation appeals to food manufacturers because it changes fats that are ordinarily liquid into a more solid state—for example, bar margarines which closely resemble butter. It also helps retard the process by which fats become rancid. But as hydrogenation reduces the number of double bonds, the beneficial unsaturated fats are transformed into saturated fats—the kind that elevate serum cholesterol.

Essential Fatty Acids

As with the nine essential amino acids that cannot be synthesized by the body, two families of fatty acids appear to be essential; they must be obtained from food. One group is based on linol*eic* acid—an eighteen-carbon chain with two double bonds. The second group is based on linol*enic* acid and includes eicosapentaenoic acid (*eye-co-sa-pen-ta-ee-no-ick*), or EPA, as well as several longer polyunsaturated fatty acids. This second group of essential fatty acids makes up the omega-3 family—so named because the first double bond is three carbons removed from the nonacidic end of the molecule—commonly found in fish oils.

Essential fatty acids are important for the formation of prostaglandins: crucial hormones unknown until about twenty years ago. These hormones help regulate a variety of biological activities, including the function of blood platelets—substances implicated in the long-term development of atherosclerosis as well as in heart attacks, strokes, and sudden cardiac death.

Cholesterol is essential in the human body; it is a major component of cell membranes and is necessary for the production of numerous hormones (including the sex hormones) as well as of vitamin D (much of which is made by the skin). It is also used by the liver to make bile acids that ensure that fats are properly absorbed from the intestinal tract.

Diet and Serum Cholesterol Levels

The type and amount of cholesterol present in the blood are the most important risk factors for coronary heart disease that can be altered by life-style. Age, gender, and familial inheritance are of great influence, but unalterable. Blood pressure and tobacco use, other risk factors affected by life-style, are also important, but persistent high serum cholesterol levels are more ruthless in the unswerving path they chart toward coronary atherosclerosis.

Many people assume that dietary cholesterol is *the* crucial ingredient determining one's serum cholesterol levels. While it is true that dietary cholesterol plays a modest role, its impact on serum cholesterol is, ironically, not as dramatic as that of either total fat intake or the proportion of saturated fat consumed. Studies show that increased dietary cholesterol does raise serum cholesterol levels somewhat. But these effects are easily masked by changes in total fat intake and by the polyunsaturated:saturated fat (P:S) ratio, factors that produce changes of much greater magnitude in cholesterol in the blood.

At present, then, the dietary factors known to affect serum cholesterol levels are these:

- Total level of dietary fat. The higher the dietary fat level, the higher the serum cholesterol level.
- The ratio of polyunsaturated to saturated fats. The higher the P:S ratio (more polyunsaturated than saturated fats), the lower the serum cholesterol level.

These factors are widely accepted by medical scientists. The Paleolithic evidence supports them as well. The diets of Paleolithic peoples had much lower levels of total fat and higher P:S ratios than do the diets of most Americans.

- Dietary cholesterol. It raises serum cholesterol levels to a modest extent.

This relationship is also widely accepted, but the magnitude of the effect is disputed. Late Paleolithic peoples generally obtained as much or more cholesterol from their diets as do affluent Americans.

- Monounsaturated fats. Their role is controversial.

Present in many foods, but especially in olives and peanuts, these fats were thought until recently to have little direct effect on serum cholesterol levels. There is no question that substitution of monounsaturated for saturated fat (for example, olive oil for butter) is desirable, but whether high monounsaturated olive oil is superior to high polyunsaturated safflower oil is now being debated.

Research on monounsaturated fats is very active, but still at an early stage. It may be that mono- and polyunsaturated fats will eventually be grouped together and that an unsaturated:saturated (U:S) ratio will some day replace the P:S ratio. Alternatively, the unique contribution of monounsaturated fats may be recognized in a new ratio that includes all three fats—polyunsaturates:monounsaturates:saturates (P:M:S).

Most Paleolithic humans ate a higher proportion of monounsaturated fat relative to saturated fat than do today's Americans, but less than do today's Mediterranean people. They could never have consistently matched the large quantities of olive oil consumed year-round by today's Italians and Greeks. Table X compares these diets.

- Omega-3 long-chain polyunsaturated fatty acids. Some, such as eicosapentaenoic acid (EPA), seem to lower serum cholesterol levels

---

TABLE X.

Consumption of Saturated and Unsaturated Fats

	P:M:S	P:S	U:S	Fat as Percent of Total Calories
Current American diet	7:19:16	7:16	26:16	40
American Heart Association "Prudent" diet	1:1:1	1:1	2:1	30
High monounsaturated Mediterranean diet	1:7:3	1:3	8:3	30
Paleolithic diet	7:8:5	7:5	3:1	20–25

more than would be expected simply on the basis of their effect on the dietary P:S ratio.

This was initially observed in Greenland Eskimos and has been confirmed by subsequent studies in Japan, Oregon, and the Netherlands. This effect is under intense investigation. These special fatty acids have other physiological properties as well, some beneficial and some not. Late Paleolithic diets would have included more of these than Americans normally consume, but considerably less than do the Eskimos.

• Dietary fiber. The soluble fiber present in beans, fruit, vegetables, and oat bran (but not in wheat bran) seems to lower serum cholesterol levels.

This work is relatively new, and there is not yet an overall consensus concerning its importance. The magnitude of the effect appears to be modest. The diets of Paleolithic humans contained considerably more fiber, overall, than is typical of Western diets and a higher proportion of their fiber was soluble in nature.

Functions of Fat

Like cholesterol, fats are essential to the normal functioning of the human body. Polyunsaturated fatty acids, for example, are the building blocks of prostaglandins—hormones that regulate a wide variety of body functions. Also, they are essential structural components of nearly all the membranes of the cell, both internal and external. And of course, fats also provide and store energy.

At 9 kilocalories per gram, fat provides more than twice the energy of either protein or carbohydrate, each of which has only about 4 kilocalories per gram, so it is more efficient for the body to store energy as fat. In addition some energy is deposited as glycogen (animal starch) in skeletal muscle and in the liver. For the most part saturated, rather than polyunsaturated, fatty acids are stored in adipose tissue. Also called depot fat, these deposits are found in various sites around the body, especially within the abdominal cavity and in subcutaneous tissues, where they provide thermal insulation as well as energy storage.

The fat-storage pattern of free-living mammals other than humans is fairly uniform. Marine mammals such as whales and seals do have considerable amounts of subcutaneous fat, stored primarily for insulation, but there is relatively little difference either in the amount or in the distribution of this fat among individuals within a species. Compared to humans, whose body fat can vary between 2 and 60 percent of total body weight, the range of body composition in wild animal species is relatively narrow.

Modern affluence has played havoc with human body composition, turning a once moderately uniform range into an extreme one. Today, people similar in age, height, and sex can differ widely in the amount of storage fat they carry. Obesity, once confined to people of high socioeconomic status, has finally become an "equal opportunity" employer: Just about everyone can get the job. Indeed, high-energy foods can now be obtained with so little physical effort that a large majority of society can accumulate almost unlimited amounts of depot fat, a pattern as estranged from that of other mammals as it is from our own genetic heritage. In fact, it is in the animals kept by humans—including those overfed in zoos—that this pattern finds echoes in nonhuman species.

Protein and Fat in Domesticated Meat

One thousand generations ago our ancestors consumed meat that was nutritionally different from the meat we eat today. Some of the animals they hunted no longer exist: mammoths, woolly rhinoceros, and giant sloths. Others—horse, deer, musk ox, and bison—do exist, but are rarely found in our diets. Dramatic differences, to be sure, but they pale when compared to the changes humans have foisted on the natural world since then; through genetic selection, we have bred animals to live lives unprecedented in animal existence.

The earliest "manipulation" could barely be called that. During the Late Paleolithic, some human groups established unique relationships with herd animals, especially reindeer and caribou near the glacier and gazelles in the Near East. They became "protoherders"—something like the Lapps—protecting the animals from predators and, in turn, harvesting them selectively for food. Hides, bone, antlers, intestines, and stomachs were also used as raw material for clothing, tools, weapons, implements, and utensils.

The first systematic domestication of animals did not take place until a few thousand years later, around 8,000 years ago in the Near East. Once established, however, the advantages of animal husbandry became so apparent that only a few thousand more years passed before sheep, goats, pigs, and cattle could be found on early farms scattered widely throughout the globe.

With domestication, it became possible to change the characteristics of herds by selecting animals with desirable traits and breeding them. Smaller, more docile animals were favored because they were easier to manage; good wool and milk producers were also chosen. With time, domesticated animals began to diverge more and more from their wild ancestors, so much so that they are archaeologically distinguishable simply on the basis of their bony remains; domestic forms are smaller and less robustly constituted.

About two hundred years ago, more "scientific" approaches to animal breeding and feeding became common. The goal was to achieve rapid weight gain during growth, together with the efficient and economical conversion of grain into tasty, well-marbled, tender flesh. In the past fifty years, these goals have been achieved with ever-more-sophisticated technology; concentrated semisynthetics are now part of many animals' food supply, antibiotics and hormones are used to promote growth, and "confinement" methods are employed for the sake of "production." Animal husbandry has turned into a branch of agribusiness, converting domestic animals into obese parodies with nutritional properties vastly different from their wild forebears.

The production of veal provides an instructive, if unappealing, example. Veal, the meat of young calves, is favored for being pale and tender, much more so than the meat of older calves who have begun to eat grass. To maximize its "production," calves are placed in stalls 1'10" wide and 4'6" long, where they are tethered so they cannot turn around. During their thirteen to fifteen weeks in these stalls, they are fed liquid diets based on nonfat milk powder supplemented with fat, minerals, vitamins, and sometimes hormones and antibiotics. In order to maximize their consumption of feed, they are given no water; their thirst can only be quenched by consuming more of the liquid diet. The buildings are kept warm, partially to minimize caloric loss for heat production, but also to encourage thirst. Activity is further reduced by keeping the barns dark for twenty-two out of each twenty-four hours. The results? With minimal movement, no exercise, and maximal consumption of highly concentrated calories, the meat is very tender—and very fatty.

Chickens, pigs, sheep, and cattle are raised in analogous ways. Aside from the residue of pesticides, hormones, antibiotics, and other chemicals found in this meat, animals we eat today are much fatter (and their fat much more saturated) than were the wild animals our ancestors ate. For example, 100 g (3.5 oz.) of choice sirloin steak has approximately seven times more fat than a similar portion of bison, and two and a half times the number of calories. Lamb loin has eight times more fat than wild goat and nearly three times the number of calories. When meat from forty-three wild game species is compared with the beef, ham, pork, and lamb commonly consumed in the United States, the same pattern emerges; wild game contains more protein than fat, while domestic meat contains more fat than protein. (See Table XI.)

Furthermore, since wild animals have relatively more structural than storage fat, more of their fat is unsaturated than saturated. When wild animals are compared with domestic animals, a pattern emerges which is shown in Table XII.

Clearly, the meat we now eat is much less healthful than the lean and relatively unsaturated meat eaten by our hunting and gathering forebears. The effect this change has had on our health is evident in some of the main "diseases of civilization"—especially those linked to atherosclerosis. To protect ourselves against the detrimental effects of high saturated-fat diets then, we have to select our meats with great care. (Guidelines and specific recommendations are presented in Chapter 6, "Hunting and Gathering in the Supermarket.")

Sources of Fat and Cholesterol

Dietary fat, like protein, can come from animal or plant sources. Most commercially available red meat contains between 20 and 30 percent fat and between 15 and 20 percent protein (the remainder is moisture). Fat, therefore, provides nearly 80 percent of the calories in meat. Most of this fat is saturated—from three to twelve times more saturated than polyunsaturated. The meat our Paleolithic ancestors ate, in contrast, had one-sixth as much total fat and contained one-tenth the saturated fat. Whether fatty or lean, however, the cholesterol content of their meat would have been roughly similar to ours because cell membranes—whether muscle or fat—contain comparable amounts of cholesterol.

It is unfortunate, in terms of our health, that our palates are so attuned to fat. Our attraction—if not craving—for it (seen in our profusion of chocolates, cookies, fried foods, and well-marbled meats) rivals our attraction for sugar, suggesting that we may have not only a sweet tooth but a "fat tooth" as well. The grading system established by the U.S. Department of Agriculture reflects these purely cultural "values," giving its highest grades to beef with the highest fat content. (See Table XIII.) This is the opposite of what the ratings would be if they were based on health considerations alone.

Poultry and fish are generally much leaner than are red meats, and their fat is less saturated, with more nearly equal proportions of saturated and polyunsaturated fat. Certain fish—mackerel, salmon, and cod—also have high levels of essential fatty acids in the linolenic family, which are scarce in other foods. As a rule, shellfish are very low in total

TABLE XI.

Protein and Fat Content of Selected Meats

100 Gram Portion	Grams of Protein	Grams of Fat
Domestic Meat		
Prime lamb loin	14.7	32.0
Ham	15.2	29.1
Regular hamburger	17.9	21.2
Choice sirloin steak	16.9	26.7
Pork loin	16.4	28.0
Wild Game		
Goat	20.6	3.8
Cape buffalo	—	2.8
Warthog	—	4.2
Horse	20.5	3.7
Wild boar	16.8	8.3
Antelope	—	3.0
Beaver	30.0	5.1
Muskrat	27.2	4.1
Caribou	—	2.4
Moose	—	1.5
Kangaroo	—	1.2
Turtle	26.8	3.9
Opossum	33.6	4.5
Wildebeest	—	5.4
Thomson's gazelle	—	1.6
Kob (waterbuck)	—	3.1
Pheasant	24.3	5.2
Rabbit	21.0	5.0
Impala	—	2.6
Topi	—	2.2
Deer	21.0	4.0
Bison	25.0	3.8

From Eaton and Konner, op. cit. Dashes indicate that figures are not available.

TABLE XII.

Percentage of Polyunsaturated
Fats in Selected Meats

	Polyunsaturated Fatty Acids as % of all Fatty Acids
Domestic Meat	
Beef	2.0
Pork	9.6
Lamb	2.7
Veal	4.2
Chicken	17.0
Wild Game	
Cape Buffalo	30.0
Eland	35.0
Hartebeest	32.0
Giraffe	39.0
Kangaroo	36.0
Warthog	43.0
Caribou	22.0
Grouse	60.0

Domestic Meat section of Table XII from Watt, B.K., Merrill, A.L., *Composition of Foods*. Agriculture Handbook No. 8, U.S. Dept. of Agriculture, Washington, D.C. 1975
From Eaton and Konner, op. cit.

fat, and usually have more polyunsaturated than saturated fat; their cholesterol content, however, is variable, and in some cases—shrimp, for example—is even higher than that of red meat, fish, or poultry.

Dairy products provide levels of fat that vary according to the cream—or butterfat—content. Milk directly from the cow is high in saturated fat (66 percent saturated, only 4 percent polyunsaturated) and high in cholesterol. Removing or reducing the butterfat creates lower fat products (for example, skim milk, low-fat yogurt, buttermilk, and low-fat cottage cheese) with less—or almost no—fat and less cholesterol.

Except for avocados and olives, most fruits and vegetables have so little fat that their contribution to our daily fat intake is minimal. A

TABLE XIII.

U.S. Department of
Agriculture Grades of Beef

Grade	Percent Fat (by weight)
Prime	46
Choice	40
Good	34
Standard	27

person would have to eat a pound of oranges or two pounds of potatoes (without butter or sour cream) to ingest a gram of fat—less than the amount in a mouthful of high-grade beef. Oils can be extracted from some vegetables, such as corn, as well as from seeds, legumes, and flowers. Oils derived from plants contain no cholesterol, but they can vary dramatically in degree of saturation. Safflower (78 percent polyunsaturated), sunflower (69 percent), corn (62 percent), and soybean (61 percent) oils are largely polyunsaturated. Olive (77 percent) and peanut (48 percent) oils are largely monounsaturated, whereas coconut (92 percent), palm kernel (86 percent), and palm (51 percent) oils are largely saturated.

Grains, except for wheat germ, are also low in fat and contain almost three times more polyunsaturated than saturated fat. Not nuts, though. These have high fat levels—between 35 and 70 percent by weight. And the type of fat varies dramatically. Coconuts have forty-five times more saturated (92 percent) than polyunsaturated (2 percent) fat. Walnuts—with six times more polyunsaturated than saturated fat—are at the opposite pole. Peanuts—with almost twice as much polyunsaturated as saturated fat—are somewhere in the middle.

We have already discussed the P:S ratio, which has been established as a shorthand technique to represent the proportions in which polyunsaturated and saturated fats are found in specific foods. When equal amounts are present, for example, the ratio is represented as 1:1. If polyunsaturates comprise 20 percent of the fat and saturates twice as much at 40 percent, the ratio is unfavorable at 1:2; if the proportions are reversed, the ratio is represented as 2:1 and is favorable. (An informal way to estimate the saturation of fat is to put it in the refrigerator; the harder it gets, the more saturated it is. For example, safflower oil remains clear liquid, peanut oil turns cloudy, and butter gets hard.

Although most margarines begin with polyunsaturated vegetable oils, hydrogenation makes them more solid as well as more saturated; still, margarine melts faster than butter at room temperature.) The P:S ratio is the usual way proportions of fat are expressed, but in some cases we have included additional data in the form of a P:M:S ratio to designate the relative amounts of monounsaturated fats as well. Thus, peanut oil with 34 percent polyunsaturated, 48 percent monounsaturated, and 18 percent saturated fatty acids can be represented as PMS = 34:48:18, or—very roughly—3:5:2.

Cholesterol is found only in foods of animal origin, largely in cell membranes. Egg yolk, brains, and organ meats (liver and kidneys) are the most concentrated sources. Butter, shellfish, and high-fat cheeses, such as cream cheese, also have high levels. Poultry, red meat, and fish have moderate levels; and low-fat dairy products—skim milk, low-fat yogurt, and low-fat cottage cheese—have very little. The game meat our ancestors consumed, having about the same amount of cell membrane, had about as much cholesterol as does the red meat we eat today. (See Table XIV.)

Fat in the Current American Diet

Between 1910 and 1976, the consumption of fats in the United States increased by about 25 percent so that, currently, fat makes up about 42 percent of the calories consumed by average Americans. Of this fat, more than twice as much is saturated as polyunsaturated. This level of fat consumption is unprecedented in human evolutionary experience, and results in diseases that kill us, but that are uncommon in countries where fat represents a much smaller proportion of the diet. In rural Japan, for example, only 10 to 12 percent of daily calories come from fat (with a P:S ratio of approximately 1:1) and the prevalence of coronary heart disease among the Japanese is only a small fraction of ours.

For some of us a moderately high-fat diet can still be associated with low risk of atherosclerotic disease, but only if the P:S ratio is sufficiently high. Yugoslavs living on the Dalmatian Coast, for example, have fairly high fat diets: 32 percent of their total calories. This fat, however, is relatively high in polyunsaturates and low in saturates: 7 percent polyunsaturated, 16 percent monounsaturated, and 9 percent saturated. Their favorable P:S ratio of 7:9, and perhaps also their high monounsaturate level, seems to help keep their rates of atherosclerotic heart disease in check. The American diet, with 42 percent fat—almost twice as saturated as theirs (a P:S ratio of 7:16)—provides no such protection.

The Finns, in contrast to the Yugoslavs, show the detrimental effect

TABLE XIV.

Cholesterol Levels in Selected Foods

Food Item	Cholesterol mg per 100 g Portion
Eggs	
Whole	550
Yolk	1,600
White	0
Brains	2,000
Organ Meats	
Liver, chicken	630
Liver, calves	440
Kidney	800
Sweetbreads (veal)	800
Butter	220
Shellfish	
Oysters	39
Lobster	112
Shrimp	130
Crab	90
Clams	31
Scallops	41
Cheeses	
Cheddar	105
Cream cheese	110
Low-fat cottage cheese	5
Poultry	
Chicken, dark meat	80
Chicken, light meat	58
Turkey	82
Duck	89
Red Meat	
Beef	76
Lamb	71
Pork	74
Veal	71
Game (avg. of four species)	67

(Continued on next page)

TABLE XIV.   *(Continued)*

Cholesterol Levels in Selected Foods

Food Item	Cholesterol mg per 100 g Portion
Fish	
Tuna	46
Salmon	40
Flounder	46
Milk	
Whole	14
Heavy (whipping) cream	137
Skim	2
Low-fat Yogurt	5

From *Composition of Foods*, Agriculture Handbooks, Nos. 8–1 through 8–14 (Washington, D.C.: U.S. Department of Agriculture, 1976–86); G. A. Laveille, M. E. Zabik, and J. K. Morgan, *Nutrients in Foods* (Cambridge, Mass.: The Nutrition Guild, 1983).

of a high saturated-fat diet on coronary health. Although they eat slightly less fat than Americans do (39 percent), saturated fats outnumber polyunsaturated fats 7 to 1 (a P:S ratio of 1:7); historically, they have had one of the world's highest rates of coronary disease (appreciably higher than that in the United States). Whether this high rate was dietary or genetic in origin was at first unclear, but recent studies have shown that diet modification made a major difference. Finns who were able to lower their total fat intake while increasing their proportion of polyunsaturated fat experienced a significant decline in the rate of coronary heart disease.

Recommendations for Fat Intake

What should our goals be? Many authoritative health agencies now recommend that 30 percent of our total calories come from fat, with equal proportions coming from each of the three types: polyunsaturated, monounsaturated, and saturated. They further recommend that dietary cholesterol be limited to no more than 300 mg a day (one egg provides 250 mg). The Pritikin diet, in contrast, recommends a much lower proportion of dietary fat—10 percent or less of total calories—and that cholesterol intake be kept as low as possible—well under 300 mg per day. This pattern is similar to that now found in many Third World countries where the prevalence of fat-related diseases is very low.

Late Paleolithic humans must have obtained, on average, between 20 and 25 percent of their calories from fat. Of this, polyunsaturates exceeded saturates; a typical P:S ratio might have been 7:5 (which can also be expressed as P:S = 1.4:1). Both values—the low total fat and the high P:S ratio—would have been applauded by groups such as the Senate Select Committee on Nutrition, the American Heart Association, and the American Diabetes Association, if not by advocates of the Pritikin diet. However, these same authorities would not have been pleased by our ancestors' cholesterol intake; their heavy reliance on game means they averaged about 500 mg of cholesterol a day. Of course, this was probably quite variable; depending upon the actual amount of meat available for consumption, the range could easily have been between 300 and 1,000 mg. Recent hunters and gatherers, with diets (and general life-styles) resembling those of Late Paleolithic humans, have extremely low *serum* cholesterol levels despite their high levels of *dietary* cholesterol. (See Table XV.)

How do these people, living much as our remote ancestors did, main-

---

TABLE XV.

Serum Cholesterol Values of Hunters and Gatherers

Population	Country	Average Serum Cholesterol Value
Hadza	Tanzania	110
Eskimos	Canada	141
San (Bushman)	Botswana	120
Aborigines	Australia	139
Pygmies	Zaire	106
Caucasians	United States	210

Modified from S. B. Eaton, M. J. Konner, and M. Shostak. "Stone Agers in the Fast Lane: Chronic Degenerative Diseases in Evolutionary Perspective." *American Journal of Medicine* 84 (1988): 739-49.

tain such low serum cholesterol levels? (Levels which approach those found in nonhuman primates: rhesus monkeys, 111; and baboons, 105 mg/dl, respectively.) Clearly, factors other than the total amount of cholesterol in their food are at work. If, as many medical scientists believe, these factors are dietary—low total fat and low proportion of saturated fat—then the intake of cholesterol in this dietary environment poses fewer risks for them than it does for us. The experience of the Masai—lion-hunting pastoralists who live along the Kenya-Tanzania border in Africa—emphasizes this point. Their warriors consume from 600 to 2,000 mg of cholesterol each day, yet their serum cholesterol levels remain low, generally ranging from 115 to 145 mg/dl. The Masai's heavy milk consumption is probably a factor in this case, since careful experimental studies have shown that milk, especially skim milk, can lower serum cholesterol levels. Still, their example adds to the evidence that dietary cholesterol, by itself, has a relatively limited influence on serum cholesterol levels.

A 1987 study of South African egg-farm workers is also illuminating. These workers, naturally, eat a great number of eggs, so that their average cholesterol intake is over 1,200 mg each day. Nevertheless, because fat provides only 20 percent of daily calories, and because the P:S ratio of their diet (0.8) is somewhat better than ours, their serum cholesterol levels average 180 mg/dl—significantly lower than those of most Americans, although higher than those of hunters and gatherers.

These findings suggest that for those of us able to match the total amount of fat (20 percent fat) and composition (a high P:S ratio) of the Paleolithic standard, a more relaxed attitude about dietary cholesterol may be justifiable. For those of us not able to do so, however, dietary cholesterol levels assume greater significance and should not exceed 300 mg per day.

MINERALS

Virtually all ninety-two of the naturally occurring elements found on earth are also present in human tissues. Some (such as hydrogen, oxygen, carbon, nitrogen, and sulfur) occur as organic material, the carbon-based molecules that are the very essence of animal life. Others occur as inorganic minerals—free elements or ions—which are necessary, in varying amounts, for normal biological function. Some minerals—such as sodium, potassium, calcium, and phosphorous—are needed in large quantities, over 100 mg a day. Other minerals—micronutrients such as iron, iodine, zinc, selenium, chromium, and copper—are necessary only in trace amounts, but are nonetheless vital to normal functioning.

Sodium and Potassium

There are two main environments inside our bodies: the intracellular fluid within cells and the extracellular fluid outside them. Potassium is the chief mineral constituent within cells. Sodium, the chief mineral outside cells, creates a bath of salty fluid resembling the seas within which the earliest life forms evolved. Since multicellular organisms first appeared in those salty oceans nearly a billion years ago, all forms of animal life have shared delicate regulatory mechanisms for maintaining appropriate levels of sodium and potassium in the fluids surrounding and within their cells.

To become terrestrial, creatures had to "learn" to conserve sodium—to recreate the extracellular "ocean" within the boundaries of a multicellular body. That this process is similar in life forms as diverse as reptiles, birds, and mammals indicates how ancient the adaptation is and how critical it was for our remote amphibian ancestors; it enabled them to abandon the high-sodium ocean for the sodium-poor land. Once on land, potassium was available in greater quantity than was sodium. It was more abundant in the food our mammalian ancestors ate and continued to be so for over 200 million years. This is still the case for free-living, nonhuman mammals today. Even Paleolithic humans probably consumed at least ten times more potassium than sodium each day.

Today, only contemporary hunters and gatherers and others in traditional societies maintain this dietary relationship; their high-potassium, low-sodium diets nicely complement the human physiological mechanisms designed to avidly conserve sodium. The benefits are also clear; their blood pressure remains low throughout their lives—a benefit probably achieved by our Paleolithic ancestors as well.

But for most of us, modern processing and preserving techniques have inverted this balance. In contrast to wild game and uncultivated plant foods, which almost invariably contain more potassium than sodium, most of what we eat contains more sodium than potassium. Fresh corn, for example, contains 280 mg of potassium and less than 1 mg of sodium per 100 g portion. An equal portion of canned corn has lost much of this potassium (it has 97 mg) and has gained 235 mg of sodium. It gets worse as corn is processed further; corn flakes, for example, have 1,005 mg of sodium per 100 g! It is much the same for other foods. Potato chips have 250 times more sodium than the same amount of baked potato; dill pickles have 238 times more sodium than a cucumber; and cured ham has sixteen times more sodium than fresh pork.

Processing also commonly leaches out potassium; 100 g of fresh grapes contain 158 mg of potassium, while an equal amount of reconstituted grape juice has only 34 mg. This is also true for hominy grits with one–twenty-fifth the potassium of fresh corn, and for canned peas with one-third the potassium of fresh peas. This list could go on and on, including most foods we eat: cakes, breads, cereals, hot dogs, and, yes, even apple pie. (See Table XVI.)

No other free-living mammals have consistently eaten this way. We are the "guinea pigs" in a novel nutritional "experiment." And the preliminary results are not encouraging. Essential hypertension (high blood pressure) is experienced by 10 to 20 percent of the population. Other risk factors are important, to be sure—insufficient dietary calcium, obesity, inadequate physical exercise, and overconsumption of alcohol—but excessive sodium and minimal potassium lead the way. Increasing our potassium intake may ultimately be part of the solution. Animal experiments have shown that increased dietary potassium reduces the tendency of excessive sodium to induce hypertension. Even in animals with well-established hypertension, high-potassium diets prolonged average length of life.

How much sodium should we be getting? The only consensus among health-care professionals is that we now get too much. Paleolithic humans probably obtained less than 1 g a day, equal to slightly more than 2.5 g of table salt—about ⅓ teaspoon! The Yanamamo Indians, living in the tropical rain forests of Brazil and Venezuela, consume even less, about 250 mg a day. Their lives are physically strenuous, and the climate is hot and humid, yet they get along very well with less than one-tenth the average American's sodium intake. Unlike most of us, their blood pressures remain consistently low throughout their lives, and there is no clinical hypertension. The Yanamamo, called "the fierce people" because of their warlike nature, are similar to many other low-salt cultures. Whether they are Arctic Eskimos, Australian Aborigines, Solo-

---

TABLE XVI.

Sodium and Potassium Levels of Selected Foods

	Sodium (mg)	Potassium (mg)
Hot Dog	1,100	220
Vension Steak	65	385
Apple Pie	110	80
Apple	1	301

mon Islanders, or Kalahari San (Bushmen), people who habitually consume less than a gram of sodium a day do not develop high blood pressure.

Hypertension is not a dramatic illness, but it promotes the development of atherosclerosis, is a potent cause of kidney failure, and is the leading risk factor for stroke. Once acquired, high blood pressure can be controlled by medications, but these are expensive and can have undesirable side effects. Also, they have to be taken for the rest of one's life. The alternatives: to "retrain" our taste buds and to hone our abilities to discriminate low-salt fare from among the ubiquitous high-salt foods surrounding us, tasks not easy, but well worth the effort.

Calcium

Calcium is the most plentiful mineral in our bodies. Nearly 99 percent is in our bones and teeth, but the relatively small amounts dissolved in our body fluids are crucial for nerve conduction, muscular contraction, maintenance of cell membrane function, heart action, and blood clotting, along with many vital intracellular regulatory activities. Because of its importance, the level of calcium in body fluids is carefully controlled by two hormones (one that increases and one that decreases the amount taken from our bones) and by vitamin D, which increases calcium absorption from the intestines.

Calcium in bone acts as a vast reservoir for all the body's calcium needs. Although there is considerable disagreement among experts, the most commonly recommended daily requirements range between 800 and 1,600 mg. But most Americans fail to obtain even the minimal 800 mg from food. When this happens, our bodies take what they need from bone. Yet if this fail-safe mechanism is relied on for too long, the bones robbed of calcium eventually weaken and deteriorate.

Osteoporosis—the clinical manifestation of these weakened, fragile bones—afflicts about 25 percent of postmenopausal women and a smaller proportion of older men. It contributes to the occurrence of over a million fractures each year, most commonly of the spine, hip, and wrist. Spinal fractures can lead to loss of overall height and to an accentuated humplike curve of the backbone—the "dowager hump" often seen in elderly women. Hip fractures are especially serious; complications resulting from this injury are fatal in up to 20 percent of cases.

During childhood, youth, and young adulthood the combination of abundant calcium intake and extensive physical exercise (especially resistance exercise) favors bone formation, maximizing bone mass within genetically determined limits. After about age thirty, bone mass begins to decline. The rate of decline is determined by a number of factors. Exercise—especially vigorous, weight-bearing exercise—and dietary calcium tend to retard bone loss; hormonal factors—especially low estrogen levels in postmenopausal women—tend to promote it. Estrogen supplementation can slow bone loss. Calcium supplementation on its own, however, is not as effective as it is in conjunction with exercise, since it seems to have less independent effect than exercise and estrogen.

Nevertheless, few of us get enough calcium. Even the levels recommended by health professionals are lower than those considered appropriate for nonhuman primates and other mammals. It is constructive to consider that animals like elephants, rhinos, and gorillas obtain sufficient calcium from their exclusively herbivorous diets to build and maintain massive skeletons.

Phosphorus

Authorities currently debate how much phosphorus is needed in our diets—not the absolute level, but how much relative to calcium. Most recommend a 1:1 calcium to phosphorus intake, but both greater and lesser ratios have been advocated. Our human and prehuman ancestors probably consumed more phosphorus than calcium, since all meat and a majority of uncultivated plant foods contain more phosphorus than calcium (leafy vegetables and berries are exceptions). From an evolutionary perspective, then, our current average consumption of phosphorus (estimated at 20 to 50 percent more phosphorus than calcium) is probably in the desirable range. Phosphorus-to-calcium ratios appreciably greater than this (as sometimes occur in people who drink too many diet soft drinks, most of which are rich in phosphorus) may interfere with calcium absorption and contribute to the development of osteoporosis.

Iron

Iron is an essential nutrient, present in all cells of the body. It is the key component of hemoglobin—the oxygen carrier found in red blood cells—where about 70 percent of all our iron is found. The rest is stored, chiefly in the liver, spleen, and bone marrow where it can be called upon whenever needed. Iron is a trace element needed only in very small amounts; its Recommended Dietary Allowance, or RDA, of 18 mg per day for premenopausal adult women and 10 mg per day for men is not very much when compared to the recommendations for other nutrients. Nevertheless, its deficiency is the most common cause of anemia throughout the world, and even in the United States iron deficiency is the "number one" nutritional disease.

Although common enough in food, iron is so poorly absorbed that it has to be consumed in considerable quantity and in the "proper" nutritional environment. Iron found in animal foods—especially red meat, organ meats, and fish—is absorbed most efficiently, yet even from these sources only between 15 and 30 percent is absorbed. Even worse are the most iron-rich plant foods—green leafy vegetables, dried fruits, dried beans and peas, molasses, and whole-grain cereals—with only a 5 percent absorption rate. The presence of vitamin C and other organic acids increases iron absorption, but some dietary substances—oxalic acid in spinach, tannic acid in tea, and antacids—actually cause interference. This means that iron will be absorbed less well from a meal with tea as the main beverage than from one with orange juice.

It is unlikely that our hunting and gathering ancestors experienced much iron deficiency, because iron-rich meat was prominent in their diets and their vegetable foods provided vitamin C to enhance iron absorption. In the United States, however, iron deficiency is common, especially among women. About 20 percent of menstruating women and about 50 percent of pregnant women are deficient. (Women using oral contraceptives are generally less vulnerable because of decreased menstrual bleeding; but those using intrauterine devices commonly have increased menstrual bleeding and thus have extra need for iron.)

American men fare better—only about 3 percent are iron deficient—but among children, especially those between twelve and twenty-four months of age, fully 30 percent are deficient. During their first six months, infants are protected by stores of iron accumulated before birth, but because milk contains little iron, they become vulnerable with time. Older children, especially adolescents experiencing rapid growth, are also vulnerable. Among adults, iron deficiency often strikes vegetarians, people on strict low-caloric diets, and junk food "addicts" (people who obtain most of their calories from foods of little nutritional value).

Chronic iron deficiency can eventually lead to anemia. Occurring in nearly 10 percent of American women, anemia produces fatigue, weakness, reduced physical performance, and decreased productivity. Iron supplementation is usually recommended for those most vulnerable: infants, adolescents, pregnant women, women with exceptionally heavy menstrual flow, and frequent blood donors. However, it is advisable to have a simple blood test taken before starting supplementation because it is quite possible to consume too much. If the body absorbs more iron than it needs, it has no means—other than bleeding—of eliminating it, so toxic levels can build up in the liver, pancreas, and heart.

Zinc

Zinc is a micronutrient with many functions. It is necessary for synthesis of both DNA and RNA; it is required for proper tissue growth and wound healing; and it is a component of several pancreatic enzymes used in digestion. In children, zinc deficiency results in failure to grow properly and experience normal sexual maturation. In adults, deficiency produces lack of appetite and slow wound healing.

Meat, liver, eggs, poultry, and seafood are excellent sources followed by whole grains and milk. For average Americans the RDA is 15 mg, but it has been suggested that higher allowances be recommended for people on high-fiber diets, which tend to decrease zinc absorption. Megadoses, however, can be harmful. They can lower beneficial HDL levels; depress absorption of copper from the intestinal tract; and cause nausea, vomiting, and anemia as well as bleeding from the stomach.

Iodine

Iodine is a trace element needed in extremely small amounts; even so, human diets frequently contain too little. Goiter (a prominent enlargement of the thyroid gland at the base of the neck) is the most common manifestation of its deficiency, and was recognized in Egypt 5,000 years ago. Even at that remote date, seaweed was known both to cure goiter and to prevent it. Its active ingredient: iodine.

The difficulty in procuring enough iodine is that the farther one goes from the ocean, the less available it becomes. Areas where deficiencies are most common include the Great Lakes region of North America, the Alps, and the Andes mountains. Iodine deficiency was probably the most common, and perhaps the only, mineral deficiency suffered by Paleolithic peoples, and at that only by those living far from the sea. If present at birth, iodine deficiency can be especially devastating, causing cretinism, a syndrome characterized by delayed growth and mental retardation.

After absorption, dietary iodine is transported to the thyroid, where it is both stored and used to make thyroid hormone. So avid is its absorption that very little is necessary for prevention of deficiency: about 35 to 50 mg per year, or about 100 to 150 micrograms a day. The best natural source is seafood; the iodine content of vegetable foods depends on the iodine content of the soil in which they grow. The primary source for most people in our society is iodized salt.

Selenium

Selenium, another trace mineral, has been the subject of recent speculation. Does it or does it not influence our risk of cancer? According to some researchers, its capacity to protect us against cancer is so dramatic that daily supplements are recommended for just about everyone. Others recognize its potential importance, but are less effusive.

Selenium's best understood function is to prevent or at least minimize a type of cellular damage called peroxidation, which, whether naturally occurring or chemically induced, can lead to cancer. In animal experiments, selenium has repeatedly reduced the number of cancers produced by various cancer-causing chemicals. Since the evidence in humans is less clear-cut, the National Academy of Sciences has remained cautious.

Red meat was probably the main source of selenium for Paleolithic peoples, since cereal grains, generally the best vegetable source, were rare in human diets before agriculture.

Chromium

Experience with patients requiring prolonged intravenous feeding as their sole source of nutrition has shown chromium to be necessary for the normal metabolism of glucose. Interacting with insulin at the cell membrane, it seems to aid the entry of glucose into the cell. Since tissue concentrations of chromium typically decline with advancing age, this may contribute to the development of adult-onset diabetes.

Our foods—calorically concentrated and low in nutrient density—apparently fail to maintain our body's stores of chromium. The wild game and uncultivated vegetable foods our ancestors ate had only slightly more chromium content, but because these foods had relatively low energy density, more total food was eaten to meet daily energy needs. As a result the chromium intake of our hunting and gathering ancestors would likely have exceeded ours.

Copper

Copper is another essential trace mineral. Although examples of its deficiency in humans are rare, animal experiments suggest that prolonged exposure to diets containing much more zinc than copper can elevate serum cholesterol levels. This observation argues against "unilateral" dietary zinc supplementation.

Summary

Winding one's way through the dizzying array of continually changing reports on the role of minerals in human health is a frustrating task. Our knowledge has so many gaps that each new finding seems isolated, just one more random piece in an intricate, complex puzzle. No wonder nutritional research so often ends up contradicting itself. Low levels of selenium in foods have been associated with higher cancer rates in the United States, but not in New Zealand; high-fiber diets have at once been blamed and exonerated for preventing absorption of minerals. Claims that one or another "magic mineral" prolongs life and enhances sexual vigor come and go so rapidly it is hard to keep count—or even remember, after the initial furor subsides—even though the cash register at the health food store is ringing.

Amid this confusion, how are we to proceed? Once again, the knowledge of our past can be a useful, if not unerring, guide. After all, our bodies were designed, and continue to be designed, to function optimally with minerals obtained through the variable diet available to hunters and gatherers. If this had not been the case, the human line would long since have faltered. But it did not. Hunters and gatherers, consuming a wide range of plant and animal life—wider than that consumed by any people who followed, until recently—adequately met their needs for all the micronutrients essential to human life.

Today, we are fortunate in being able to match, if not exceed, this range, with foods from around the world available throughout the year. Our task, amid this smorgasbord of plenty, is to learn to choose foods that optimize our health; foods with nutritional properties similar to those consumed by our preagricultural ancestors. Yet the realities of twentieth-century life sometimes justify veering from our ancestral path. Some supplementation, for example, can be worthwhile. Consider calcium. Paleolithic peoples met their calcium requirements with much greater ease than we do, so calcium supplementation is probably justified. (Guidelines on how to make dietary choices and a discussion of supplementation can be found in Chapter 6.)

Science will continue, of course, to provide additional pieces of the human health puzzle from one year to the next. Trace minerals still not well understood—chromium, zinc, copper, silicon, and selenium, for example—may be among the areas where breakthroughs occur. Our prediction is that most of these findings will recapitulate the experience of the past. Our task in the present, then, is to learn from both the past and the future.

VITAMINS

Vitamins are organic, carbon-containing compounds found in minute quantities in plants and animals. They are needed in infinitesimal amounts in human metabolism. Since most cannot be manufactured by the body, they must be obtained from diet. (Exceptions are vitamin D, which is synthesized by the skin in the presence of sunlight, and some of the B vitamins, which can be synthesized by intestinal bacteria.) They are classified as a group not because of common chemical structures or physiological functions, but because they do not fit into other categories; neither carbohydrates, proteins, fats, nor minerals, they are nevertheless vital for human life.

Discovered relatively late—in the early 1900s—vitamins are divided into two groups: fat soluble and water soluble. The fat-soluble vitamins—A, D, E, and K—are absorbed from the intestinal tract only if fat is present in the meal. They can be stored—to a greater or lesser extent—in the fat cells of our body, so a backup exists if dietary intake is insufficient. Daily intake is therefore less crucial than it is for water-soluble vitamins. However, because they are stored, toxic levels can build up if fat-soluble vitamins (other than vitamin E) are consumed in excessive amounts, although this usually happens only when people take massive supplemental doses.

Water-soluble vitamins—the eight B vitamins and vitamin C—are not stored (except for vitamin B_{12} which is stored in the liver and kidneys), so daily replenishment is necessary. Since they dissolve in water, they leach easily from foods during soaking or boiling. They are also quite fragile—sensitive to heat and light—and are readily destroyed by careless processing, improper storage, or any form of prolonged heating. Megadoses of these vitamins are rarely harmful; when consumed in excess, they are excreted in the urine.

Paleolithic hunters and gatherers, consuming a wide variety of nutrient-rich game and wild vegetable foods, are unlikely to have commonly developed vitamin deficiencies. Nor have recent hunters and gatherers developed them. As much as three pounds of plant foods are eaten each day soon after they are gathered—with little processing, washing, or cooking—so maximum utilization of vitamins is the rule, not the exception. Their foods—green leafy vegetables, peas and beans, nuts, seeds, fruit, and very lean meat—so parallel current recommendations for the best sources of vitamins and minerals that their diets look like "wish lists" for contemporary health advocates.

However, the long-standing relationship between humans and vitamins changed with the beginning of agriculture, when the range of foods narrowed along with the supply of vitamins; cultivated vegetables frequently proved nutritionally inferior to the wild strains from which they were bred. Only in the twentieth century have abundant food resources, vitamin enrichment, and vitamin supplementation enabled large numbers of people in "advanced" countries to reach levels of dietary vitamin intake approaching the high Paleolithic standard.

Vitamin A and Beta-carotene

Also called retinal because of its role in forming visual pigments in the retina, vitamin A occurs in two forms: as the vitamin itself and as precursors, called carotenes. (Of ten different carotenes, beta-carotene is the most active.) Along with malnutrition caused by inadequate dietary protein, and anemia caused by inadequate dietary iron, vitamin A deficiency ranks as one of the most common serious deficiency diseases. It is a leading cause of blindness in many parts of the world.

Vitamin A has many functions. It aids vision in dim light; it affects normal bone formation; and it helps maintain the body's epithelial surfaces. In this last role, it is thought to help prevent epithelial cancers from developing in the lungs or urinary bladder. Research has shown that people with habitually low intake of vitamin A are more prone to lung cancer than people with normal or high intake. This is true even for smokers; those with low serum levels of beta-carotene are apparently four times more likely to develop lung cancer as are those with high levels.

Both vitamin A and beta-carotene occur naturally in liver, dairy products, most yellow vegetables, tomatoes, some green leafy vegetables (especially broccoli and spinach), and many fruits. The RDA for vitamin A is 5,000 International Units for adult men and 4,000 for adult women. Beta-carotene, biologically less active, if used as a substitute, requires three times the intake of vitamin A. Because vitamin A can be stored in the body, chiefly in the liver, continued excessive intake (ten to one hundred times the RDA) can be toxic. Cases of acute vitamin A toxicity have occurred in Arctic explorers who ate polar bear liver, which contains extremely high concentrations of vitamin A.

A similar case may have affected a person who lived 1.6 million years ago. Paleontologist Alan Walker of the Johns Hopkins Medical School believes that a *Homo erectus* skeleton found in Kenya in 1973 shows pathological signs of chronic vitamin A overdose (hypervitaminosis A). He reasons that as humans in this time period became more effective hunters, they may have consumed excessive amounts of vitamin A by eating large quantities of liver, especially from carnivores.

Vitamin D

Rickets is a bone disorder observed in children living in countries where smog and overcast skies are common. Debate once raged over whether its cause was dietary deficiency or lack of sunlight. Both answers ultimately proved correct. Vitamin D is available in foods such as milk, eggs, liver, and fish; it is also produced by the skin after exposure to sunlight. (It is the only vitamin made by the body; it could be considered a hormone as logically as a vitamin.) Rickets was probably rare among Paleolithic peoples. Its relevance to human history is more recent—a classic "disease of civilization." Its causes? Clothing and indoor living combined with domestic and industrial smoke, which literally block out the sun.

Vitamin D, also called calciferol, helps regulate calcium and phosphorus levels in the blood, facilitates calcium absorption from the intestines, and promotes normal formation and maintenance of bones and teeth. The RDA is 400 International Units. People who drink milk and who have some exposure to sunlight are unlikely to need supplementation, but older people confined indoors may. Megadoses, from five to one hundred times the RDA, taken over a long period of time, can promote the formation of kidney stones.

Vitamin E

Vitamin E—also called alpha-tocopherol—is a vitamin in search of a deficiency disease. Although essential for certain animals, its necessity for humans has not yet been established. Its role as an antioxidant, however, is intriguing. Because it prevents substances from reacting with oxygen, it has been touted as an anti-aging as well as an anti-cancer compound, especially for cancers of the breast and lung. Since oxidation can chemically convert susceptible substances—such as polyunsaturated fats—into toxic ones, people following diets with high proportions of unsaturated fats, like the Paleolithic diet, might profit from supplemental vitamin E. In animals, selenium and possibly vitamin C can substitute for vitamin E when its intake is low.

The RDA for vitamin E is 15 International Units for men and 12 for women, but people whose diets are high in polyunsaturated fats might want to double that amount. Fortunately, vitamin E is widely distributed in foods so that, except for junk-food enthusiasts, most Americans' diets provide an adequate supply. The richest sources are vegetable oils, especially oils pressed from seeds (like corn and sesame), as well as peanuts, soybeans, wheat germ, whole-grain cereals, liver, eggs, fresh greens, and dried beans. Unlike fat-soluble vitamins A and D, megadoses up to one hundred times the RDA of vitamin E, while not recommended, show little if any evidence of toxicity. Contrary to recent advertising claims—unfortunately—vitamin E has no proven effect on sexual potency or responsiveness.

The B-Complex Vitamins

Vitamin B was initially thought to be a single, water-soluble essential nutrient; only several years after its discovery was it found to represent a number of independent factors which, although chemically unrelated, usually occur together in the same foods. The B vitamins along with vitamin C are easily destroyed by improper storage or cooking. People experiencing physical stress—injury or illness—often need more than normal amounts owing to increased tissue requirements.

Thiamine (Vitamin B_1)

Rice polishing—removal of the outer coating of the rice kernel in order to make white rice—was introduced during the seventeenth century. Thereafter, beriberi—a disease affecting the heart and nervous system—became widespread throughout Southeast Asia. The connection between rice polishing and the disease, however, was not made until 1890 when Christiaan Eijkman, a Dutch physician, noted that beriberi was common among wealthy Indonesians who ate polished white rice but rare among peasants who continued to eat unrefined brown rice. Following his hunch, Eijkman gave discarded rice hulls to his beriberi patients. They promptly recovered, confirming his hypothesis that the disease represented a deficiency disorder. A few years later, in 1912, Casimir Funk isolated the responsible agent, thiamine. Funk's discovery, chemically an "amine," was also clearly "vital" for beriberi patients; accordingly he coined the word *vitamine* which has since been shortened to *vitamin*.

Thiamine is required daily. Because little is stored in the body, even short periods of deprivation can cause symptoms of deficiency. The RDA is between 1 and 1.5 mg. Few foods supply thiamine in large concentrations, but pork, yeast, nuts, legumes, whole grains, oysters, dried beans, and leafy vegetables are reasonable sources.

Megadoses of thiamine have revealed no known toxicity, but because it functions in conjunction with the other B vitamins, an excess of one might adversely affect the efficacy of the others.

Niacin

Around the turn of the century, pellagra—a disease that began with a skin rash and often progressed to mental illness and death—was common among poor people in the southeastern United States whose diets were based largely on cornmeal and molasses. Inspired by the role thiamine played in beriberi, Dr. Joseph Goldberger of the U.S. Public Health Service became convinced that pellagra was also a deficiency disease; in 1937, he discovered that niacin deficiency was the basis of this disorder. The little niacin corn has is mostly "bound"— which means it cannot be absorbed. It also lacks tryptophan—an essential amino acid that the body could otherwise convert into niacin. Plagued by this double deficiency, people relying heavily on corn developed pellagra.

Widespread niacin supplementation eradicated the disease in the United States by 1945, but it remains endemic in other populations throughout the world, especially in very poor areas. In Western nations, alcoholics, food faddists, and drug addicts are most susceptible to deficiency. The RDA for niacin is between 10 and 20 mg a day, depending on the amount of tryptophan in the diet. Tryptophan is converted into niacin at a rate of sixty parts tryptophan to one part niacin; people who eat considerable quantities of animal protein each day, like Paleolithic hunters and gatherers, can obtain nearly all the niacin they need from this source alone. Niacin is widely distributed in foods, especially whole-grain cereals, lean meat, peanuts, fruit, and most vegetables.

When recommended in megadoses (up to three hundred times the RDA) for its cholesterol-lowering properties, it is more properly considered a drug than a vitamin and, like other drugs, can exhibit undesirable side effects.

Folic Acid

Folic acid is necessary for synthesis of DNA and RNA—nucleic acids which form the genes as well as the protein-manufacturing apparatus of each cell. Since folic acid deficiency impairs DNA synthesis, cells that need constant replacement—such as red blood cells and those that form the intestinal lining—are especially dependent on its presence in adequate amounts. This is true as well for rapidly reproducing cancer cells, and some anti-cancer drugs have been developed which inhibit folic acid activity; by interfering with its availability, cancer cells are rendered less able to manufacture DNA and thus proliferate less readily.

The RDA for folic acid is very small: 400 micrograms. It is widely available in foods, especially in peas, beans, nuts, whole grains, green leafy vegetables, asparagus, and oranges. Small amounts are synthesized by intestinal bacteria, and these alone may be enough to meet our normal daily requirements. Clinical folic acid deficiency, therefore, tends to occur only in unusual dietary circumstances: in people with intestinal absorption disorders; in junk-food "addicts"; in those who, like many elderly, subsist primarily on canned foods, tea, and toast; and in alcoholics.

Megadoses of folic acid have not been associated with negative effects, but doses greater than .1 mg (the legal, nonprescription maximum) per day can mask pernicious anemia, a vitamin B_{12} deficiency.

Vitamin B_{12}

Vitamin B_{12} is the largest and most structurally complex of all the vitamins—the only one that contains an essential mineral, cobalt. Like folic acid, it is necessary for normal synthesis of DNA and RNA. Cells which grow quickly—in the bone marrow and intestinal tract—are therefore most readily affected by B_{12} deficiency, but slow-growing central nervous system cells are also quite susceptible because it helps maintain myelin sheaths surrounding nerve fibers.

Unlike other water-soluble vitamins, vitamin B_{12} is stored in the liver and kidneys in quantities large enough to meet the body's needs for months. When the stores are used up in the context of inadequate dietary B_{12}, a lethal form of anemia—pernicious anemia—accompanied by a slow degeneration of the spinal cord can result. Vegans—people who eat no meat or dairy products—are most vulnerable to vitamin B_{12} deficiency. Deficiency, however, can also result from other conditions, such as surgery or inflammatory bowel disease, which impairs intestinal absorption. It is also caused by an inadequate supply of "intrinsic factor," a protein secreted by the stomach, without which the absorption of vitamin B_{12}, the "extrinsic factor," is greatly reduced. In the 1920s the complex pathophysiology of pernicious anemia was worked out; since then intramuscular injections of B_{12} have essentially eliminated the condition.

The RDA for vitamin B_{12} is only 3 micrograms. Unlike the other B vitamins, it does not occur in vegetable foods. Animal foods—meat, dairy products, and liver—are the best sources. While B_{12} injections are life-saving in pernicious anemia, they have no effect on other anemias or nonspecific ailments.

Vitamin C: Ascorbic Acid

Scurvy, a disease which was often fatal until about two hundred years ago, is characterized by bleeding gums, musculoskeletal aches, fatigue, and emotional lability. Chronicled as early as 400 B.C. by Xenophon, a Greek historian and soldier, it appears and reappears throughout the historical record. During the Crusades many Christians fighting to win the Holy Land from the Muslims died of scurvy; during the Age of Discovery, it became the leading cause of disability and death among sailors; and as recently as the nineteenth century, infants fed on newly introduced powdered or canned milk instead of breast milk contracted it.

Although the role citrus fruits play in preventing scurvy was suspected as early as 1720, it was not until 1747 that James Lind, a Scottish surgeon, proved that they could both cure it and prevent it. When Captain James Cook included sauerkraut and as many fresh vegetables as possible in his crew's ration on his trips of exploration (1770s), only one out of 1,000 sailors died from the disease; without such dietary measures, more than half of them probably would have. It took until 1802, however, for the British admiralty to become convinced. Then, daily rations of lemon or lime juice became compulsory for British sailors, earning them the nickname "limeys." The active chemical, ascorbic acid, was isolated only in 1928.

Despite its importance to health and the popular interest it excites, the exact function of ascorbic acid, also called vitamin C, is not well known. It is necessary for the formation of collagen, the main protein of connective tissues, and thus is essential for maintaining the structural integrity of blood vessel walls. Since vitamin C is readily absorbed and is stored to a moderate extent, deficiency usually develops only after long-term and severe dietary deficiency. Except for humans and other primates, most animals are capable of synthesizing ascorbic acid.

The RDA has been set at 60 mg for adults, but nursing mothers require more and additional amounts may be indicated during periods of increased physical stress: when undergoing surgery, after sustaining a burn, or when combating infection. Smokers and women on oral contraceptives may also need more. The best sources for vitamin C are fresh fruits and their juices, especially oranges, strawberries, grapefruit, melons, and papayas. Raw or minimally cooked vegetables—broccoli, tomatoes, cauliflower, green peppers, leafy green vegetables, turnips, and potatoes—are also good sources. Rose hips, the seed pods of the rose flower, however, are not of any greater superiority; their popular reputation is derived from their use as a vitamin C source in England during World War II, when citrus fruits were in extremely limited supply.

There is no doubt about vitamin C's role in preventing scurvy, but controversy surrounds its possible role in combating other physical conditions, especially the common cold. Two-time Nobel Prize winner Linus Pauling has consistently argued, despite vehement opposition, that in doses up to fifty times the RDA, it does. Others interpret the studies differently, challenging his conclusions. When the smoke settles on this argument, it is possible that vitamin C may actually prove beneficial for some people in lessening the severity, if not the frequency, of the common cold; but it will, in all likelihood, work—if at all—in ways less dramatic than have been claimed.

Another purported vitamin C effect—its possible role in the prevention of cancer—is also intriguing. At issue is the effect vitamin C may have on cancer-causing chemicals called nitrosamines, the end products of a conversion that takes place in the intestines. Nitrites—found in cured meats such as hot dogs, luncheon meats, bacon, and ham as well as in other foods—are altered by intestinal bacteria into nitrosamines. Since vitamin C has been shown to reduce this conversion, it could *theoretically* be able to decrease the incidence of gastrointestinal malignancies such as gastric cancer.

Paleolithic humans generally consumed over seven times the currently recommended amount of vitamin C, but even these high levels are considerably lower than those advocated by today's vitamin enthusiasts. At present, self-prescribed, chronic megadoses are unwarranted and unjustified. For some people they may even be detrimental to health.

Summary

The vitamin requirements of our late Paleolithic ancestors were readily provided by wild game animals and uncultivated vegetable foods. Their foods were low in energy density and rich in nutrients, including vitamins. To meet their caloric needs, they consumed greater weights of food each day than we do, and they processed and cooked them (or, in many cases, did not cook them) in ways that minimally affected the vitamins. Their lives progressed in an essentially vitamin-abundant nutritional environment.

With the exception of chronic hypervitaminosis A in early *Homo erectus*, excessive vitamin consumption has no known prehistorical precedent. What is evident from the past is that our physiology is capable of, if not actually designed for, functioning with vitamin-intake levels somewhat greater than those we now maintain, but nowhere near the megadose levels advocated by various health faddists.

CHAPTER SIX

HUNTING AND GATHERING
IN THE SUPERMARKET

If mammoth steak and uncultivated vegetables were sold in today's supermarkets, we might find it simple to recreate the nutritional patterns of our ancestors. But, of course, they are not. And, while wild game is increasingly available at specialty stores and chic restaurants, its cost makes it prohibitively expensive as regular fare (except for hunters with large freezers). Even organically grown vegetables—fresh, whole, and produced without use of chemical fertilizers—are different from those of the Cro-Magnons. They are the product of thousands of years of agricultural modification.

Is it possible, then, to emulate the past? By applying the concept of *equivalency*, it is not only possible but, in some respects, fairly easy. This approach recognizes that although the specific dietary fare of pre-agricultural humans is out of our reach, foods encompassing comparable nutritional elements are not. Aurochs steak, for example, high in animal protein and low in fat, and containing more potassium than sodium, can be nutritionally matched by a similar portion of poultry or fish. And despite botanical differences, wild plant foods, generally high in food value and low in calories, have nutritional parallels in many cultivated varieties.

Equivalency allows for considerable flexibility. When anatomically modern humans first became widespread, dairy foods (except of course for mother's milk) did not exist; animals would not be domesticated for close to 25,000 years. Even wild grains, abundant in many locations, required such arduous processing that more easily utilized plant resources were eaten instead. But this doesn't mean we should refuse dairy products and grains. These modern foods are excellent and versatile nutritional sources.

The approach we offer here, then, is one that incorporates what *is* available today to create a diet comparable to the Paleolithic one. With modest effort, the rewards are likely to be great. After all, the nutritional environment of our past is the one our genes "know" best; it promotes optimal operating conditions for our physiology and biochemistry.

GOALS

Energy Sources

Despite wide regional and seasonal variation in dietary pattern, most preagricultural people obtained 20 to 25 percent of their daily calories from fat. Their protein and carbohydrate intake, however, varied widely depending upon whether game or plant foods predominated. But within this broad range, the most common pattern probably provided an additional 40 to 50 percent of daily calories from carbohydrates and 25 to 35 percent from protein.

To consume comparably high levels of protein today would be expensive and might, over the course of our longer average life span, prove harmful to our kidneys. A balance of 60 percent carbohydrate, 20 percent protein, and 20 percent fat—a pattern well within the broad Paleolithic range—therefore makes more sense, accommodating the realities of twentieth-century life with the patterns of the past.

Fats

One of the most salient features of Paleolithic nutrition is that people not only ate much less fat than we do, but the fat they did eat was more polyunsaturated than saturated. The diet of most Americans, in contrast, is in reverse of this pattern. Our ancestors must also have eaten a higher proportion of monounsaturated fat relative to saturated fat.

While health authorities currently recommend that we lower our saturated-fat intake, they usually go only so far as to advise equal consumption of saturated and polyunsaturated fats. But this recommendation falls short of the pattern that prevailed for most of the past 2 million (or more) years. More in keeping with this past would be to have polyunsaturated and monounsaturated fat each exceed the amount of saturated fat in our diet.

Nutrient Density

Another striking feature of our ancestors' food was its high nutrient density. Calorie for calorie, their food provided more protein, vitamins, minerals, and fiber than the comparatively empty calories of the energy-dense diets so prevalent in the West today. A pound of venison steak, for example, contains 572 calories and supplies 95 g of protein; a pound of frankfurters contains more than twice the calories (1,402), but less than two-thirds the protein (56.7 g). Similarly, a pound of apples contains about 242 calories, fewer than one-fourth the calories in a pound of apple pie (1,161 calories). Although the amount of calcium and iron in the two are nearly equal (29 vs. 36 g and 1.3 vs. 1.4 mg, respectively), the apples provide two and a half times·more fiber and five times more vitamin C than does the pie.

Foods of the past—physically bulky and dense in nutrients—were also generally low in calories. To obtain 3,000 calories a day meant an intake of nearly five pounds of food. Today, five pounds of some of our rich foods, such as devil's food cake, can yield 9,000 calories—the equivalent of the daily calorie requirement of three large active men! Calorically concentrated but nutritionally depleted foods should be reduced in our diet in favor of bulky, filling, and more nutritionally dense fare.

Micronutrients

Our preagricultural ancestors obtained more vitamins from their foods than we generally do from ours. They consumed more iron, more than twice the calcium, far less sodium (under a gram a day), and considerably more potassium than sodium. Their food also contained more essential fatty acids—particularly long-chain, omega-3, polyunsaturated fatty acids currently being studied for their possible role in preventing heart disease. However, they probably consumed lower levels than do the often-mentioned Eskimos—and also less than the doses being evaluated in most experimental studies.

Carbohydrates

Honey, their only refined carbohydrate, was such a treat that our ancestors withstood discomfort and even danger to procure it. Still, before the domestication of bees, it was obtainable only seasonally (from two to four months a year), so the great majority of carbohydrates came from bulky, high-fiber fruits and vegetables. In order to approach this pattern we should limit sugar and finely milled flours, and replace them with foods that provide chiefly complex carbohydrates. Our intake of non-nutrient fiber needs to be augmented. The typical Late Paleolithic human obtained from 100 to 150 g daily—an amount similar to that consumed by today's rural Africans. In Western nations a goal of 50 to 100 g/day seems feasible; whereas a target of 100 g/day or more would require a major—and probably unattainable—readjustment of current dietary patterns. To date the experimental evidence pertaining to high fiber diets and mineral malabsorption is contradictory and inconclusive. The high fiber content of our ancestors' diet was balanced by an abundance of calcium, other minerals, and vitamins. Americans who consume 50 to 100 g of fiber daily need to increase their intake of micronutrients at the same time—in line with this chapter's suggestions. The proportion of soluble, fermentable fiber (from fruits, vegetables, beans, and oats) should nearly equal that of insoluble fiber from sources like wheat bran.

Balancing Macronutrients

In order to evaluate the foods we eat, we need to know the relative contributions of carbohydrates, proteins, and fats. This is determined not by weight alone, but by the proportion of calories each nutrient contributes. To calculate this contribution, simply count 4 calories for each gram of protein or carbohydrate and 9 calories for each gram of fat. A food that contains 20 g of carbohydrate, 8 g of protein, and 8 g of fat—chili con carne, for example—does not have a carbohydrate:protein:fat caloric distribution of 20:8:8 (which would be fairly close to the Paleolithic standard), but rather one of 80:32:72, which is quite undesirable. Of course, we can't achieve the ideal ratio in every food; some foods will depart from it markedly, but the total balance can be redressed with better ones.

A convenient if imperfect approach is to make sure carbohydrates make up at least half the diet, and then consider only protein and fat. As long as calories from protein exceed those from fat, a food is likely to be nutritionally acceptable. Regular and low-fat yogurt are good examples. Regular yogurt contains 12 g of protein and 9 g of ft; low-fat yogurt contains 8 g of protein and 2 g of fat. If only the relative weights of protein and fat are considered, there might be some question as to which is nutritionally superior. However, when the calorie relationships are calculated, the Paleolithic answer is clear. Regular yogurt, with a fat:protein distribution of 81:48, has almost twice as many calories coming from fat (81) as from protein (48); low-fat yogurt, with a fat:protein ratio of 18:32, has almost twice as many calories coming from protein (32) as from fat (18).

Priority Levels

To achieve a modern version of the Paleolithic diet, we need a hierarchy of nutritional principles so that when, as often happens, a given food meets some but not all criteria, it is possible to determine which nutritional factors take precedence. There are three levels.

Level A—Highest Priority
Total Fat Content: Since fat is implicated in the development of both cardiovascular disease (heart attack and stroke) and cancer, total fat content is probably the single most important consideration. If two food items differ in fat content, the one with less fat is almost always the better choice.

Polyunsaturated vs. *Saturated Fat (P:S ratio):* Fats that are more polyunsaturated and/or monounsaturated are preferable. (More simply stated, the lower the proportion of saturated fat, the better.)

Level B—Moderate Priority
Sodium and Potassium: The less salt (sodium chloride) the better. (People with borderline or high blood pressure should probably place sodium reduction at the top of the priority list.) Since potassium can partially offset sodium's adverse effects, foods with more *potassium* than sodium are preferable.

Fiber Content: The more the better. It is possible to get too much fiber in the form of pure bran supplements, but with regard to actual foods, the more fiber the better.

Cholesterol Content: If total fat is at 20 percent or less of total calories consumed and if polyunsaturated fat exceeds saturated fat, then controlling cholesterol intake is less critical. Few studies show that cholesterol in the diet, *independent of saturated fat,* is a major determinant of serum cholesterol levels. Nevertheless, when given a choice, foods containing less cholesterol should generally be chosen.

Calcium Content: High-calcium foods are better choices.

Level C—Supplemental Priority
Carbohydrate:Protein:Fat Ratio: With other priorities satisfied, a carbohydrate:protein:fat pattern of 60:20:20 is ideal.

Caloric Content and Nutrient Density: Foods providing fewer calories and greater bulk are better choices. However, a plan combining exercise with the preceding priorities will usually prevent obesity without special attention to calories.

MATERIALS

While foods today are not as uniformly healthful as were those eaten by Stone Age foragers, we are more than compensated by the impressive diversity and range of items from which to choose. Reproducing most features of our ancestors' nutrition with modern fare is therefore relatively easy.

Meat and Fish

Our preagricultural ancestors ate more red meat than most of us do or should eat today. As we have seen, however, their meat was low in total fat, with a high proportion of polyunsaturated fat.

The nutritional properties of wild game are best matched by poultry, fish, and shellfish. These foods generally have little fat, and sometimes even less than is found in wild game, while their protein is complete and of good quality. Turkey and chicken—with skin removed because of its high fat content—are the poultry of choice, especially the white meat which has less fat than the dark meat. Although wild ducks and geese are comparatively lean, their domestic cousins are quite fatty, another nutritional consequence of domestication. The very leanest cuts of red meat—round steak, flank steak, and chopped meat with 15 percent or less fat—can be included occasionally, but even with these cuts, avoid marbling and remove all visible fat. Unfortunately, meat this lean is expensive, difficult to find, and even when available, still has about double the fat of wild game. Extremely lean chopped meat can be custom ordered, however, even in large supermarkets, by buying precut steak or roasts and asking butchers to grind them. Be sure to request all visible fat be removed before grinding. This is an extremely expensive way to buy chopped meat, but think of what we spend on our health in other ways. Furthermore, by increasing our demand for healthier meat, we will eventually bring its price down to affordable levels.

Fish—also, unfortunately, expensive—are generally low in fat and have especially low levels of saturated fat. Some fish such as mackerel, salmon, and cod are also excellent sources of essential fatty acids, including the long-chain, omega-3 polyunsaturated fatty acids which are thought to protect against atherosclerosis. Furthermore, most fish have fairly low levels of cholesterol. Be careful, however, where your fish come from. Many states now issue warnings and monitor levels of chemical contaminants, such as PCBs (polychlorinated biphenyls), in their fish supply and these should be heeded. To lower the intake of contaminants in fatty fish, remove the skin and discard the darkest—and fattiest—tissues; along the sides, the back, and the belly. Broiling, baking, or grilling will reduce the fat content further.

Shellfish contain almost no fat and are excellent, although again expensive, sources of protein. Crab and especially shrimp have more cholesterol than poultry or red meat; oysters, clams, and scallops have levels comparable to those of fish. The other shellfish have intermediate cholesterol values.

Organ meats like liver and kidneys are relatively low in fat but high in cholesterol, while brains are not only high in fat, but have more cholesterol than any other source. Specialty meats like bacon, sausage, frankfurters, and luncheon meats (in addition to containing many additives) are also high in fat and cholesterol. Pork sausage, for example, provides six times more calories from fat than from protein, while bacon provides up to twenty times more. With the exception of liver and kidneys, which can be eaten in moderation, these meats should be avoided.

Hot dogs and luncheon meats—the most commonly consumed types of meat in the United States—seem inexpensive. But they provide so little protein (16 percent of their calories come from protein and 81 percent from fat—mostly saturated) that the protein itself is actually quite expensive compared with poultry or fish. Furthermore these foods contain extremely high levels of sodium along with nitrites—preservatives implicated in causing cancer.

Fruits, Vegetables, and Nuts

It's hard for a diet to contain too many fruits or vegetables (except for a handful of high-fat items such as avocados and coconuts). These food sources provide a wide variety of vitamins and minerals as well as fiber, especially in its soluble form. High-fiber vegetables include peas, beans, spinach, carrots, artichokes, broccoli, brussels sprouts, and potatoes; high-fiber fruits include dates, figs, raisins, bananas, pears, apples, raspberries, blackberries, and loganberries. Vegetables and fruits eaten raw are better fiber and nutrient sources than those cooked, dried, or frozen.

One group of vegetables—the cruciferous family—has gained special distinction: They have been recommended by the American Cancer Society for their possible cancer-preventive benefits. Cabbage, broccoli, brussels sprouts, cauliflower, collards, kale, mustard and turnip greens, rutabagas, turnips, and radishes are in this category. In addition to containing antioxidants that may block the formation of cancer-causing substances, they also are excellent sources of fiber, vitamins, and minerals.

Nuts are generally high in fat—it constitutes from 40 to 70 percent of their weight and even more of their caloric contribution. For some recent hunters and gatherers, such as the !Kung San of Africa's Kalahari Desert, nuts are a dietary staple, and remains at preagricultural living sites indicate that they were also popular among many Late Paleolithic peoples. Including them in our diets, however, requires discretion. Some, especially cashews and coconuts, are unacceptably high in saturated fat. Walnuts, sunflower seeds, and to a lesser extent pecans, hazelnuts (filberts), and almonds, have good polyunsaturated to saturated fat ratios and can be eaten with moderation, as can peanuts which have mostly monounsaturated fat. (Special care should be taken, however, to avoid nuts that are moldy or have been improperly stored; aflatoxin, a common mold found on these nuts, especially on peanuts, is one of the most potent carcinogens known. Also, nuts should not be salted; a can of salted peanuts, for example, contains a drastic and, for hypertensive individuals, dangerous salt overload.)

Avocados and olives are also exceptionally high in fat. But while the fat of avocados is largely saturated, that of olives is largely monounsaturated. Olive oil is therefore preferable to butter and lard as a cooking oil, and its use may be one reason why Mediterranean peoples tend to have less atherosclerosis than northern Europeans, who have traditionally used the more saturated animal fats in their cuisine.

Fresh vegetables and fruits are nutritionally superior to canned or otherwise processed varieties. Frozen foods are somewhere in between; most have added salt and, with fruits, added sugar, but otherwise their nutrient properties are fairly comparable to those of fresh produce. When you are buying frozen fruits and vegetables, check ingredients for sugar, salt, and other additives. Except for low-sodium products, cut back on canned vegetables whenever possible.

In the remote past, vegetables and fruits were eaten raw, roasted, or otherwise minimally processed—not doused with salt, fats, and sauces. Fruits and vegetables today can also be enjoyed—even more than ever—without added flavorings. Unlike wild foods, cultivated varieties have been bred for texture, flavor, and sweetness. With experience many people find that they appreciate, and even prefer, the broad variety of subtle unadorned flavors—much as a veteran taster develops an increasingly sophisticated appreciation of wine. When condiments *must* be added, however, use vegetable oil margarine instead of butter;

skim milk is preferable to nondairy creamers; and low-calorie sweeteners can be used sparingly instead of sugar.

While some food value is necessarily lost between the harvest and the grocery shelves, plenty is still left for us to extract—as long as we are careful to minimize the further destruction of nutrients. This can be accomplished in various ways: (1) shop in stores with rapid turnover of fresh produce; (2) shop frequently and buy only what will be used quickly; (3) buy only whole, not precut produce; (4) discriminate for freshness—choose produce in plastic, nearest the refrigeration coils or on the bottom, not the top, of the pile; (5) don't cut, chop, or peel anything before it is ready to be used; (6) cook vegetables whole whenever possible, cut to serve; (7) rinse, rather than soak, vegetables to be washed; (8) cook vegetables quickly—steaming or microwaving—rather than slowly boiling, and cover to reduce cooking time.

Improperly handled fresh produce may be less nutritious than properly handled frozen foods. Avoid packages with frost on the outside since this indicates the food has been thawed and refrozen. Transfer packages from the store to your freezer, which should be at 0° F (or 32° *below* freezing).

Dairy Products and Eggs

Although preagricultural people had no milk products after early childhood, that is not reason enough for us to avoid them. But we do have to be careful. Along with beneficial calcium and protein, they also contain high levels of saturated fat and cholesterol, and their lactose is a problem for people with lactase deficiency. Avoid products made from cream or whole milk, including butter, most cheeses, cream cheese, ice cream, and sour cream.

Dairy foods most compatible with a Paleolithic dietary regimen are ones with little or no butterfat: skim milk, cultured buttermilk, low-fat cottage cheese, and low-fat yogurt. (Yogurt and other cultured milk products are usually tolerated by those with lactase deficiency.) A number of studies have shown that while high-fat dairy products raise the serum cholesterol level, low-fat dairy products can actually lower it.

Eggs are eaten by contemporary hunters and gatherers whenever possible and were almost certainly eaten by Paleolithic people as well. But it was harder to find nests of wild fowl than it is to pick up a dozen eggs at the supermarket, so our ancestors did not have access to comparable quantities. Since eggs are high in total fat (more of which is saturated than polyunsaturated) and are exceptionally high in cholesterol, consumption should be restricted. Eggs as a separate dish (such as deviled eggs, eggs for breakfast, and egg salad) should be served rarely and only when half or more of the yolks are discarded. (These can be called "eggs light.") Egg substitutes are acceptable. Egg whites—almost pure protein—can be used in most recipes in the ratio of two whites for each egg.

Breads and Cereals

Before 20,000 years ago, people seldom ate cereal grains, but their excellent nutritional properties make them, like low-fat dairy products, compelling foods for today. Care has to be exercised in their selection; many commercial breads and cereals, made from highly refined flour, have lost most of their original fiber and some of their nutrient value. Minimally processed whole-grain breads and cereals should therefore replace refined varieties. Oats (especially oat bran) and whole-grain cornmeal are good sources of soluble fiber; wheat bran is the best source of insoluble fiber, but dark rye flour, pearled barley, and whole wheat also furnish significant amounts.

Fats and Oils

The less fat the better, of course, and what there is should be predominantly polyunsaturated and monounsaturated. Avoid butter, cream, lard, chocolate, coconut, and palm oil. Soft margarines made from vegetable oils—safflower, sunflower, soybean, or corn oil—with minimal hydrogenization and high proportions of polyunsaturated fat should replace butter. Better still, skip spreads altogether. For cooking, liquid vegetable oils as well as olive oil should be used, but avoid highly saturated coconut and palm oils. Safflower-oil or soy-oil mayonnaise, available in many areas, is lower in saturated fat and cholesterol than most regular mayonnaises. Vegetable oil sprayed sparingly on cooking pans is better than butter or margarine; half a teaspoon of vegetable oil spread with a paper towel is as effective, cheaper, and avoids additives.

Prepared Foods

A shopper born before the Industrial Revolution and magically transported to a large modern supermarket might find the meats, fish, poultry, vegetables, fruits, grains, and flour familiar but be dumbfounded by row upon row of prepared foods. Dehydrated, canned, or frozen varieties, mixes for sauces, puddings, cakes, cookies, muffins, and biscuits, ready-made breads, cereals, pastries—all promising tasty, picture-perfect fare with little or no preparation, time savers to fit our fast-paced lives. Yet hidden beneath these mouth-watering, package-wrapper pictures are high levels of saturated fat, cholesterol, sodium, and sugar and calories—along with reduced levels of calcium, potassium, and dietary fiber.

Nevertheless, few of us are ready to bypass all prepared products, nor is it imperative that we do. A number of prepared foods are reasonably healthful; others might even be considered Paleolithic. To figure out which is which we have to become astute label readers. Most packaged foods contain a list of ingredients, ordered according to quantity or weight. If whole wheat flour appears first, for example, the product contains whole wheat flour in greater quantity than any other ingredient. If sugar comes next, sugar content will be high. But if salt comes last, that doesn't necessarily reflect an acceptable level since even unhealthy levels of salt weigh relatively little.

The same is true for other additives such as emulsifiers, flavor enhancers, antioxidants, preservatives, and artificial colorings and flavorings, which are also listed toward the end. It is difficult—and, in many cases, impossible—to distinguish those that are potentially harmful from those that are neutral or even beneficial. Until the effects of these additives are better understood, products with long lists of unpronounceable ingredients should probably be avoided when possible. But freshness is especially essential in food products without preservatives!

Eating molds on grains or breads, for example, can be far more hazardous than ingesting small quantities of chemicals added to prevent their growth. Aflatoxin, formed by certain molds which grow on grains and nuts, is one of the most potent cancer-causing agents known.

Whole wheat (or other whole-grain flour) should replace refined flours. (Be alert: "Wheat flour" is not the same as "whole wheat flour." Check ingredients to see which comes first.) Cut back on all sugars, whether white or brown, syrups, and, yes, even honey, since they are essentially equivalent in their overall nutritional poverty. (Molasses has some mineral content, but not enough to matter.) Most vegetable shortenings are better than animal fats (such as butter or lard) but not always. Palm, palm kernel, and coconut oils, although cholesterol free, are more highly saturated than butterfat. As we have seen, hydrogenation—a manufacturing process that solidifies oils—unfavorably alters the P:S ratio by turning polyunsaturated fats into saturated ones, and should be avoided. Partially hydrogenated shortenings, however, are less harmful than fully hydrogenated ones.

Some products include a chart showing the nutritional information per serving on their labels. This usually gives the weight, in grams, of protein, carbohydrate, and fat in a standard serving. Products with little fat in relation to protein and carbohydrate are optimal, providing the closest "fit" to the Paleolithic pattern. Don't be fooled, however, by seemingly small differences: Canned tuna packed in water, for example, derives 94 percent of its calories from protein while tuna packed in oil derives 66 percent of its calories from fat (and only 34 percent from protein).

A breakdown of polyunsaturated and saturated fats is another optional listing. (This is especially helpful in choosing margarines, since their relative proportions of polyunsaturated and saturated fat vary considerably.) Other label newcomers are cholesterol and/or sodium. Even special carbohydrate information is sometimes provided, which may compare complex carbohydrates (such as starch) and simple sugars (such as sucrose, maltose, and fructose). Label reading can detect dramatic differences; Shredded Wheat, for example, is less than 1 percent sugar, whereas certain alternatives (such as Sugar Smacks and Apple Jacks) are over 50 percent.

One has to approach label reading with caution, however, since the language used is often misleading. Consider terms like "sugar-free" (which means, there is no sucrose even though other forms of sugar, such as "corn sweetener," may be present) and "light" (which can refer to color, taste, sodium content, texture, or to reduced calories). "Natural" actually has no legal meaning and can be used despite the presence of preservatives, artificial flavorings, and other additives. Some foods may have no ingredient labeling at all; they may be full of fat, salt, and sugar but if they are made according to a recipe considered "standard" by the FDA, they are not required to list their contents.

Beverages

Water was the beverage of preagriculturalists, but today few of us drink it plain. An ideal thirst quencher, it has few, if any, rivals. It has no calories; it is essentially free; it is available worldwide; and, it doesn't "speed up" or "slow down" our metabolism or nervous systems. No other beverage is so unabashedly and unequivocally "Paleolithic." Others can, however, be incorporated into a Paleolithic nutrition scheme.

Skim milk, for example, is an excellent choice, with fourteen times more protein than fat. Low-fat milk up to 1.5 percent fat also contains more protein than fat. At the 2 percent level, however, the balance begins to change: Fat (largely saturated) now contributes more calories than protein. Whole milk is the least acceptable, with twenty times the fat and seven times the cholesterol of skim milk. Since all milk is rich in calcium, low-fat or non-fat varieties are preferable (except for people with lactase deficiency). Milk-based drinks like cocoa, malted milk, and hot chocolate should be avoided since they are usually made with whole milk to which flavorings rich in fat, sugar, and calories have been added.

What about tea and coffee? Are they hazardous to our health? Various studies have implicated coffee as a cause of pancreatic cancer, as a cause of birth defects, as increasing the risk of fatal cardiac arrhythmias during heart attacks, as a contributing factor in gastric and duodenal ulcers, and as an elevator of serum cholesterol levels. Other studies have disputed these findings. Tea has also been questioned, although to a lesser extent than has coffee. For now, at least, moderate use of either beverage does not appear to be harmful to health. However, since most of our ancestors functioned in a largely caffeine-free environment, caffeinated drinks should probably be held to a minimum.

Many herbal teas are also acceptable, but some contain herbs that can be quite dangerous to health. For example, lobelia can depress breathing, wormwood can cause convulsions, and sassafras or comfrey may be carcinogenic. Herbal tea remedies containing coltsfoot, mistletoe, and pennyroyal are also potentially dangerous. Other herbal teas (such as those made with senna) may be safe in small quantities, but not in large. Given the difficulty of identifying levels in various sources and people's individual reactions, it is hard to specify safe levels. As a rule, choose fully labeled teas packed by well-known companies and avoid those sold by weight in health food stores.

Unsweetened fruit juices such as grapefruit and, especially, orange juice, contain fair amounts of potassium, very little sodium, and are good sources of vitamins A and C. Unsalted tomato juice is also an excellent beverage. However, what Americans are primarily drinking are not natural juices and water, but soft drinks. Laden with sugary calories and devastating to our teeth and to our waistlines, these thirst-quenching wonders are being substituted for nutritionally valuable fare. Diet varieties have other problems. Noncaloric, they often contain excessive phosphorus (which at high levels can interfere with absorption of calcium from the intestinal tract) along with a wide array of chemical additives including saccharin, which has been shown to induce cancer in laboratory animals. Obesity, however, is such a serious risk to health that for those most vulnerable, moderate consumption of low-phosphorus, diet soft drinks can be considered an acceptable alternative to calorie-rich juices, although water is preferable (and more Paleolithic!).

We do not know whether or not alcoholic beverages were available to preagricultural people. Honey and fruits with high sugar content undergo natural fermentation, so it is possible that there was seasonal access to intoxicating drinks. None of our ancestors, however, could have obtained year round the 7 to 10 percent of total calories from alcohol that Americans on the average do.

There is also some question as to whether moderate drinking (1 to 2 standard-size cocktails, or cans of beer, or glasses of wine a day) is beneficial to health. Some studies have shown a correlation with increased life expectancy, the supposed result of alcohol's tendency to elevate levels of "good" HDL-cholesterol. However, more recent analyses have shown that the HDL-cholesterol affected by alcohol is only a subfraction of HDL, one that has a neutral, not positive, effect. The apparent benefit may be coming from other factors. People who drink in moderation are likely to be psychologically healthy—being neither overly rigid (like some teetotalers) nor self-destructive (like many heavy drinkers). Overall, they constitute a group more likely to practice good health habits.

Present average levels of alcohol consumption are incompatible with a Paleolithic perspective. Even moderate drinking has been shown to increase the risk of breast cancer and, of course, can result in unnecessary fatalities—from fires, drownings, and especially auto accidents. Occasional, moderate (subintoxicating) consumption is a practice many of us may judge worth continuing, but beyond this level the risks far outweigh the benefits.

Supplements

The estimated micronutrient intake of our preagricultural ancestors was greater than most of us obtain today. But they did not consume megadoses—levels recommended by many of today's vitamin and mineral enthusiasts—except on rare occasions when a particular type of food, such as baobab fruit or carnivore liver, was in extraordinary yet temporary abundance. Following our ancestral dietary pattern should eliminate the need for additional vitamins and minerals; however, modest supplementation is unlikely to be harmful, and, given our often imperfect nutritional diligence, may insure against lapses. Amounts should approximate the Recommended Dietary Allowance (RDA) for ascorbic acid, the B-complex vitamins, B-carotene (in preference to vitamin A), and vitamin E; diets high in calcium require no extra vitamin D.

Calcium is probably the mineral most in need of supplementation. Since relatively few of us reach the average Paleolithic daily intake of over 1,500 mg, a supplement of 400 mg may be considered (except for people with a history of kidney stones). Other minerals can be added but, again, not much above the RDA amounts; iron (especially for women), magnesium, iodine, chromium, selenium, zinc, and copper are especially important. (Zinc and copper should be in the proper ratio since supplemental zinc, without copper, may adversely affect HDL-cholesterol levels.) Except for the water-soluble vitamins, the body has stores of most vitamins and trace minerals that are adequate for a period of weeks or months. Thus there is no need to panic about dropping below the RDA on a day-to-day basis. Fluctuations in the diet of our ancestors made it necessary for them to evolve chemical cushions against temporary deprivation. Most American diets provide enough micronutrients to forestall classic deficiency diseases, but the amounts necessary for optimal health are as yet undetermined. The relative abundance our ancestors obtained may ultimately prove more appropriate for humans than are today's recommended allowances.

While taking extra vitamins and minerals may merely provide nutritional insurance for most of us, our need for supplemental fiber is probably greater, since most Americans get far too little. Eating a wide variety of fruits, vegetables, and whole-grain products can help ensure that we adequately meet our needs, but modest supplementation—one or two tablespoons each of wheat bran and oat bran added daily to one's food—is inexpensive and probably helpful. Fiber pills, however, are expensive, unnecessary, and inefficient—a health-food hype that contributes only trivial amounts of complex carbohydrates better supplied by food and by added bran.

Whether or not supplements of long-chain, omega-3 polyunsaturated fatty acids (like eicosapentaenoic acid, or EPA) should be taken is controversial. Some studies suggest that supplementation may help prevent atherosclerosis; others point out that EPA may have an undesirable anticoagulant effect. Eskimos, who obtain large quantities of these fatty acids from fish, have little coronary artery disease, but they frequently die of strokes (which probably result from brain hemorrhage rather than from atherosclerotic blockage). Our remote ancestors almost certainly had more of these fatty acids than we do, but not as much as the Eskimos. Minimal supplementation may be in keeping with their experience, but it is too early to make firm recommendations. In the meanwhile it seems simpler to eat more fish.

COOKING TECHNIQUES

Recent evidence suggests that the earliest user of fire was probably *Homo erectus* living 1.4 million years ago. Roasting, baking, and steaming (water is poured over hot stones as at a Polynesian luau) are techniques used by recent hunters and gatherers and are probably ancient. While all cooking procedures affect the nutrient content of food, these traditional techniques are relatively healthful. Baking and roasting reduce the fat content of meat while steaming (in contrast to boiling) minimizes vitamin loss. Furthermore, none of these methods add fat. Recently studied hunters and gatherers do not fry their food, chiefly because they lack appropriate cooking vessels.

Baking, roasting, and steaming are the cooking techniques of choice. Deep-fat frying is out, as is grilling or barbecuing at high temperatures—these methods can create carcinogens. Nonstick pans should be used to cut down on fat or oil. Or, oil can be spread lightly with a paper towel. Vegetable oil sprays now available achieve the same result mechanically, but contain preservatives.

With poultry, remove skin and visible fat. Defat gravies with a bulb syringe or skimmer. In preparing very lean meat (such as wild game) reduce cooking time by 20 percent—lean meat cooks faster and can quickly become tough. A meat thermometer will help.

MEAL PLANS

How can we employ twentieth-century materials to meet Paleolithic nutritional goals? We have available an abundance of food choices; by picking and choosing carefully, a great variety of meals is possible. Some of our favorite combinations are the following.

Breakfast

Emphasize juices, fresh fruit, whole-grain cereals without added sugar, and whole-grain toast or muffins. Use skim milk for hot beverages, caffeinated or not. Fruit and chopped nuts (especially walnuts) add variety to cereal and make sugar unnecessary.

Breakfast is a good meal for adding extra wheat and oat bran to boost fiber content. Low-sugar jams or fruit conserves are preferable to margarine (and certainly butter) on toast or muffins; muffins made with dates or berries require no spread. If margarine is used, it should be made with vegetable oils and have a high proportion of polyunsaturated fat. Fish lightly sautéed in vegetable oil provides protein and is a good substitute for sausage, bacon, or ham. Eggs with half or more of the yolks discarded can be scrambled, prepared as an omelet with vegetables, or used to make whole wheat or buckwheat pancakes or waffles. Use unsweetened applesauce or fruit conserves in place of butter and syrup.

Recommended Choices	Comments
JUICE AND FRUIT: Orange and grapefruit juice; other fruit (fresh)	Use fresh or frozen, not canned. Good sources of vitamin C and potassium. Fresh fruit provides more fiber and has a better calcium:phosphorus ratio.
Tomato juice	Use only the low-sodium variety. One of the few instances in which a canned vegetable product is acceptable, but making juice from fresh tomatoes (in season) in a blender is preferable.
TOAST OR MUFFINS: Made from whole wheat, oatmeal, bran, etc. CEREALS: Hot or cold oat-based (e.g., oatmeal, Familia, etc.) or whole wheat (e.g., Wheatena, Maltex, Shredded Wheat, etc.)	Oat-based breads, cereals, etc., provide appreciable soluble fiber; those based on whole wheat are good sources of insoluble fiber. All are low in fat and have favorable P:S ratios, as well as more protein than fat. Choose products (or recipes) with no added sugar or salt.
PANCAKES AND WAFFLES: Buckwheat or whole wheat	Use recipes that call for little fat (especially saturated fat) and require few egg yolks.
FROZEN FISH FILLETS: Without batter-coating	Extra protein; pan-fry using vegetable oil spray or light coating of vegetable oil.
UNSWEETENED APPLESAUCE	A topping for pancakes and waffles.
JAMS OR FRUIT CONSERVES: Low-sugar varieties only; blackberry, raspberry, strawberry, apricot, etc.	Use in place of margarine for toast or muffins. Source of fiber, including some soluble fiber.
ENGLISH WALNUTS	Ten times more polyunsaturated than saturated fat; use as condiment for cereals.
DRIED FRUIT: Raisins, unsugared dates, prunes, figs	Good sources of iron and fiber; high protein-to-fat ratio; available year-round; but high in calories: use as a condiment. If allergic avoid varieties with sulfite preservatives.
SKIM MILK	Excellent calcium source; excellent protein:fat ratio.

Lunch

When possible bring lunch from home. Sandwiches should be made with whole-grain bread or whole-grain pita (no added fat). Tuna (water-packed, low-salt—or you can rinse the salt off yourself), chicken (preferably white meat), or turkey (white meat) are good choices. A container of salad or low-fat cottage cheese or yogurt with fruit can complement the sandwich or become the main course, depending on its size. Sliced raw vegetables add extra fiber and vitamins. For dessert, fresh fruit is nutritious and convenient. Water, skim milk, and juice are ideal beverages; unsweetened iced tea or coffee (with or without caffeine) are also acceptable.

Recommended Choices	Comments
SANDWICHES: Tuna, salmon, chicken, or turkey on whole wheat, oatmeal, or pita bread.	Provides considerable protein and some fiber. Garnish with lettuce and tomato. Use vegetable oil margarine or low-fat mayonnaise if absolutely necessary.
RAW VEGETABLES: Carrots, celery, tomatoes, cucumber, broccoli, cauliflower, turnips, etc.	Good sources of soluble fiber, low in fat; cruciferous vegetables and carrots have possible anti-cancer effects.
SALADS: Chicken, crab, tuna, salmon, calamari, low-fat cottage cheese, etc.	Moderate amounts of protein and more protein than fat. Use low-fat mayonnaise if necessary. Use raw vegetable garnishes.
DESSERTS: Fruit—apple (with skin), pear, unsugared dates, grapes, figs, plums, orange, banana, etc.	Fairly good sources of fiber, especially dates and figs, much of it soluble. All provide far more potassium than sodium. Oranges are an excellent vitamin C source.
Yogurt—use low-fat, low-sugar varieties	Excellent source of protein and calcium; attractive for people who have difficulty digesting milk sugar (i.e., lactose deficiency).

Dinner

Dinners can begin with salads and whole-grain breads or rolls (without margarine if possible), pasta, or hearty, *noncream* soups such as minestrone and lentil. A chilled fruit soup makes a nice variation. For the main course try to develop twenty or more different low-fat dishes based on poultry, legumes, fish or shellfish, and game or comparably lean meat that appeal to your particular taste and then alternate among them. Serve one or two vegetables, especially yellow or orange ones (sweet potato, some winter and summer squashes, and carrots) and those in the cabbage, or cruciferous, family: cabbage, broccoli, brussels sprouts, turnips, bok choy, among others. Develop a repertoire of low-fat desserts including fruit and low-fat yogurt. Water, herbal teas, or skim milk are acceptable beverages.

Recommended Choices	Comments
SOUPS:	
Vegetable (lentil, split pea, minestrone)	Low in sodium and fat.
Fruit (cold cherry, cold cantaloupe)	
Boullion (defatted, low salt beef or chicken)	
Fish (tomato based, not creamed)	
SALADS:	
Chicken, turkey, seafood	Good protein sources; use low-fat mayonnaise if absolutely necessary.
Cottage cheese with fruit	Extra protein; use low-fat variety.
Pasta	Whole wheat is best.
Beet	
Tabouli	A good source of insoluble fiber.
Fruit	Fat-free; a good source of vitamin C and soluble fiber.
BREAD AND ROLLS:	
Whole grain varieties	Good fiber sources; eat without spread or use vegetable oil margarine if absolutely necessary.

MAIN DISHES:
Fish and shellfish
Poultry (chicken, turkey—without skin)
Wild game or comparably lean domestic meat (if available)

Baked, broiled, roasted, or pan-fried with minimal vegetable oil or cooking spray. No deep-fat frying. Excellent protein sources with minimum fat compared to most red meat. Cook game and lean meat at low temperatures. Reduce fat with gravy skimmer or bulb syringe. Discard all visible fat.

VEGETABLES:
Baked potato

Best with skin; delicious without spread; vegetable oil margarine acceptable, but no salt or sour cream.

Cauliflower, broccoli, brussels sprouts, bok choy, kale, collards, etc.

Cruciferous vegetables with possible anti-cancer effects; steam, don't boil.

Carrots, sweet potato, squash

Excellent sources of vitamin A and beta-carotene; possible cancer-preventing effects; steam.

English peas, lima, kidney, and pinto beans

Excellent sources of soluble fiber; good protein-to-fat ratio.

DESSERTS:
Fruit
Low-fat yogurt
Fruit smoothies
Ice milk
Ice-fruit bars

Low in fat and salt.

Snacks

From the Agta of the Philippines to the Aché of Paraguay, recent hunters and gatherers do not restrict themselves to three meals a day; like us (and presumably like our remote ancestors as well) they have their meals but they also snack—the bane of weight control for most of us. We can turn our propensity for snacking into a strength instead of a weakness, however, by snacking on good food: all fruits; most raw vegetables; low-fat yogurt and cottage cheese; fruit juices and applesauce; low-fat crackers, especially fiber crackers; low-fat cookies; and skim milk.

Snacking has been part of the human and higher primate experience for millions of years; as long as snacks fall within Paleolithic nutritional guidelines (and you don't have to worry about the extra calories), there is no reason to eliminate them. They can even supplement nutrients that might otherwise be deficient in the day's regular meals.

| Possible Choices | Nutritional Parameters | | | | |
| | Grams | | % Total Calories | | |
	Protein	Fat	Protein	Fat	Carbohydrate
Low-fat cottage cheese (½ cup)	12.0	1.0	62	12	22
Low-fat vanilla yogurt (1 cup)	11.0	4.0	21	17	62
Raw carrot (1 whole)	0.8	0.1	10	3	87
Raw cherries (10 whole)	0.9	0.2	7	3	90
Plum (1 whole)	0.3	0.1	4	2	94
Banana (1 large)	1.5	0.3	5	3	92
Skim milk (8 oz.)	8.4	0.4	40	5	56
Rice cakes (1 whole)	1.0	0.0	11	0	89
Oatmeal raisin cookies (2)	3.3	2.3	10	16	74
Whole grain crisp breads (1 slice)	1.0	1.0	14	31	55
Some Snacks to Avoid					
Premium vanilla ice cream (½ cup)	1.7	10.8	4	64	32
Brownie with nuts	3.3	15.7	5	55	40
Candy bar*	4.7	11.6	8	43	49
Potato chips (2 oz.)	4.5	22.5	5	59	36
Plain doughnut (1)	2.7	11.3	6	58	36
Cheese crackers (3)	2.8	5.3	9	40	51

*Chocolate-coated fudge, peanuts, caramel

A SAMPLE DAY'S NUTRITION

How do these guidelines work during a hypothetical day? Can we successfully recreate a Paleolithic nutritional pattern using foods available in twentieth-century supermarkets? Table XVII provides an analysis of the nutrients in a variety of Paleolithic meals and snacks that might be consumed by an imaginary American over the course of one day.

Measured against Paleolithic nutritional priorities, this day's food has an acceptably low level of fat (19 percent of the day's total calories) and an appropriate polyunsaturated to saturated fat ratio (P:S = 1.35). It provides more than enough calcium and iron, even for pregnant or nursing women. It has too much sodium (2,765 mg *vs.* a goal of 1,000 mg or less), however, reflecting the pervasive presence of salt in our foods; none was added at the table.

These meals and snacks provide somewhat more protein (26 percent of the day's total energy intake) and correspondingly less carbohydrate (55 percent of total energy) than recommended by the guidelines, although these levels are well within the Paleolithic range. Dietary fiber (64 g) is also within the target range, although more is insoluble than would have been in our ancestors' diets. (A tablespoon or more of oat bran added to cereal or used in cooking in place of breadcrumbs—as a topping or filling, for example—can supplement soluble fiber intake.)

Energy density is relatively low, except for the oatmeal cookies and blackberry jam. Cholesterol content is also low—less than might be expected for a diet providing so much protein. Total caloric intake is well within acceptable limits for a physically active male; a physically active female could have the same foods, but would have to limit her portions by about 20 percent.

SODIUM AND HYPERTENSION

While this hypothetical day's meals and snacks contain less sodium (2,765 mg) than would be consumed in one day by a typical American (about 4,500 mg), it is about three and a half times more than what our remote ancestors obtained from their food (about 700 mg/day). It is also more than what recent hunters and gatherers and other traditional people obtain from theirs. Although the high levels of calcium and potassium ($K = 2.5$ Na) should reduce the risk of hypertension, the level of sodium is still far outside the Paleolithic range. It could be reduced by eliminating most commercial breads (which add over 500 mg) and by omitting dairy foods (another 1,500 mg!). Since Stone Age people had no milk and made little use of grains, such measures are eminently Paleolithic.

For most of us, however, the value of dairy products and whole-grain foods outweighs their drawbacks. People with blood pressure at or below 130/80 and who do not have a strong family history of high blood pressure, can safely eat according to the guidelines in this chapter. For those with gradually rising blood pressure, with some degree of hypertension (at or above 135/85), or with a strong family history of high blood pressure, a more rigorous sodium-reducing dietary program (and perhaps additional therapy) may be needed, as determined by a phy-

TABLE XVII.

One Day's "Paleolithic" Food Consumption

Item	Protein	Fat	Carbohydrate	Fiber	Calories	P:S	Calcium	Sodium	Potassium	Cholesterol	Vit. C
	Grams						Milligrams				
Breakfast, 6:45 A.M.:											
Oat bran cereal (3.5 oz.)	21.0	7.0	56.0	4.2	385	3.5:1.7	60	0.0	490	0	0
Wheat bran (1 tbsp.)	1.5	0.4	6.0	4.0	20	0.2:0.1	20	0.0	106	0	0
Skim milk (1 cup)	8.4	0.4	11.9	—*	86	0:0.2	240	126.0	360	8	2.5
Raspberries (½ cup)	0.8	0.3	8.4	5.0	35	0.6:0	15	1.0	112	0	15.0
Whole wheat toast (2 slices)	5.2	1.6	23.8	4.2	122	0.4:0.2	50	264.0	135	0	Trace
Blackberry jam (1 tbsp.)	0.1	—	14.0	1.1	50	—	4	2.5	18	0	0.5
Orange juice (1 cup)	1.7	0.2	28.5	0.7	122	0:0.2	33	2.0	600	0	145.0
Total	38.7	9.9	148.6	19.2	820	4.9:2.2	422	395.5	1821	8	163.0
Snack, 10:30 A.M.:											
Pear (1 unpeeled)	1.1	0.7	25.1	5.0	100	0.7:0	12	3	195	0	6
Water (1 cup)											
Lunch, 12:30 P.M.:											
Whole wheat bread (2 slices)	5.2	1.6	23.8	4.2	122	0.4:0.2	50	264	135	0	Trace
Turkey, light meat no skin (100 g)	32.9	3.9	—	—	176	0.9:0.9	1	82	411	92	0
Lettuce (½ cup)	0.3	0.1	0.8	0.5	4	0.1:0.1	12	3	89	0	28
Tomato (2 slices)	1.4	0.1	2.9	0.7	13	0.1:0	6	2	120	0	11
Low-fat vanilla yogurt (1 cup)	16.0	4.8	22.0	—	200	0.2:2.8	480	203	429	20	4
Apple (1 unpeeled)	0.3	0.8	20.0	2.8	80	0.8:0	10	1	110	0	6
Water (2 cups)											
Total	56.1	11.3	69.5	8.2	595	2.5:4.0	559	555	1294	112	49

Item	Grams				Calories	P:S	Milligrams				
	Protein	Fat	Carbohydrate	Fiber			Calcium	Sodium	Potassium	Cholesterol	Vit. C
Snack, 5:30 P.M.:											
Low-fat cottage cheese (1 cup)	31.2	4.4	8.4	—	204	0:2.8	225	920	422	20	0
Raisins (2 tbsp.)	0.4	—	14.0	1.5	52	—	11	4	128	—	Trace
English walnuts (2 tbsp.)	2.2	9.6	2.4	2.4	98	6.2:1.0	12	Trace	75	0	0
Water (1 cup)											
Total	33.8	14.0	24.8	3.9	354	6.2:3.8	248	924	625	20	0
Dinner, 7:30 P.M.:											
Beet salad	2.9	0.4	15.9	8.4	71	0.1:0.2	15	100	652	0	8.0
Whole wheat roll (1)	2.6	0.8	11.9	2.1	61	0.2:0.1	25	132	67.5	0	Trace
Corn oil marg..rine (1 tbsp.)	0	11.0	0	—	100	5.0:2.0	2	95	2	0	0
Chicken breast fricassée	31.7	3.9	26.8	5.2	262	1.0:2.0	70	216	856	72	7.0
Brussels sprouts, no margarine or salt	4.2	0.4	6.4	8.8	36	0.1:0.1	32	10	273	0	87.0
Skim milk (8 oz.)	8.4	0.4	11.9	—	86	0:0.2	240	126	360	8	2.5
Plums (3; 100 g)	0.5	Trace	17.8	2.1	66	—	18	2	229	0	2.0
Total	50.3	16.9	90.7	26.6	682	6.4:4.6	402	681	2439.5	80	106.5
Snack, 11:00 P.M.:											
Oatmeal raisin cookies (4)	3.2	7.7	36.8	1.0	204	2.0:2.0	11	81	185	0	Trace
Skim milk (8 oz.)	8.4	0.4	11.9	—	86	0:0.2	240	126	360	8	2.5
Total	11.6	8.1	48.7	1.0	290	2.0:2.2	251	207	515	8	2.5
Grand total	191.6	60.9	407.4	63.9	2841	22.7:16.8	1894	2765.5	6889.5	228	327

Percent of Total Calories: Protein 26%; Fat 19%; Carbohydrate 55%. P:S = 1.35.

*—means negligible

Source: Leveille, G. A., Zabik, M. E., Morgan, K. J. Nutrients in foods. Cambridge, Mass.: The Nutrition Guild. 1983.

Anderson, J. W. Plant fiber in foods. Lexington, Ky.: HCF Diabetes Research Foundation, Inc. 1986.

Human Information Service. Composition of foods. Agriculture Handbooks Nos. 8-1 through 8-14. Washington, D.C.: U.S. Dept. of Agriculture. 1976-1986.

Watt, B. K., Merrill, A. L. Composition of foods. Agriculture Handbook No. 8. Washington, D.C.: U.S. Dept. of Agriculture. 1963.

sician. Once blood pressure reverts to normal levels, the protocols presented here will again be appropriate.

EATING OUT

Eating out is usually fun, and the average American does so about 190 times a year, according to one estimate. But eating out while maintaining a Paleolithic diet presents a challenge. As an invited guest in other people's homes, or in restaurants or cafeterias, you have to be an astute forager, discriminating carefully within the field of offerings. When meals (other than brown-bag lunches) are eaten away from home rarely, you can be somewhat less stringent; even hunters and gatherers had occasional times of excess—when a large cache of honey was found or when an especially fat animal was brought back. But when eating out is routine, diligence has to be the rule.

Meals at other people's homes often start with appetizers, from the mundane—chips, cheese dips, cheese boards with crackers, or salted nuts—to the elaborate—assorted canapés, bacon-wrapped asparagus tips, miniature pies and quiches, or slightly warm Brie cheese in flaky pastry dough. Consider the following situation.

ACT I, SCENE I

  Setting: A small, intimate gathering.
  Action: Your host (or hostess) approaches graciously, with a smile, urging you to try a tasty (albeit a highly fatty and salty) delight described, perhaps, as a prized recipe.
  Response: You take one of whatever is offered and comment positively on it. (Do not refuse or lecture on its nutritional evils. Health can be maintained without becoming a social outcast.)
  Outcome: Audience applause.

In a setting where you have more control over what you eat, your hardest job will be to control what you choose. A small sample of the most tempting dishes should be balanced by larger portions of more acceptable fare: fresh vegetables (without the dip), fruit, Scandinavian-style flat crackers, or a moderate helping of shrimp. Remember, at dinner it will probably be even more difficult to avoid nutritionally undesirable foods, especially if you've had a drink, so don't use up your "margin" on the before-dinner snacks.

As for alcohol, many carbonated drinks with a twist of lemon or lime look enough like the real thing that no one but the host or hostess may know for sure—and, anyway, in these days of health consciousness you might be surprised at how many other guests are drinking the same. Alternatively, wine and beer, especially reduced-calorie beer, contain less alcohol than most hard-liquor drinks. Spritzers made of wine and carbonated water are even better. Alternating alcoholic drinks with sparkling water (seltzer and some natural mineral waters do not have added salt, whereas club soda does) or flavored carbonated drinks, diet or regular, is also effective.

When dinner is served, take some of everything, if necessary, but take larger portions of more nutritionally sound foods. Politely refuse second helpings of unhealthful dishes—without lecturing on why—and double up on the healthful ones. (Joggers who endlessly discuss mileage, routes, and shoes at social gatherings quickly bore all but other dedicated joggers; talk of nutrition while eating someone else's food is at least as deplorable if not more so.)

Only restaurants that offer healthful choices should be patronized. Whether in fast-food places or the most fancy restaurants, nutritionally sound fare can usually be found. Fast-food menus may include low-fat and low-salt items: salad bars with fresh fruits and vegetables, sliced turkey or chicken sandwiches on whole wheat buns, baked potato without butter or sour cream, and unbuttered corn. Even fried chicken, *with skin and batter removed,* can be relatively low in fat.

Of course expensive doesn't necessarily mean healthful either. Foods served in elite restaurants contain about the same proportions of fat, salt, and sugar as do typical fast-food choices. Many restaurants are beginning to cater to the changing palates (and rising consciousness) of their clientele, making available a number of Paleolithic meals alongside the higher-fat and higher-salt ones. The challenge, then, in the four-star restaurant as in the burger chain, is to learn how to choose: to order tasty dishes that adhere reasonably closely to Paleolithic nutritional guidelines.

Unsalted fish, melon, and fruit cocktail are acceptable appetizers. Salads with an oil and vinegar or reduced-calorie dressing are better than the same salads with cheese- or cream-based dressing. (Ask for dressing on the side so that you can control the amount used.) Clear, tomato, or bean-based soups can be ordered instead of creamy ones. Poultry and fish are good entrées; veal is somewhat fatty but preferable to other red meats. Most restaurants will broil or bake an entrée on request instead of frying it and will prepare foods with margarine or vegetable oil rather than with butter. The skin of poultry can be removed after it is served, and sometimes the chef will remove it before cooking if requested to do so. Heavy gravies and sauces should be replaced by tomato- or wine-based ones. Ask for margarine rather than butter for vegetables; better still, eat the vegetables *au naturel*. (Many restaurants also stock low-fat or skim milk and salt substitutes; if they don't, ask them to.) Fruit, yogurt, or sherbet can replace high-fat sweets. Most restaurants offer decaffeinated coffee and sometimes decaffeinated or herbal teas. Hot water and lemon is a refreshing alternative—and a request that no longer surprises waiters and waitresses. If the conversation is making you doze, regular coffee is also acceptable, but pass up coffee drinks loaded with hot whole milk, whipped cream, and sugar.

DIETING, WEIGHT LOSS, AND BODY COMPOSITION

Cave and rock wall paintings found in Europe, Africa, and Australia depict slender people. Recent hunters and gatherers are also lean and well muscled. The Aborigines of Australia, the Cuiva of Venezuela, the Aché of Paraguay, and the Hadza of Tanzania—all with adequate food sources—do not have to "diet" to maintain appropriate body composition. (In fact, members of such societies show no obesity until they adopt Western ways.) Yet the way they maintain appropriate body weight and composition is a lesson for us in our generally overweight society.

In many respects Late Paleolithic life was an extremely advantageous adaptation; it was in this context that humankind flourished, ultimately populating the globe. As an economic base it has seemed secure enough so that some have described this life-style as "the original affluent society." Although this captures a degree of truth as far as social and economic equality goes, it falls short in describing what it is like to be completely dependent on the vagaries of the natural world. Periodic food shortages, for example, have been observed among all recent hunters and gatherers. Depending on local geographic and ecological conditions, these may occur every ten to fifteen years or more frequently, as often as several times a year. Shortages also vary in intensity; only rarely are they famines severe enough to cause death. More often they are mild, limiting the amount of food available and causing modest losses of weight. In fact, archaeologists have shown, for several temperate climates, that signs of nutritional stress in bony remains were less for hunters and gatherers than they were for the agriculturalists that succeeded them.

Paradoxically, the existence of periodic food shortages throughout evolution is a key to understanding our human propensity to gain weight. Since such shortages were ubiquitous, people who efficiently stored extra calories as fat during times of plenty better withstood times of scarcity, passing this characteristic on to their offspring who passed it forward through the generations, ultimately to us. But in the present the benefit has become a liability; because continuous food surplus without famine was so rare for hunters and gatherers and even for most agriculturalists, we have not had time to develop adaptive responses to cope with it.

Our bodies today simply haven't "learned" that there is no longer an advantage to carrying extra weight. We are still essentially Late Paleolithic hunters and gatherers, and our appetite-control centers continue to operate as if the food surplus may come to a crashing halt at any time. We persist in storing up against that eventuality and, because the shortages fail to materialize, we become obese. Fat people in Western society are stocking up for a famine that never comes.

It is unlikely that there was much human "fatness" until the Late Paleolithic, about 20,000 years ago. Then a variety of factors—population growth, intergroup competition, territorial demarcation, and resource pressure—spurred the development of social complexity. Mobile egalitarian bands gradually evolved into sedentary, socially stratified tribes, replete with status hierarchies. Late Paleolithic "Venus" statuettes found in a number of sites in Europe—small figurines which realistically depict obese human females—may reflect class, wealth, and power—people whose needs were attended to by others. With agriculture, status hierarchies became more elaborate and rigid, and the privileged—who benefited from the skills and services of the less privileged—had even greater access to resources. That is, as long as resources existed. Agriculture is also risky, dependent as it is on climate and rainfall—even more so than is foraging, which has at its base a wide variety of indigenous uncultivated plants with proven ability to survive environmental extremes. For agriculturalists, then, fat was still a form of insurance.

But not today, when the vast majority of people living in Western societies have access to unlimited calories throughout their lives. Fat has finally become egalitarian. Anyone can have it. As a result, its relation to social class has reversed. It is now a hallmark of lower status, while the advantaged have money, time, knowledge, and energy to concentrate on being slim. This transfer of obesity to the poor is occurring at the same time as obesity's harmful health effects are becoming well documented.

A PALEOLITHIC APPROACH TO MAINTENANCE OF BODY COMPOSITION

The Paleolithic Prescription offers a way to promote health and prevent disease. It is not a manual for the treatment of illness and it offers no magical insight as to how overweight people can effortlessly and quickly become slim. The experience of the human past, however, does suggest a direction, offering guiding principles that can help us do battle against a pervasive twentieth-century ill.

Consistency

Our ancestors maintained their trim yet muscular physiques through a lifelong pattern of Paleolithic eating and exercise. They did not do or eat the same things every day. But, averaged over the course of a few months, their activities and diet would seem remarkably consistent from year to year; and so, consequently, would their bodily composition. In Western nations body weight typically increases between the ages of twenty and sixty; at the same time the proportions of fat and lean tissue gradually change—the former increasing, the latter decreasing.

Throughout most of human history average people did not steadily gain weight with age. Studies of recent traditional societies show people maintaining fairly constant body weights from ages twenty to forty, after which weight very gradually declined. The body weight of recent hunters and gatherers does fluctuate, but this is short term, usually annual, with small weight losses resulting from seasons of shortage offset by small weight gains during seasons of abundance. Estimated weight loss for the !Kung San during the dry season, for example, is between 2 and 7 percent of total body weight (between one and eight pounds). These fluctuations, however, balance out over the year and do not translate into steady lifelong patterns of weight gain. Modest short-term weight fluctuation is well within the Paleolithic experience and is probably easily accommodated by our genetic makeup.

Exercise

If you have a runaway appetite, run with it! In other words, exercise enough to accommodate your appetite. Physical exertion was a constant feature of Paleolithic existence; every aspect of life required considerable muscular effort—a far cry from our sedentary lives today. Aside from promoting strength and endurance, physical activity promotes "high-energy through-put"—a state of efficient energy utilization. It also tends to lower the body weight "set point." Not least of all, of course, it burns calories.

Most Western weight-loss-advice marketers emphasize caloric restriction. To buffer us against this rather unpleasant prospect, endless variations on the how-to theme have arisen. Fructose is the panacea! No, others claim, liquid protein is. No, no, no; it is carbohydrates that need to be slashed. No! It's protein. No! It's fat. Grapefruit is the key. Diet pills! Nearly all approaches are designed for the short haul—just long enough for you to recommend the plan and buy the book—and nearly all have dismal records of long-term success.

Enter exercise—an increasingly popular facilitator of weight loss and weight maintenance—to quiet the cacophonous crowd of diet advisers. Experimental studies show that people who increase their level of exercise, especially their aerobic fitness, generally lose weight without dieting. Even a small daily caloric deficit maintained over a fairly long period does it. For example, burning off an additional one hundred calories a day in exercise without changing one's eating pattern can result in a loss of ten pounds within a year. Also, dieters who exercise lose fat while they conserve or actually build muscle. Sedentary dieters, in contrast, lose both fat and muscle.

Periodic Shortages

Obesity is, literally, a condition for which an ounce of prevention is worth a pound of cure. For this reason regular assessment of our body composition is necessary.

Once adult stature is attained, body fat should not exceed 15 percent for males or 25 percent for females, regardless of age. Your initial body composition determination should probably be performed by a health professional; thereafter "do-it-yourself" skinfold thickness or body girth measurements can acceptably monitor your percentage of body fat.* Once you have established a track record and have reached an acceptable level, determinations need be made only occasionally. If you gain weight or at any time think your level has changed, more frequent monitoring should be reinstated.

What should you do when body fat exceeds these guidelines? You should do voluntarily what our ancestors were forced to do: Create a temporary food shortage by reducing caloric intake and increasing phys-

---

*Acceptably accurate, low-priced ($11.95 to $21.95) skinfold calipers with instructions for use can be obtained from Creative Health Products, 5148 Saddle Ridge Road, Plymouth, Michigan 48170; phone: (313) 453-5309 or 455-0177.

ical exertion. Can this food shortage concept be practically applied today? The following examples illustrate how it can.

Example 1

Suppose you are a woman thirty-five years old in fairly good shape, exercising moderately, and eating sensibly. Nevertheless, you are a little heavier than you would like. You are 5'5" tall and weigh 135 pounds. On testing, your proportion of body fat is found to be 30 percent. First, you need to make some simple calculations:

- If you weigh 135 pounds and 30 percent of your weight is fat, then 40.5 pounds (135 times .30) is fat and 94.5 pounds (135 − 40.5) is lean body mass. With a lean body mass of 94.5 pounds, what should your weight be?
- Aiming for an overall body composition of 25 percent fat, multiply your lean body mass by 1.33. (If you are aiming for 20 percent fat, multiply your lean body mass by 1.25.) Your target weight is therefore 125.7 pounds (94.5 × 1.33), or about 125 pounds.
- This means you need to lose 10 pounds of fat from your body weight of 135 pounds. To lose 1 pound, you need to expend 3,500 calories. To lose 10, a calorie deficit of 35,000 (10 × 3,500) will be necessary. Calculating the loss over a three-month period (90 days), about 390 calories per day need to be eliminated (35,000 divided by 90).

To ensure that the weight lost is mostly fat, exercise will have to be increased at the same time that calorie intake is cut back. Remember, this exercise is in addition to, not a substitute for, your regular exercise patterns. Still, it doesn't have to be very much. Twenty minutes of swimming (at 50 meters/minute) or jogging (at 11 minutes/mile) expends about 200 calories. That leaves 200 calories to be made up by decreased food intake. That's only half a piece of cake, or half a slice of pie, or a small dish of ice cream (for those still eating these kinds of foods). For more sensible eaters it might mean a handful fewer nuts, a whole-grain muffin uneaten, or a glass or two of water exchanged for juice.

When the three-month shortage period is over, you should be about ten pounds lighter. How much fat will you have actually lost? It can vary, but it is unlikely that all the weight lost will have been fat. Nevertheless, by losing weight in the context of increased exercise, you will have lowered your proportion of body fat; you'll probably also feel and look better, too. You can now begin eating and exercising as before, according to the general nutritional and exercise practices described here, in order to maintain your weight and body composition at the new levels.

Don't be too disappointed, however, if on retesting, your proportion of body fat hasn't reached 25 percent or less. With prudent eating and exercise, you will make steady progress—each year coming closer to your goal—until you attain it. Whether you achieve this level after one shortage period or several is less important than the trend you establish. You should aim for a consistently decreasing proportion of body fat, in contrast to the pattern of increase experienced by most Americans.

Example 2

Suppose you're a fifty-year-old man who has let himself go. You are 5'9" tall, weigh 200 pounds, and your proportion of body fat is also 30 percent. The difference is, of course, that body fat for males should be no greater than 15 percent of body weight.

At age fifty the first step is to have a general medical checkup by a physician interested in disease prevention, especially preventive cardiology. If you receive medical clearance to follow the diet and exercise program outlined here, your first six months should not include shortages. After your body becomes familiar with the program, your shortage experience will be similar to the example just outlined:

- If you weigh 200 pounds and 30 percent of your weight is fat, then 60 pounds (200 × .3) is fat and 140 pounds (200 − 60) is lean body mass. With a lean body mass of 140 pounds, what should your weight be?
- Aiming for an overall body composition of 15 percent fat, multiply your lean body mass by 1.175. (If you are aiming for 10 percent fat, multiply your lean body mass by 1.11.) Your target weight is therefore 164.5 pounds (140 × 1.175), or about 165 pounds.
- This means you need to lose 35 pounds of fat from your body weight of 200 pounds.

Short of drastic dieting, it is not feasible to plan on losing thirty-five pounds in three months. The general approach in your case—a combination of dieting plus increased exercise—will be similar to the first example, but the overall strategy will require modification. The total deficit required can be estimated at 122,500 calories (3,500 calories/pound × 35 pounds) and a reasonable approach for achieving this deficit might be to anticipate a series of shortages, each of two months' duration. The intervening periods might last two to three months each and would be intervals of Paleolithic exercise and nutrition expected to maintain or slightly improve the body composition achieved by the preceding period of shortage. When a 122,500-calorie deficit is divided, say, into six parts, each will require a 20,500-calorie shortfall during two months (60 days), or about 340 calories per day. This is slightly less daily deficit than was required for the earlier example, so the necessary physical exertion and dietary restriction will be even less demanding.

Unless you maintain the proper attitude, however, long-term adherence to the protocol may be psychologically difficult because the realization of your goal is likely to require a long haul—a year or more. Again, you need to focus on progressive improvement, not on the ultimate end point. You will want to have periodic redeterminations of your body composition, partly to maintain your enthusiasm and partly because the nature of the weight lost during each shortage period cannot be predicted with absolute accuracy; it may consist entirely of fat, it may consist of both fat and lean tissue, or there may be fat loss while lean body mass is actually increased.

Suppose that after your first shortage period you're found to weigh 194 pounds—just 6 pounds less after sixty days of significant effort! You could easily become depressed about such slow progress. Furthermore your new body composition evaluation still shows 26 percent fat—a discouragingly long way from the desirable 15 percent figure. But there's another way of looking at your progress:

- If your new weight is 194 pounds and 26 percent is fat, then your fat content is 50.44 pounds (194 × 0.26) or about 50.5 pounds.
- Since your original fat content was 60 pounds, you've actually lost 9.5 pounds of fat (60 − 50.5).
- Your current lean body mass is 143.5 pounds (194 − 50.5), and since your starting lean body mass was 140 pounds, you've gained 3.5 pounds of lean tissue at the expense of fat.

That first shortage period actually produced a 9.5-pound fat loss while you were adding 3.5 pounds of bone and muscle. Those are pretty encouraging results—the kind that generate determination to do as well or even better in the future. You're on your way!

Summary

The Importance of Body Composition

Body composition is a more meaningful concept than body weight. People who are heavy because of "excess" lean body mass (for example, professional football linemen, shot-putters, and bodybuilders of both sexes) are generally healthy and fit, whereas people who are heavy because of excess fat are generally out of shape and at high risk for disease conditions ranging from diabetes to hypertension. To look better physically, it therefore makes more sense to think about improving body composition than only about "losing weight." Improved body composition helps one feel more attractive at the same time as it creates superior fitness and, therefore, health. Men should aim for 15 percent or less of their body weight as fat, regardless of age; women, between 20 and 25 percent, also regardless of age. (Lowering one's body fat below 5 percent for males or 15 percent for females, however, is not recommended. It has been associated with decreased sex drive for men and cessation of menstrual periods for women.)

Reasons for Monitoring Body Composition

Body composition should be monitored by *periodic evaluations*. For those actively working on changing their level, testing can follow each shortage period, because weight loss can occur in one of several ways:

1. Pure fat loss with no significant change in lean body mass: acceptable, but not ideal.
2. Loss of fat and lean body mass: the typical result of most weight loss plans. Although the loss of weight will be welcomed, it is, statistically, apt to be temporary. It will more likely endure if accompanied by increased exercise, especially resistance-type exercise (such as weight training).
3. Loss of fat while increasing lean body mass: the ideal pattern.

The Long-term Approach

To achieve and maintain appropriate body composition, one's efforts need to be directed at the long term—*a lifelong approach*, not a one-time-only crash program.

Periodic Food Shortages

Throughout human evolution, body composition was affected by *periodic food shortages*. These were generally limited in duration (one to three months), involved both a decrease in caloric intake and an increase in caloric expenditure, and were superimposed upon the normal Paleolithic routine of diet and exercise. Applying this situation to the twentieth century, certain concepts stand out:

1. Combining food restriction with additional exercise is essential. Conventional diets, emphasizing caloric restriction, usually wind up re-

ducing levels of physical exercise—one action thus offsetting the other. Exercise helps maintain and often increases lean body mass while fat is being lost.

2. The division between caloric restriction and added exercise is a flexible one and should be determined according to individual need. For example, an increase in daily energy expended beyond a typical 100–200 calories/day can be emphasized when body fat levels are high and when general fitness is poor; an increase in daily caloric restriction beyond a 100–300 calories/day can be emphasized when daily exercise is nearly adequate but caloric intake is excessive.

3. Shortage periods should emphasize protein, complex carbohydrate, and low-calorie foods with high-nutrient density. Fat should be reduced as much as possible—a pattern typical for shortage periods of recent hunters and gatherers. The calorie deficit can be accomplished by choosing lower-calorie foods, by eating less per meal, by having fewer and lower-calorie snacks, or by eliminating an occasional meal altogether.

Preliminary Medical Evaluation

For people forty years or older, overweight and out-of-shape, a preliminary medical checkup is recommended before embarking on the exercise and diet program outlined in this book. In particular, a heart examination should rule out potentially dangerous arrhythmias—a necessary prerequisite for vigorous aerobic exercise—while routine tests of blood pressure, cholesterol, HDL/LDL, and glucose levels should eliminate the need for specific dietary or drug regimens.

Alternating two-month shortage periods with longer (three- to four-month) phases of basic Paleolithic eating and exercise will reverse the typical age-related American trend toward ever-increasing body fat and ultimately produce an acceptable—and thereafter stable—body composition. This long-term program does not sound glamorous, but it works. And it is much less important to achieve dramatic *temporary* weight losses than to establish dietary and exercise patterns that become a permanent way of life.

NUTRITION IN PERSPECTIVE

During the past decade, "fitness" seems to be everywhere. At every time of the day runners, joggers, cyclists, or walkers can be seen on the roads, trails, and tracks. Swimming pools have had to allot more lanes to lap swimmers. Sales of weight-training equipment are at an all-time high. Aerobic classes and health clubs are booming. Amateur tennis leagues report steadily increasing membership. And racquetball is said to be the fastest-growing sport of all time.

Unfortunately, healthful eating has not been met with comparable enthusiasm. True, health food stores abound and sales of vitamins have skyrocketed, but many of these products are unnecessary or even harmful, and most people still obtain the majority of their nutritional information from quick-weight-loss diet books. Many of us know the number of calories in a banana, but don't know a saturated fatty acid from a simple sugar.

Diets come and go. Some, like those of Drs. Yudkin and Atkins, are based on restricting carbohydrates. Others, like those of Nathan Pritikin and some advocates of vegetarianism, aim at cutting down fat and protein. Still others, like Dr. Kempner's Rice Diet or various liquid-protein-supplemented diets, emphasize specific dietary components to the exclusion of nearly all others. Such conflicting advice has bred more confusion than weight loss. Yet the diet our bodies adapted to during human evolution is very different from any of these fads and fashions.

How to approximate this diet and fit it into the realities of modern life has been the thrust of this chapter. It is not an especially difficult task, although it does mean reorienting ourselves to a new repertoire of food experiences. The basic principles are simple. We should aim at a pattern that provides 60 percent of our calories as carbohydrate, 20 percent as protein, and 20 percent as fat. Carbohydrate should be mainly complex, with little simple sugar and abundant dietary fiber. Protein should come primarily from animal sources which, in our society, means poultry, seafood, and low-fat dairy products; vegetarian protein-balancing is an acceptable alternative. The goal is a low-fat, low-sugar, low-sodium, high-fiber, high-calcium regimen that provides an adequate level of both macro- and micronutrients while avoiding the harmful features of the typical twentieth-century diet.

With few exceptions Paleolithic nutritional principles encompass dietary guidelines proposed by many physicians and scientists. Without giving much thought to the past or trying actively to reassess it, these scientists have found themselves immersed in it, unaware that the past has caught up with them. That nutritional science and anthropology are finally converging should not be surprising. After all, evolution put our physiology into motion in the first place.

CHAPTER SEVEN

THE FIRST FITNESS FORMULA

The current American exercise boom is not without its detractors. There are at present no unequivocal long-term medical investigations proving that regular exercise significantly prolongs life. Worse, exercise can sometimes be harmful. Jim Fixx, the exercise guru who helped popularize running for millions of Americans, suffered a fatal heart attack during a morning jog when he was just fifty-two years old. And his has not been the only exercise fatality. Athletes from Pheidippides, purportedly the original marathoner, to Olympic oarsman John B. Kelly, Grace Kelly's brother, have died as an immediate consequence of their activity. Furthermore, exercise commonly produces minor musculoskeletal injuries. Heel pain, sore knees, stress fractures, and shin splits are all more frequent in runners, and other forms of exercise produce comparable orthopedic ailments.

To be sure, these detractors have *their* detractors, who cite studies published in eminent medical journals proving the clear overall advantages of exercise. Amid the claims and counterclaims, few mention a not-so-current, yet overriding and ineluctable evolutionary consideration: Our genetic constitution has been selected to operate within a milieu of vigorous, daily, and lifelong physical exertion. From the first appearance of vertebrate life on earth almost until the present century, our ancestors have been active and strong—"athletic" before organized games created athletes. The exercise boom is not just a fad; it is a return to "natural" activity—the kind for which our bodies are engineered and which facilitates the proper function of our biochemistry and physiology. Viewed through the perspective of evolutionary time, sedentary existence, possible for great numbers of people only during the past century, represents a transient, unnatural aberration.

EXERCISE IN EVOLUTIONARY PERSPECTIVE

There is little doubt that strenuous physical activity has been part of human and prehuman ancestral life for millions of years. Paleontological and comparative biological evidence, studies of contemporary nonindustrial people, and animal investigations all make this clear. Since bones respond to the forces exerted on them by attached muscles, detailed analysis of human remains can assess an individual's muscular strength during life. Specifically, this analysis entails measuring the cross-sectional diameter, shape, and cortical thickness of long (limb) bones, the area of joint surfaces, and, especially, the prominence of sites where tendons attach muscles to bones.

Ancient human remains examined in this way show that our ancestors, from the earliest australopithecines (3 million years ago) to truly modern people (30,000 years ago), were strong, much stronger in fact than most people alive today. The earliest modern humans were much like current professional athletes, both men and women, whose strength generally greatly exceeds that of the average person.

With the beginnings of agriculture, however, a decrease in human muscular development becomes noticeable. Even though farmers work longer hours than hunters and gatherers, their peak-effort levels—the maximum energy they expend during the most demanding times—are generally less. This observation anticipates conclusions held by current exercise physiologists: Relatively short periods of intense muscular effort, such as carrying heavy loads of meat back to base camps, or in our era weight training, produce far greater strength and muscularity than do much longer periods of submaximal effort required in occupations such as farming.

Not all areas of the world experienced the transition from foraging to farming at the same time. Yet whenever and wherever the changeover occurred—whether 10,000 years ago in the Middle East or merely 1,000 years ago in parts of North America—the remains of the preceding hunters and gatherers indicate greater muscularity than do the remains of the succeeding agriculturalists. Given the consistency of these findings, the generally lacklustre muscularity of today's humans reflects our changed conditions of life rather than genetic evolution. A more recent demonstration of this same phenomenon—basic human plasticity—involves professional football players. Most teams introduced regular resistance exercise (weight training) into their programs ten to fifteen years ago—one reason why National Football League (NFL) players are now measurably stronger than were their predecessors.

Paleolithic hunters and gatherers were nevertheless susceptible to injuries and degenerative changes much as we are today. Indeed, the prevalence of degenerative ("wear and tear") arthritic changes in their bony remains exceeds that found among people living in agricultural and industrial societies today. Of course, such arthritic involvement cannot be considered healthy—it results from much more and harder exercise than even we recommend—but it does indicate that vigorous physical exertion has long been part of human existence.

Aerobic fitness is another aspect of overall health. Clearly, people who rely on their own muscles for locomotion will be more aerobically fit than people who depend on the internal combustion engine. Yet unlike strength-building activities, endurance-and-stamina-building activities (such as running and walking long distances) leave no direct skeletal evidence. Fortunately, other means of inferring ancient human aerobic fitness are available.

First, endurance-related activities generate considerable heat. The long-standing human need for dissipating heat is reflected in a number of exceptional physiological mechanisms. We are one of a very few animals that sweat—a much more efficient means of heat release than is the panting found among carnivores such as wolves or lions. We are also among a relatively small number of essentially hairless terrestrial mammals; exposed skin allows heat to escape readily, especially during rapid movement like running, when airflow over the skin increases. Given these two unusual physiological adaptations, it is clear that heat-generating aerobic activity has been integral to human life since we separated from the apes.

Second, assessments of aerobic fitness among recent hunters and gatherers as diverse as the Eskimos in the Canadian Arctic and the Aché of the Paraguayan forest confirm that their endurance far exceeds that of average people in the West. The same has been found true for rudimentary horticulturists, simple agriculturalists, and pastoralists, all of whom are more aerobically fit than are most people in the affluent West. Unlike strength and muscularity, which apparently decreased with the Agricultural Revolution, human aerobic fitness has probably been maintained throughout our more recent past. Indeed, the societal upheaval which can be credited with drastically reducing human stamina and endurance levels is the Industrial Revolution, at most two hundred years old. Fortunately, there is no reason to think that this decrease is genetic. Aerobic fitness in Westerners who exercise regularly and vigorously often equals or exceeds that of average people living in traditional societies.

While there are important differences between the exercise patterns of recent hunters and gatherers and those of Late Paleolithic humans, their experiences nevertheless are parallel in enough ways to allow inferences about our past. Even people living in other preindustrial and, in some cases, preliterate societies offer insight into the health status of our more remote ancestors. Such people include *rudimentary horticulturists* such as the Chimbu, Wabag, Bomai, and Yongamuggl of New Guinea, the Kren-Akorore and Yanamamo of South America, and the Kwaio and Aita of the Solomon Islands, *simple agriculturalists* from remote areas of Mexico, Africa, and Central America, and *pastoralists* such as the Samburu and Masai from Kenya and the Bedouin Broayas from North Africa. On a continuum of physical activity—with people in today's industrial societies at one end and people of the Paleolithic at the other—these traditional groups are considerably closer to our Paleolithic ancestors than they are to ourselves. Historically documented preindustrial societies provide additional points of reference.

The Iroquois Confederacy, for example, was made up of linguistically related tribes of rudimentary horticulturists. They lived along the Iroquois Trail, which extended about 240 miles (from what is now Albany to the vicinity of Buffalo in western New York). Iroquois runners usually traveled this distance in four days, but in exceptional circumstances, they made the trip in under three, sometimes traveling 90 miles in one day.

Other runners, those living in the more complex pre-Columbian states of Central and South America, typically worked in relays—something like the Pony Express in the United States of the late 1850s, only without horses. These runners were capable of remarkable feats: Within twenty-four hours of Cortes's landing at Chianiztlan on the Mexican coast in 1519, runners had described to Montezuma, 260 miles away in Mexico City, Cortes's ships, men, guns, and horses. The historian William H. Prescott relates that these same runners regularly supplied Montezuma's kitchen with fresh fish from the Gulf of Mexico.

Another group of relay runners traversed the greatest pre-Columbian road system: the 2,500-mile South American "Inca Highway." Post shelters were placed at roughly 2-mile intervals along the entire length, and relay runners ran each 2-mile segment at top speed. Messages were sometimes carried as far as 150 miles a day through the difficult terrain of the Andes Mountains.

Today, the most celebrated traditional runners in North America may be the Tarahumara Indians of northern Mexico. The rugged, mountainous region makes aerobic fitness a requirement for a people who practice simple corn farming and goatherding. Their traditional men's sport is a form of kickball, played as often as possible—sometimes originating spontaneously, as at parties, and sometimes organized as multiday events in which villages compete against each other. These games can cover as much as two hundred miles and continue through the night, with runners carrying torches. The route traverses crags, hollows, rock-strewn ridges, and mountain streams and usually consists of multiple circuits, sometimes as many as forty. (Tarahumara women also race, but with a hoop instead of a ball. They run in bright shawls and flowing skirts using long wooden forks to keep the hoops rolling forward.) These impressive endurance feats are also reflected in daily life. Tarahumara runners have been observed to carry forty- to sixty-pound loads at a steady trot over rough terrain, sometimes for more than fifty miles a day.

Perhaps the most formidable Indian runners are the Ge-speaking log racers of eastern Brazil: the Kraho, Timbira, Sherente, Krikati, and Pukobye. These rudimentary horticulturists live in circular villages arranged around spokelike plazas; the pattern resembles a giant wagon wheel. They construct tracklike paths extending out from the villages, sometimes ten miles long and as wide as a country road. Along these wilderness paths, teams of relay runners, usually men fifteen to fifty-five years of age, carry logs that weigh from one hundred to two hundred pounds in races that are part sport, part ritual, and part test of strength and manhood. (During role reversal ceremonies, women sometimes carry lighter versions of the logs.) Ethnographer Curt Nimuendaju described one such race, observed during the 1930s:

Four men from each team lift their own log to the first racer's shoulder and all immediately dash off in the direction of the village. Yelling and inciting the racers to greater efforts the Indians bound deer-like to the right and left of the log-bearer's path, leaping over tufts of grass and low steppe bushes. After a distance of about 150 meters, a fellow team-member runs up to the log bearer who, without stopping in his course, dexterously twists his body around so as to transfer his load to his mate's shoulder and the race continues without the least interruption. Thus it goes on madly down the slopes of hills in the torrid sunshine of the shadeless steppe, across brooks and uphill again in the burning, loose sand that unresistingly yields to the feet. Again and again a new substitute rushes up to relieve a racer as soon as his pace begins to slacken. After a few kilometers (some races are 10 miles long) the panting runners, bathed in perspiration, urge one another on with forced, hoarse cries and, toward the end of the race not a man can carry his load further than 30 meters so that there is a constant change of log bearers. On finally reaching the village the leading team takes the nearest radial path to the central plaza where the log can at last be dropped and the runners can begin to recapture their breath.

Kim Hill is a contemporary anthropologist who studies Amerindian foragers: the Cuiva in Venezuela, the Mashco-Piro in Peru, and, especially, the Aché of Paraguay. His adventures are reminiscent of a real-life Indiana Jones (the anthropologist protagonist of *Raiders of the Lost Ark* and *Indiana Jones and the Temple of Doom*). Like the cinema hero, some of Hill's adventures have been life-threatening, some amusing, and many enlightening. One of the latter involved a 50-yard race arranged between Hill, a 10.2 sprinter in college, and the men and boys of an Aché band. Over half of the Aché were able to beat him, whereas it is unlikely that a comparable group of American men and boys would include even one 10.2 sprinter.

Similar descriptions of the strength and fitness of traditional people have been recorded from the Arctic to the Equator, from the deserts of Africa and Australia to the most remote Pacific islands. Details differ, but the main thrust remains: People who live much like our preindustrial ancestors did are strong and fit. Some of the data are precise and scientific; some are more observational. Where scientific documentation has been possible, the results have been impressive. Maximum oxygen uptake values (the best measure of aerobic fitness) for these groups are nearly 50 percent greater, on average, than they are for typical Americans. Similarly, leg strength (for example, thigh extension) of Alaskan Eskimos is more than 50 percent greater than that of Americans matched for age and weight.

EXERCISE AND HEALTH

At one time exercise enthusiasts made outrageous claims concerning the health effects of regular physical exertion, especially long-distance running. For example, they flagrantly asserted that no one who had once completed a marathon had ever suffered a fatal heart attack. Most people, including physicians, were doubtful of such statements, and subsequent experience has supported their skepticism.

However, while the health benefits of exercise have limitations, and a relationship among exercise, disease prevention, and longevity has not been unequivocally established, numerous well-designed studies have shown that both aerobic and resistance exercise beneficially affect human anatomy and physiology. And, while not completely definitive, the best long-term investigations do suggest that regular exercise—when begun in moderation and continued in accordance with one's known health profile—can decrease the likelihood of disease and prolong life.

STAMINA PLUS STRENGTH

Popular fitness literature in the United States promotes idealized stereotypes. Runners' magazines are illustrated with lithe men and women effortlessly and gracefully participating in runs ranging from six to fifty miles. The accompanying text details weekly training schedules totaling fifty, seventy, and sometimes over one hundred miles. Bodybuilding publications show men with startlingly defined, bulging muscles and women with muscularity unprecedented in prior female experience. The legendary training routines of bodybuilding champions are outlined; some have lifted more than a total of 25,000 pounds during one single session. Competitive swimmers often cover 10,000 yards a day during the course of double or even triple pool workouts.

The champion performers in each of these activities (and in others ranging from bicycling to basketball) are role models for thousands or even millions of less-proficient followers. But for nonparticipants, such champions—whether pencil-thin ultramarathoners or gargantuan power-lifters—represent stereotypical, freakish extremes. Our Paleolithic ancestors are less familiar but more natural role models. Their daily activities promoted both strength and endurance. They more closely resembled versatile decathlon athletes than they did specialized distance runners or weight trainers.

To understand better the demands of this ancient world, imagine life among Paleoindian hunters and gatherers 11,200 years ago in the western part of what is now the United States. The countryside is unspoiled, beautiful, and lush, the climate chilly and moist. Winds blowing from the mile-thick glacial ice to the north cool the air, bringing enough rainfall to produce a lush cover of vegetation. The lower and wetter areas are forested, while the higher land, except for the wooded lake margins and river valleys, is open, covered with grass, low-growing shrubs, and wildflowers. These green meadows are home to abundant grazing herd animals: wild horse, antelope, and bison. Mammoths are also plentiful and dwarf the others. Some stand twelve feet at the shoulders and have tusks twice as long as those found on today's elephants; their shaggy coats—coarse and reddish—make them appear even bulkier.

Spring has come, the time mammoths migrate to their summer feeding grounds. Scouts placed along their usual migration route saw a small herd heading north along the lakeshore earlier that day and have run into camp to report their findings. That evening, the hunters sit by the fire, carefully checking their equipment. They examine their spears: stone points four to five inches long, with parallel sides curving together to form a pointed tip, like the end of a bayonet. The sharp, symmetrical edges cut at least as cleanly as modern steel scalpel blades, except near the base; here the edges are dulled to prevent the lashings, which hold the stone tips to the wooden shaft, from being severed. The shafts themselves are jointed so that the stone tip and foreshaft will separate from the main shaft after an animal is struck.

Their spears are of two sizes: larger lancelike ones for thrusting or stabbing, and smaller javelinlike ones for hurling. These smaller ones are used together with spear throwers, or atlatls: stout sticks eighteen to twenty-four inches long with a turned-up hook at one end. When the butt end of the spear is engaged by the atlatl's hook, the hunter grasps the atlatl to hurl the spear. Having in effect extended his arm, he increases the range and striking power of his throw. The rest of the hunting kit—stone knives, hammer stones for sharpening damaged blades, spare projectile points, animal hides, lengths of sinew, torch materials, and fire drills—is also checked.

As the hunters work, they debate tactics for the hunt. They decide to meet the mammoths where their customary trail passes close to the swampy lakeshore. The hunters will break into groups, waiting ahead, behind, and on the land side of the trail. On signal, they will attack the mammoths from all three sides. They may not wound or kill any this way, but they hope to drive one or more into the adjacent swampy ground to become mired or at least greatly hindered by the mucky footing.

Early the next morning, twelve men, aged fourteen to fifty, leave camp, walking the four miles to the ambush site almost without noticing. They choose hiding places along a 250-yard stretch of marsh and wait in the low bushes, some with unlit torches and smoldering embers, others with hides, all with spears. As the mammoths approach, anticipation and excitement rise. The hunters light their torches, then remain motionless. Then, a wild yell erupts as the leader leaps into the open, waving a flaming torch. He runs to head off the oncoming herd—a huge old bull, four adult females, five younger animals (two males and three females), and three calves. Other hunters join, shouting, flapping hides, and waving torches. Bewildered at first, the older mammoths recover. Trumpeting angrily, they rally together and charge, scattering the hunters in their path. Females herd their calves along, and juveniles are swept up by the stampede. But amid the confusion, one young male turns away from the hunters and blunders toward the marsh. The hunters immediately converge on this single animal as the remainder of the herd breaks away and proceeds in its original northward direction.

The isolated animal is trapped: An impressively large though still immature male is driven into the marsh, as torches, flapping hides, screams, and spearpoints direct its way. Its movements become greatly impeded while the hunters now stand no more than fifty feet away, casting their javelins with deadly effect. The great beast trumpets shrilly, flailing about in rage with its trunk and enormous tusks, towering above its tormentors. Because of its wounds and its frantic effort to maneuver through the boggy mire, the animal steadily weakens. At last, a young hunter leaps to a patch of solid ground near the mammoth's exposed flank and drives home a thrusting spear. The animal staggers, then collapses onto its side in the swamp, twenty feet from the marsh edge.

A juvenile, yet the exposed upper side accessible for butchering represents a huge quantity of meat. The hunters work efficiently, removing as much of the hide in one piece as possible. Their stone knives work fast, capable of skinning the carcass at least as quickly as can contemporary steel knives. They discard the feet and lower portion of each leg, cut the haunches and shoulders into manageable sections, and carry them to dry land, where they are stacked on fresh-cut branches. Other choice cuts—the rump, pelvis, and back—are also carried to shore. The rib cage is opened, exposing the chest and abdominal cavities. The intestines are a special prize. Emptied of content, they can be used as storage containers or cut into sinew for sewing, lashings, and thongs. On shore, a fire is blazing. Portions of the tongue and liver are already being roasted, an impromptu feast before the return trip. There is so much meat that several trips will be needed. The men take turns—two at a time—guarding the meat while others hike back and forth the four miles to base camp, carrying loads of from forty to eighty pounds on each homeward journey.

With mammoths now extinct, such an account must be, of course, partly conjecture. Yet observations of recent hunters and gatherers—including Mbuti Pygmy elephant hunters—confirm that comparable levels of physical exertion are often required by their hunting expeditions. Although ambush or trapping techniques similar to that described above are widespread, tracking is also common. Hunters of today have formidable observational skills, stunning to Westerners, which enable them to pick up and follow the faintest trail of game animals traveling individually or in small groups.

Tracking can take several hours, with hunters proceeding at a steady jog or walk, although they may come to a complete halt if an animal's trail becomes especially difficult to follow. Once an animal is sighted, movement must be stealthy and decisive. Depending on wind conditions, they may have to circle the animal, moving rapidly and carefully, facing downwind. Ready, they stalk quietly, then crouch or even crawl until they reach a strategic position. If several hunters are together, they will fan out to cover escape routes. As soon as one hunter gets close enough to cast his spear (perhaps fifty yards with a spear thrower), a throw is made, if possible, from concealment. A second throw will be attempted if the first is a miss and the animal is uncertain about the location of its attacker. If the throw results in a nonfatal wound or misses altogether, the hunter will chase the prey toward the other hunters so that additional spear casts may be made.

Depending on the depth of a wound, it may take hours, a full day or even longer, before an animal succumbs. A wounded animal is usually easy to follow—it moves relatively slowly and may leave a trail of blood—so trackers can close in fairly quickly. The trail may be a mile or less, but it may also be ten miles or more, so hunters must press on rapidly to ensure that carnivores or other scavengers do not rob them of their reward.

Once the animal is killed, it is butchered. If conditions are favorable and the animal is especially large, the entire group may move to the kill site, living there until the meat is gone. Otherwise, the meat will be carried back to camp. One hunter may stay with the kill, waiting for others to return with additional help (men, women, and even older children). If alone, the hunter will try to secure from scavengers whatever he can't carry. The loads carried by adult hunters such as the !Kung San who themselves are small (averaging 5'2" and 112 pounds) commonly range from forty-five to seventy pounds. Their pace is slow, perhaps three miles an hour, and they rest frequently, but they make every effort to complete the journey in one day; the distance involved may exceed fifteen miles.

For preagricultural people, hunting was highly valued—perhaps partly for religious reasons—so much so that they depicted it in cave and rock wall paintings found throughout the world. Yet in many locations, wild vegetable foods probably constituted the bulk of the diet. Among many recent hunters and gatherers such as the !Kung San, plant foods—gathered primarily by women—predominate over game. Working two or three days a week, !Kung women walk from two to twelve miles round trip, carrying on their return from fifteen to thirty-five pounds of plant foods, quite impressive given their small size and weight (they average 4'11" and 93 pounds). They also carry infants and sometimes young children for a good portion of the expedition (even, occasionally, both). Nor is gathering merely confined to picking fruit from easily accessible branches. Considerable energy and strength are required to dig tubers and roots, sometimes at depths of several feet through drought-hardened soil.

In addition to these physically demanding activities, adults (and children) make day trips as often as once or twice a week to visit friends and relatives living in other villages. "Nearby" camps are typically three to ten miles away, so the round trip may be as much as twenty miles. Visits to "far away" camps, however, usually involve a stay of several weeks. And when the entire band moves camp, at least several times each year, adults and older children may carry from ten to forty pounds for sixty miles or more over the course of a few days.

Even young children in forager bands have levels of physical activity that would be exceptional for children of like age in Western society. With no televisions or video games to immobilize them, no cars to transport them, and no schools to contain them physically, children growing up in hunting and gathering societies engage in vigorous physical play throughout the day. That is, unless they are otherwise physically engaged: accompanying their parents on hunting or gathering expeditions, taking day trips to nearby villages, making seasonal rounds, moving to temporary living sites near animal kills, or traveling to distant villages for longer-term visits.

PALEOLITHIC RHYTHM AND CYCLE

Most recent hunters and gatherers space their subsistence activities, a pattern we call a "Paleolithic work rhythm." Men commonly hunt from two to four nonconsecutive days a week, while women usually gather about every two or three days. Toolmaking and repair, housework, and child care are additional forms of labor, some of which (butchering meat, certain types of vegetable food preparation, gathering wood, and carrying children) are also quite physical. And dancing, a major recreation for many preagricultural people, can occur several nights a week, lasting for hours. Over time, physical activity tends to be "regularly intermittent": alternating days of intense physical output with days of comparative rest.

Work effort also varies with the seasons. Migrations of animals between winter and summer grazing areas and to well-watered regions result in different availability of game animals, often requiring separate hunting techniques. Even foods ripening at different times demand flexible foraging strategies. Dry periods on the savannas mean that roots and tubers predominate; the rainy season brings green vegetables, berries, other fruits, and beans. In some locations nuts, such as the mongongo nut of the African Kalahari and the acorns favored by California Mimok Indians, provide the staple food during part of the year.

Hunters and gatherers are typically seminomadic. The !Kung San make as many as thirty moves a year, and paleontological evidence from Greece, northern Australia, and southern France strongly suggests that prehistoric foragers were also mobile, although they may have occupied their living sites for longer periods of time. Other physically demanding tasks may have included intense harvesting of seasonally abundant food sources, such as salmon runs, along with other activities: trips to quarry flint and constructing pit traps, weirs, and stockades for specialized hunting.

Since the types of physical exertion common to hunters and gatherers, past and present, varied cyclically, it may not be mere coincidence that the most recent theories of coaches, trainers, and sports physiologists emphasize periodic variation in exercise routines as a means of maximizing training effectiveness. This pattern has also been shown to prevent boredom, overtraining, and burnout, as well as minor, temporarily disabling injuries.

TYPES OF PHYSICAL FITNESS

There are three main components of physical fitness: cardiorespiratory (aerobic) endurance, muscular strength, and flexibility.

Cardiorespiratory Endurance

Good cardiorespiratory endurance means that activities requiring stamina (such as soccer, swimming, long-distance running, and basketball) can be maintained for relatively prolonged periods. This type of fitness depends on the ability of the heart, lungs, blood, and blood vessels to take up and transport oxygen to the muscles and on the ability of the muscles in turn to use the oxygen for energy production.

The list of health benefits that accrue from maintaining aerobic endurance is impressive. People who by systematic exercise significantly improve their aerobic fitness tend to reduce their percentage of body fat, lower their blood pressure and pulse, lower their "bad" LDL-cholesterol values, increase their proportion of "good" HDL-cholesterol, lower their blood sugar and insulin levels, and lower their level of serum triglycerides.

Muscular Strength

This aspect of fitness is measured by how much force is exerted when single muscle groups contract. Muscular endurance is a related concept, and refers to how often the muscle group is able to contract (against a given resistance) before it becomes so fatigued that it no longer functions.

During the 1950s and early 1960s, the muscular strength and endurance of average young Americans were found to be significantly inferior to that of Europeans. Since that time, Americans have become more fitness conscious and Europeans relatively more affluent, so these differences have become less pronounced. In relation to preindustrial peoples, however, the reports of anthropologists, explorers, and physicians overwhelmingly agree: The strength and especially muscular endurance of people in most preindustrial societies far exceeds that of average Westerners.

Muscular strength usually peaks between the ages of twenty and thirty, and thereafter steadily declines. For many older Americans, this translates into extreme weakness, the legacy of sedentary, inactive lives. Yet, although maximum strength declines inexorably with age no matter what culture one lives in, regular exercise greatly reduces the rate of decline. Active men and women well into their sixties and seventies can actually retain physical strength greater than that of inactive thirty-year-olds. Although strength has become relatively unimportant in our society today, it is a prerequisite for many types of athletic activity. It is also important for health: Strong muscles guard against injuries, resisting forces that might otherwise cause fractures. Strong bones do much the same.

Except for swimming, all forms of exercise tend to increase bone density, but resistance training is most effective. Such training strengthens bones, ligaments, and tendons, not just muscles. Maintaining and increasing muscular strength helps prevent osteoporosis, the bony weakening that afflicts many older people, especially women. Even vulnerability to heart disease may be favorably affected. While physicians generally emphasize the importance of aerobic exercise for cardiovascular health, weight training also has a beneficial, although less-pronounced effect on serum cholesterol levels.

Flexibility

This refers to the range of motion possible at the body's joints; flexible bodies are limber, supple, and graceful. Flexibility usually peaks between the ages of ten and fifteen, and thereafter declines gradually until, in old age, we become rigid, awkward, and stiff. But Dame Margot Fonteyn, a prima ballerina who commanded the most rigorous dance roles into her late-fifties, and Martha Graham, who continued as a dance teacher and choreographer long after her performance career ended in her midsixties, serve as reminders that flexibility—even for the majority who are not dance professionals—can be maintained into maturity.

In addition to its aesthetic appeal, flexibility also promotes health. Flexibility exercises help minimize the effects of arthritis, and like resistance exercises, tend to protect against musculoskeletal injuries (such as strains and sprains). Finally, people who are strong and flexible are less likely to incur acute and chronic low-back disability, a cause of common physical discomfort and immense economic loss each year.

CARDIORESPIRATORY FITNESS

Since they participate in 25- to 150-mile races lasting up to forty-eight hours, it is little wonder that the Tarahumara Indians of the Sierra Madre Occidentale Mountains of Mexico have extraordinary cardiovascular endurance and capacity. The landscape they live in looks much like the Grand Canyon—a tangle of deep gorges and rugged plateaus. Anthropologists who have painfully negotiated the terrain like to say there are only two directions in the region: up and down. The Tarahumara are proud of their running ability. Among these wild gorges, buttes, and mesas, travel afoot is often safer and faster than by burro or horse, so running is part of their life-style. In the past, they also chased deer on foot—sometimes for days—until the prey finally toppled over in exhaustion; they pursued wild turkeys until the birds could no longer rise from the ground in flight. The Aché of Paraguay and the Agta of the Philippines are hunting and gathering groups that also run down prey—including deer and wild bearded pigs.

Such running abilities were also previously widespread among various tribes of native North Americans. The Yaquis, Apaches, Pimas, and Navajos were all noted runners as were the Mohawks of upstate New York. In Africa, the Masai, who habitually walk long distances at a brisk rate, also maintain superior cardiovascular fitness.

Aerobic activities like walking and running have been part of human life since the earliest humans appeared; there was no other means of land travel until horses were domesticated around 6,000 years ago. Of course, all that is now changed. Motor vehicles have almost eliminated the need for human ambulation, and walking, let alone running, is avoided as much as possible. Consider, for example, how much time we are willing to spend circling a parking lot to find a space that will "save" us from having to walk an extra hundred feet; now multiply this by every day in every parking lot in every town in America, and consider the total loss in our fitness.

The average number of calories expended on physical activity generally varies inversely with the degree of "civilization." Metabolic studies of Australian Aborigines who normally lived in urban environments but who returned to their traditional life-style for a three-month experimental period greatly increased their physical activity. Likewise, Masai and Bedouin pastoralists are much more physically active than people living in nearby urban centers. The same is true for rural Puerto Ricans and Ethiopians, who expend far more calories in physical activity than do their urban counterparts.

These observations confirm what common sense suggests. Today, most of us are less active by far than were agricultural and preagricultural people of the past. This profound deviation from a life-style for which we are genetically constituted has had significant effects upon our health.

HEALTH BENEFITS OF AEROBIC EXERCISE

Cardiovascular Alterations

When an otherwise sedentary person begins a program of aerobic exercise, a series of predictable bodily changes occurs, many influencing cardiovascular function. These include alterations in the blood, the heart, the nervous system, and the skeletal muscles. There is some question as to whether pulmonary function is consistently affected.

Blood
Both the total volume of blood and the total number of red blood cells increase in response to aerobic conditioning. In one study of eighteen young men and women who underwent a six-month training program, total blood volume increased an average of about 31 percent.

The Heart as a Pump
The hearts of patients in congestive heart failure are large; so are those of the aerobically fit. However, while the enlargement in the former group is a manifestation of disease—a response to reduced pumping efficiency—the enlarged hearts of the aerobically fit result from regular endurance exercise, a sign of increased capacity and extra cardiac reserve.

The consequence of increased total blood volume is that more blood enters the chambers of the heart. This extra blood stretches the cardiac muscle fibers, increasing the heart's strength and the efficiency of its contractions. An "aerobically conditioned heart" actually pumps about 20 percent more blood per beat than the same "unconditioned" heart would. Since maximum heart rate is essentially fixed (it decreases with age, but is unaffected by physical conditioning), the amount of blood the heart can pump in a minute—called maximum cardiac output—is higher. This allows greater blood flow during strenuous exertion.

Nerves

Our resting heartbeat—how fast our hearts beat when we are at rest— is largely controlled by two brain centers: One, operating via the vagus nerve, lowers the heart rate; the other, operating via the sympathetic nerves, raises it. In people who are fit, vagal tone increases, resulting in a relatively low heart rate (in one study, 18 percent lower after six months of training).

With lower heart rates and higher volume per beat, the resting cardiac output of the fit is comparable to that of the unfit. However, because the hearts of the fit beat more efficiently and at slower rates, the amount of work (in physiologic terms) expended by the conditioned heart is much less (23 percent less in a recent experimental investigation).

Skeletal Muscle

Prolonged endurance exercise increases the body's ability to produce energy. This process originates in intracellular structures called mitochondria—the "power stations" of the cells. With aerobic fitness training, the number, size, and activity of mitochondria in muscle cells markedly increase. These "enhanced" muscles, now able to extract greater proportions of oxygen from blood, are more effective at producing energy.

This has a major impact on the heart. Fewer heartbeats are necessary to supply oxygen to conditioned muscles than to unconditioned ones for similar amounts of work. For example, if a jogger has a quarter-mile uphill segment during a run, the heart will work less hard during that segment after two months of aerobic training than before training began, largely because the muscles are now able to extract more oxygen from the blood.

Lungs

The lungs of the fit similarly accommodate more air. Aerobically conditioned lungs exhale more air in one second (a test used to evaluate obstructive lung diseases such as emphysema) than do unconditioned lungs. The impact of these findings for people suffering from lung disorders is not entirely clear, but patients with pulmonary emphysema have been shown to improve their tolerance for exercise after such training was initiated. Even slight improvement can offer someone with pulmonary disability a wider range of physical options, making it easier to cope with impairment.

Coronary Arteries

The effect of physical training on coronary arteries is not well documented in people. In animals, however, exercise has been shown to increase vascular supply to the heart muscle. For example, rats that were forced to exercise developed additional capillaries to the heart, supplying it with more blood and oxygen than rats whose exercise was restricted. A similar phenomenon has been observed in nature. Wild rabbits have larger hearts and more extensive capillary networks than do domesticated rabbits confined in hutches and unable to exercise.

Comparable effects in humans have only been suggested. Traditional people with high daily aerobic activity levels, such as the Masai of East Africa and lifelong distance runners in the West, have been found on autopsy to have exceptionally large coronary arteries (especially when compared to those of average, sedentary members of our culture). However, X-rays of people engaged in exercise programs did not show similar changes in their hearts. (This may have been because systematic training only began in middle age, after coronary atherosclerosis had already set in, or because the periods of aerobic training were short, between six and twenty-four months.) Perhaps because of flaws like these in a number of studies, no firm evidence yet exists to document an increase in the vascularity of human cardiac muscle after aerobic training.

Summary

The major, proven cardiovascular benefits of aerobic exercise training include increased total body blood volume, increased efficiency of the heart as a pump (resulting in more blood flow per stroke and increased maximum output per minute), slower heart rate at rest as well as at different levels of physical exertion, and a greater capability of skeletal muscle to extract and use oxygen delivered to it for the production of energy. Taken together, these factors ensure that the heart's pumping job is easier at any given work load. With the heart pumping maximally, therefore, the muscles of a fit individual can perform more work than those of an unfit person—a result repeatedly shown by treadmill or bicycle ergometer testing. The relationship between endurance exercise training and the vascular supply of heart muscle is still unsettled; an increase has been found in animals, but has not been proved in humans. Still, there is suggestive evidence that it may occur when such exercise is part of a lifelong pattern.

Fitness Training and Diabetes

The basic problem in adult-onset diabetes is now suspected to be a decreased sensitivity of body tissues (especially muscle) to insulin. When this develops, more insulin has to be secreted by the pancreas to balance glucose released into the blood after a meal. Insulin resistance, as this condition is called, is more common in the obese and the physically unfit.

Physical endurance training increases the sensitivity of the body's cells to insulin. Studies show that the physically fit secrete less insulin after being given test doses of carbohydrates than do the physically unfit. Two possible explanations have been advanced. First, conditioned muscles are more responsive to insulin. Second, exercise increases the percentage of muscle while decreasing body fat. Since muscle—even muscle with reduced sensitivity—is more responsive to insulin than is fat, overall body sensitivity to insulin is enhanced. Exercise has always been a cornerstone in the treatment of diabetes, especially adult-onset diabetes. With studies of this kind lending additional support, programs for treating and preventing diabetes have increasingly stressed exercise in their protocols.

Exercise and Weight Loss

English playwright George Bernard Shaw is reputed to have said, "Whenever I feel the urge to exercise, I just lie down on the sofa and rest until it goes away." This attitude is widespread among obese Americans who often rationalize their disinclination toward physical activity by observing that "it would take six hours of handball, a thirty-six-mile walk, or seven hours of splitting wood to burn off the 3,500 calories needed to lose just one pound." They buttress their sedentary position further by arguing that "exercise just makes you hungrier."

In this country the approach to obesity has traditionally been through dieting: cutting down on food intake. We have an annual crop of weight-loss diet books, appetite-suppression pills, diet clubs and spas, and even surgical operations to short-circuit the intestinal tract so that less of the food eaten will be absorbed by the body. What we don't have is much success. Seventy years ago the average American ate 1,592 pounds of food a year; that figure is now down to 1,441 pounds a year. But because our daily physical activity decreased sharply over the same period of time, while caloric density—food energy per pound—increased, the average American now weighs from seven to ten pounds more than an American of similar age and height who lived seventy-five years ago.

It is true that 3,500 calories must be expended for each pound of weight lost, but those 3,500 calories do not have to be burned all at once. Without even reducing one's calorie intake at all, a ten-pound weight loss can be effected over a year's time by merely expending one hundred calories a day in exercise. That translates into a twenty-minute walk, ten minutes of jogging, or fifteen minutes of single's tennis; or thirty minutes of jogging three times a week. (See Table XVIII.)

Most Americans gain weight gradually, yet as little as a pound or two extra a year can turn into ten pounds within a few years. These one or two extra pounds can result from an imbalance between intake and expenditure of calories—even as little as ten to twenty calories a day. To expend all those ten calories in exercise would require very little physical activity; a single extension phone in the home has been calculated to "save" a typical American seventy miles of walking a year. That's the kind of saving we can do without.

Another plus for exercise: Most of the weight you lose is fat. In one experiment a group of overweight college women exercised enough to burn 500 calories a day for eight weeks (that's about fifty minutes of jogging a day). In those two months they lost an average of five pounds each, even though they had *no* dietary restrictions. Even more encouraging, analysis of their body composition showed that they had actually lost nearly twelve pounds of fat while gaining seven back as muscle.

The pattern that results from weight loss due to extreme caloric restriction (such as fasting) offers a dramatic contrast. As much as two-thirds of the lost weight can come from lean body mass (bone and muscle), while only one-third may be fat. In Chapter 3, we noted that, in Western societies, lean body mass typically decreases and fat increases with age. This pattern, however, is not "natural." It is the rule neither for people living in preagricultural societies nor among vigorously active Westerners such as Norwegian woodcutters or California distance runners. Medical studies have shown that both groups of middle-aged and older adult men have body weights similar to what they had as youths. In addition, with proportions of body fat under 15 percent, they maintained "natural" or "Paleolithic" body composition throughout their lives.

Exercise also makes an impact on appetite. Common sense tells us that the more we exercise, the more we need (and want) to eat. At

TABLE XVIII.

Caloric Expenditures for Selected Exercise Activities: Kcal/15 minutes

Activity	Body weight (lbs) 110	123	137	150	163	176	190	203	216
Aerobic Dancing (medium intensity)	78	87	96	105	114	123	134	143	152
Basketball	104	116	129	141	153	165	179	191	203
Circuit Weight Training (resistance machines)	78	89	98	107	116	126	135	144	155
Cycling (9.4 mph)	75	84	93	102	111	120	129	138	147
Jumping Rope (80 per min.)	123	138	153	168	182	197	212	227	242
Racquetball	134	150	165	182	198	213	230	246	261
Running (flat surface)									
11 min, 30 sec/mile	102	114	126	138	150	164	176	188	200
9 min/mile	146	162	180	197	215	231	249	267	284
7 min/mile	183	200	218	234	252	269	287	305	321
Squash	159	179	197	216	236	255	273	293	312
Swimming (slow crawl)	96	108	119	131	143	153	165	177	188
Tennis (singles)	83	92	102	111	122	131	141	150	161
Walking (3.5 mph)	60	68	75	81	89	96	104	111	117

Source: Modified from McArdle, W. D., Katch, F. I., Katch, V. L. Exercise physiology. Energy, nutrition, and human performance. Philadelphia: Lea & Febiger. 1986: Appendix D.

higher levels of exercise, this is certainly true; our appetite control mechanisms try to ensure that our food intake balances our energy expenditure almost exactly. Lumberjacks and others engaged in very physically demanding occupations may eat 4,000 to 6,000 calories a day. But they tend to maintain a lean, fit body composition because they need that level of calorie intake to meet their level of energy expenditure.

At very low levels of activity, however, common to many in the affluent West, the appetite control mechanism seems to get out of whack. Dr. Jean Mayer, a leading nutritionist, has shown that inactive animals eat more, not less, than animals moderately exercised. Similar results have been found for sedentary workers as compared to others whose jobs demanded physical exertion.

Just what controls our appetites is not clear, but whatever mechanisms are involved must have evolved over millions of years, fashioning the pattern we see today. Genetically, our appetites are programmed to balance food intake and energy outlay so that stable body weight and desirable body composition can be maintained.

But these controls operate most efficiently within the context of high activity levels, those typical of the past and still seen among preagricultural and other traditional peoples today. Under conditions of abundance, such people would also reduce their activity levels and overeat. But the difference is that for them, the period of abundance would be brief, whereas for us it is continuous. For most of us, sedentary lives demand such low levels of physical exertion that they barely seem to register on the appetite control scale. Regular exercise, however, helps activate our appetite control centers, making it easier not to overeat.

Aerobic Exercise and Serum Lipids

Studies show that aerobic exercise increases serum levels of HDL, or "good" cholesterol, protective against atherosclerosis. This is true for the healthy, for those known to have atherosclerotic heart disease, and even for victims of heart attack. Comparing inactive and active men makes this clear: Middle-aged inactive men have average HDL levels of about 40 to 45 (measured in milligrams per decaliter) while very active runners (for example, marathoners) have average levels closer to 65. (Joggers are somewhere in between, with HDL levels of 55 to 60, lower than marathoners but higher than sedentary men.) Studies of very limited exercise, chiefly in postcoronary patients, also show that exercise-related increases in HDL develop early in fitness training programs; this occurs even when the level of exercise is insufficient to produce other effects associated with aerobic conditioning, such as weight loss and increased oxygen uptake capacity. Since similarly beneficial, although less pronounced effects on blood lipids other than HDL have also been shown, it seems likely that aerobic fitness may be a deterrent to atherosclerosis generally and to coronary heart disease in particular.

Aerobic Exercise in Prevention of Heart Attacks

These considerations suggest that there should be a relationship between endurance exercise and longevity. To "prove" conclusively such a relationship is statistically difficult, but mounting evidence tends to confirm its existence. Dr. Ralph Paffenbarger has tracked the health and life-styles of nearly 17,000 Harvard College alumni. His data strongly indicate that, in this group at least, regular physical activity extends length of life, chiefly because it decreases the risk of cardiovascular mortality. Those alumni whose habitual activity levels required expenditures of at least 2,000 calories per week had 50 percent less risk of heart attack than did their less-energetic classmates. Paffenbarger's figures suggest that each hour of strenuous exercise—jogging, vigorous walking, bicycling, single's tennis, and so on—adds one to three hours of increased life expectancy. In other words, people who remain physically active and fit can add up to two years of life by this means alone. For the Harvard alumni this was true regardless of age and was independent of other risk factors such as smoking, hypertension, and obesity.

Another long-term ongoing investigation—the Framingham study—shows a similar inverse relationship between level of physical activity and risk of cardiovascular disease. The influence of habitual physical activity, however, was modest in comparison with that of other risk factors. On the other hand, epidemiologists at the Centers for Disease Control recently reviewed forty-three studies of the association between physical activity and coronary heart disease. Their conclusion? Lack of physical activity is as strong a risk factor for coronary heart disease as are high serum cholesterol levels, high blood pressure, and cigarette smoking.

Where does all this leave us? These studies cannot unequivocally establish a causal relationship. If we are looking for incontrovertible scientific proof that habitual aerobic exercise helps prevent heart attacks and promotes longevity, we must continue to wait for definitive experiments. However, mortality from coronary atherosclerosis declined 20 percent between 1967 and 1980—at the same time that enthusiasm for and participation in athletic activities such as jogging, cycling, tennis, and racquetball skyrocketed. Given the increasing evidence from long-term human studies and the additional evidence from physiological experiments in both animals and humans, the relationship between exercise and declining mortality is unlikely to be coincidental.

STRENGTH FITNESS

In 1805, the Lewis and Clark expedition witnessed an Indian bison kill comparable in method to that employed by Paleoindians 10,000 years before. A small herd was stampeded over a cliff into a deep, broad ravine. As the bison fell one on top of the other, dazed and injured, hunters killed those on top with spears; the others were crushed and suffocated underneath. The ravine was twelve feet wide and eight feet deep; most of the bulls weighed over a ton, yet a team of five Indian hunters pulled nearly all the bison out of the ravine onto level ground for butchering.

Feats requiring similar levels of strength and endurance have also been noted for other groups. Before their extermination in the nineteenth century, Tasmanian Aborigines were observed by British colonists to throw fifteen-foot spears a distance of 250 feet; they regularly hit animal-size targets at distances of 180 feet. The Nootka Indians of Vancouver Island, who hunted the California gray whale as late as the 1890s, harpooned these giant mammals from small, eight-man boats. As few as two of these boats would tow a whale back to shore, sometimes ten miles or more, and the boats were powered by oars, not sails.

As these examples suggest, those who developed and maintained muscular strength had a survival advantage throughout human existence. Even today, strength accounts for much in preindustrial societies. The physiques of the Masakin Quisar of Sudan's Nuba Mountains have been described as ironlike, and the muscularity of other aboriginal people from New Guinea to Alaska has been similarly praised. Everyday jobs in these communities require considerable strength. Dip-netting for fish, portaging a canoe, cutting and carrying loads of firewood—these and similar tasks performed by men, women, and even children require considerable muscular power, much more than is needed by most of us in our routine work today.

Our bodies still have the genetic potential to be strong, yet modern "conveniences" such as automobiles, power tools, and televised spectator sports have turned us into the weakest human beings of all time.

HEALTH BENEFITS OF STRENGTH FITNESS

Osteoporosis

As we in Western countries grow older, our body composition changes. Body fat typically increases and lean body mass—made up of skeletal muscle, tendons, ligaments, and bone—gradually decreases. Osteoporosis, the medical term for the phenomenon of gradually diminishing bone mass, is the most common skeletal disorder found in the United States. Vulnerable to trauma, these weakened bones may break even in the absence of apparent injury. Osteoporosis is thought responsible for at least 1.2 million fractures in the United States each year; its direct and indirect costs are estimated at over $6 billion annually.

Most fractures occur in the vertebrae of the spine. Rarely life threatening, they are nevertheless quite painful; after numerous occurrences, they can ultimately produce an exaggerated spinal curvature—the "dowager's hump" frequently seen in older women. As discussed previously, other fractures can be deadly serious. Falls and injuries that produce bruises, sprains, or merely wounded pride in younger people can cause fractures of the wrists, shoulders, ribs, or hips in older people with osteoporosis. Hip fractures are especially ominous. Fatal in from 12 to 20 percent of cases, about half the survivors have enough loss of mobility to require long-term nursing home care.

The importance of physical activity in preserving relatively normal bone density has only recently been recognized. Exercises that stress the skeleton with powerful forces (such as weight lifting) seem to be most effective in preventing osteoporosis, but almost all forms of physical exertion tend to promote bone strength. In athletes, in normal young men and women, and even in animals, such resistance exercises have been shown actually to *increase* bone mass. In an experiment involving older, postmenopausal women—the population group most susceptible to developing osteoporosis—light resistance exercise consistently produced modest increases in bone density (from 1.4 to 2.5 percent a year), while a control group who continued the typical Western pattern of sedentary inactivity lost bone mass at the usual rate.

High levels of physical activity benefit people with osteoporosis in other ways, as well. Older women in the Vilcabamba region of Ecuador, for example, also get osteoporosis, presumably because their calcium intake is so low. Yet even in these Vilcabamba women—with bone loss *more* severe than is typical for Westerners—spontaneous fractures and spinal curvature are almost unknown. Their superior muscle tone and ligament strength—products of their relatively rigorous life-style—support, protect, and compensate for their weakened bones, preventing the fractures so common among people with similar osteoporosis in our own society.

Backache

While all types of injuries are more frequent in the physically weak and inactive, lower back pain is ubiquitous in our population. Few references to chronic back disorders appear in the early medical literature, yet 70 percent of people in this country today suffer from lower back pain at some time during their lives. Back pain is second only to upper respiratory infections as a cause of time lost from work; its economic impact amounts to billions of dollars lost annually when treatment costs, disability payments, and lost productivity are taken into account.

Flabby muscle tone, limited flexibility, obesity, and poor posture are all implicated in the problem. Medical studies of patients with back pain show that 80 percent have no significant skeletal abnormality such as a slipped disk. Their discomfort stems from weakness or excessive stiffness in one or more of the muscle groups that support and control movement in the torso. Such weakness allows fairly routine stresses on the spine to produce excessive stretching or actual tearing of the attached ligaments. Training programs that strengthen abdominal and back muscles and improve trunk flexibility help prevent chronic lower back pain by guarding against repeated injury.

The relationship between back pain and physical activity was the focus of a study conducted by Drs. Hans Kraus and Sonja Weber on 423 psychoanalysts, all of whom were physically inactive during their working hours. Of the 196 analysts who participated in regular exercise during their leisure time, only 27 percent complained of back pain. Of the other 227 who were physically inactive during leisure as well as during work, 84 percent complained of back pain. In a follow-up study, the doctors prescribed therapeutic and preventive exercises for 26 of the psychoanalysts with pain. The results? Seven were relieved of pain altogether and 18 showed significant, although incomplete, improvement. Only 1 reported no improvement at all—and he had discontinued the exercises.

Musculoskeletal Injuries

More than 2,400 years ago, Hippocrates proposed exercise as a factor in healing musculoskeletal injuries. Today, nearly all rehabilitation programs recognize that resistance exercises for such injuries speed recovery and lead to stronger repair. For over one hundred years medical students have learned Wolff's Law: A bone develops the structure most suited to resist the forces acting upon it. That is, weight bearing and muscle action directly influence the size, shape, and strength of bones. It follows, then, that strength training with relatively heavy weights can increase the width and density of normal bones. Heavier bones are less vulnerable to osteoporosis and are less susceptible to breakage. Resistance training also produces stronger connective tissue supporting structures and skeletal muscles, which can then absorb and cushion stresses that would otherwise act directly on the bony skeleton. Thus the chances of fracture are reduced still further. Professional and college sports teams have learned this. They now emphasize weight training not only to improve athletic performance, but to help prevent injuries as well.

Lean Body Mass

Progressive resistance exercise can positively influence body composition in relatively short periods of time. In one experiment, a group of men around forty-one years of age lifted weights for approximately one hour, three times a week, for twelve weeks. Under no dietary restrictions, they ate as they wished. During this period their strength—assessed by weights used—nearly doubled, their lean body weight—determined by underwater weighing—increased by 4 percent, and their body fat decreased by 9 percent.

Long-term strength training also affects body size, contour, strength, and composition. The normal twenty-year-old male averages 13 to 15 percent body fat (as tested by the accepted method of underwater weighing). By age forty, fat typically increases to about 24 percent, and by age sixty, it reaches 28 percent of total body weight. (The pattern for women is similar: 27 percent body fat at age twenty, 34 percent at age forty, and 39 percent at age sixty.) In contrast, men who have actively worked with weights (wrestlers, bodybuilders, power-lifters, Olympic weight lifters, discus throwers, and shot-putters, among others) often maintain body-fat levels similar to twenty-year-olds for as long as they train; indeed, bodybuilders usually have even less body fat— around 10 percent of total body weight.

Strength Fitness and the Heart

Another of Ralph S. Paffenbarger's landmark studies involved San Francisco longshoremen. Those who performed heavy physical labor had lower mortality rates from heart disease than did workers whose jobs were less physically demanding. The work pattern for the longshore-men—which involved repeated bursts of peak effort rather than contin-uous, lower-level energy output—was more comparable to strength training than it was to aerobic exercise.

Cardiovascular Endurance

The effects of aerobic exercise on the heart are more widely recognized, but resistance exercise acts similarly. In one study, thirty outstanding weight-trained athletes (ranging from bodybuilders to discus throwers), all of whom could bench-press at least 350 pounds, were tested by bicycle ergometer. Their maximum oxygen-uptake values averaged 48.8, considerably lower than that achieved by top endurance athletes (who often attained maximum oxygen-uptake values of 75 or more), but high enough to place them in cardiovascular training authority Kenneth Cooper's "excellent" fitness category.

The effect of progressive resistance strength training on previously sedentary middle-aged men was also studied. In one experiment four-teen men about forty-one years old participated in a twelve-week weight training program. Their cardiovascular endurance, as determined by bicycle ergometer testing, improved significantly when compared with a control group. Strength training, then, also increases cardiovascular fitness, although to a lesser extent than aerobic exercise.

Serum Lipids

Although the causal relationship is not well understood, the effect is well documented: High levels of aerobic fitness lead to high levels of beneficial HDL-cholesterol. Less well known, perhaps, is the similar, although less pronounced, effect of strength training on serum-lipid levels. Previously sedentary men and women who completed a three- to four-month program of resistance exercise showed decreases in total serum-cholesterol levels, including "bad" LDL-cholesterol, and im-provement in the ratio of HDL-cholesterol to total serum cholesterol. According to the Framingham study, such improvement, if sustained, should reduce these subjects' risk of cardiovascular disease by nearly 50 percent.

FLEXIBILITY, WARMING UP, AND COOLING DOWN

While less dramatic and perhaps less crucial than cardiorespiratory and muscular fitness, flexibility is also an important dimension. As for warm-ing up and cooling down, adequate attention to these processes can be lifesaving.

Flexibility

A number of professional and college football teams now have "flex" coaches to direct flexibility conditioning for athletes. These exercises are designed to reduce the number of injuries such as muscle pulls, ligament sprains, and joint capsular tears. Since flexible muscles and joints withstand better the stresses exerted on them by vigorous physical activity, flexibility exercise is a kind of preventive medicine. It also improves athletic performance, because it increases the range of motion possible at the joints.

At present, flexibility exercises are most commonly included in the warm-up period before training or competition begins, but sports physiologists and trainers now recommend that they also (or even exclusively) be done *after* exercising, as part of a formal cool-down period.

The Warm-Up Period

Properly preparing the body for vigorous physical exertion consists of "warming up" muscles and "lubricating" joints. When blood is pumped into the muscles of the extremities, they *literally* warm up, allowing the cells' metabolic processes to proceed at higher rates; energy is produced faster, and oxygen is exchanged between blood and tissues more rapidly. Nerve impulses also travel slightly faster at higher temperatures, and the gentle movements of warm-up exercises increase the amount of synovial fluid, produced by the joints as a lubricant. Since body temperature affects body function, ambient temperature should influence the length of the warm-up. Cold days may require a fifteen-minute warm-up while on hot days, five minutes may be sufficient.

An adequate warm-up is important for at least three reasons. First, it decreases muscle soreness and minimizes the risk of injuries such as muscle pulls, ligament sprains, and lower back problems. Second, it improves athletic performance 2 to 5 percent; for those involved in competitive sports, this advantage could be the winning margin. Third, and most significant, it helps forestall the irregularities in heart rhythm that can result when vigorous exercise is begun abruptly. In one investigation such abnormalities occurred in 70 percent of forty-four normal subjects aged twenty-one to fifty-two years. As little as two minutes of warm-up, however, eliminated most of these ECG abnormalities and reduced the severity of those that persisted. Given the rare but real possibility of sudden death from cardiac rhythm disturbances, an adequate warm-up should precede every workout.

The Cooling-Down Period

Sudden death can also occur shortly *after*, rather than *during* activities such as jogging or snow-shoveling. When endurance exercise is stopped abruptly, the rate of electrical discharge by the pacemaker tissue of the heart decreases rapidly. Also, when aerobic exercise is performed in an upright position (as in running or walking) blood tends to collect—or "pool"—in the lower half of the body. When exercise is stopped, the return of blood to the heart can sometimes be reduced so that coronary blood flow falls below the level needed to provide appropriate oxygen supplies to the heart. This may be aggravated by the "surge" of the hormones adrenalin and noradrenalin that normally occurs in the immediate postexercise period. As a result, a spontaneous beat may be generated by muscle tissue in the heart ventricles, the main pumping chambers of the heart, especially when the coronary arteries supplying the heart are narrowed by atherosclerosis. Such spontaneous ventricular beats are usually harmless, but they can sometimes lead to ventricular fibrillation (a fluttering, arrhythmic beating pattern that pumps no blood) and sudden death.

These difficulties—rapid decrease in heart rate, a pooling of blood in the lower body, and adrenalin surge—can be minimized by incorporating an active cooling-down period of from five to ten minutes after exercise. Walking three to five minutes is effective, a natural end to a jog or run, providing a gradual return of physiologic processes from vigorous exertion to a resting state. But this should be followed by flexibility exercises including stretching, since muscles are maximally warmed-up, but typically "tight" after aerobic exercise like jogging.

EXERCISE RECOMMENDATIONS

We are still linked, by genetic design, to the patterns of physical activity required of our Late Paleolithic ancestors. Throughout eons of continued cultural flux, the stability of our human biology has remained almost untouched. This past can continue to serve us—an ancient, tried-and-true guide. It is in effect the original "operator's manual" for bodies whose essential features have not changed for tens, and in many ways hundreds, of thousands of years.

The basic features of the paradigm are simple:

1. High levels of physical exertion were integral to people's lives starting in childhood and lasting until old age.
2. Activities of daily life promoted both aerobic endurance and muscular strength.

3. Exercise generally occurred in short-term rhythmic patterns; days of strenuous exertion alternated with days of relative rest.
4. Activities varied according to the seasons; aerobic and resistance exercise continued throughout the year, but the specific forms of exercise varied cyclically.

These facts can be translated into guidelines appropriate for ourselves. For example, children of both sexes should be encouraged to be active through participation in sports or other forms of physical activity; these activities need to be maintained throughout youth, adulthood, and into late life. No one is too old for a properly designed, medically supervised exercise program, and many special conditions, such as pregnancy or disability, are compatible with properly planned exercise routines.

Physical training should emphasize both aerobic and resistance exercise. Many organized sports programs are designed with this principle in mind, but individually selected activities too often stress only one, not both dimensions. This kind of restriction can induce a sense of complacency while providing only half the health benefits to be derived from exercise.

The findings of exercise physiologists and physicians can help establish both aerobic and strength fitness norms appropriate for adults regardless of age. For those just beginning an exercise regimen, they can serve as goals to work toward; for those whose conditioning programs are well established, they can be used as standards to maintain. Maximum oxygen uptake capacity (VO_2 max)—the best measure of aerobic fitness—should be at least 40–50 ml/kg/min. for men and 30–40 ml/kg/min. for women. This measure—which characterizes the maximum amount of oxygen used by a person exercising at his or her peak level—is often determined by treadmill testing. The values obtained roughly correlate with a number of fitness parameters such as the distance an individual can run in a given time period, say twelve minutes. Men should be able to bench-press a minimum of their body weight and leg-press 1.5 times their body weight; for women, 65 and 100 percent of body weight, respectively, are appropriate standards.

Exercise should be alternated with rest. For preagricultural humans, a day or two of extensive and intensive combined aerobic and resistance activity was usually followed by a day or more of relative rest. For most of us today, such an exercise program is impractical, but exercise physiologists have shown that alternating days of resistance with days of aerobic exercise constitutes a near-optimal modern version of this routine. Each body system (cardiorespiratory and musculoskeletal) is able to recover during the day "off" when the other system is exercised. A three-day-a-week workout of from thirty to ninety minutes in length for each system is sufficient to provide high-level health maintenance; longer workouts generally produce diminishing returns.

Many different types of exercise are appropriate for either aerobic or resistance training. An exercise program guided by Paleolithic principles should include considerable variation in exercise mode. Bicycling, running, walking, swimming, aerobics classes, dancing, rowing, and rope jumping are all ways to increase cardiorespiratory endurance. For strength training, changing specific exercises together with varying the combination of sets, repetitions, and weights or resistance machines (a concept called periodization, developed by eastern European sports physiologists) accomplishes the same end. Such variation forestalls burnout, maintains enthusiasm, and maximizes results even as it recapitulates the past.

CONCLUSION

Three conditions for fitness and for the prevention of disease stand out: (1) avoiding harmful substances such as tobacco, excessive alcohol, and drugs; (2) maintaining sensible nutrition; and (3) getting adequate exercise. Of these, the last may seem least important because sedentary living has not, as yet, been proven to be as important a risk factor—for either heart disease or cancer—as have improper nutrition and exposure to tobacco.

However, exercise confers many psychological as well as physical benefits. Regular exercise helps promote a positive self-image even before anatomical or physiological improvements are noticeable. Nutrition is central to disease prevention, exercise is essential for wellness. The "runner's high," although transient and frequently unattained, is only one of many positive psychological effects of running and weight training that augment an array of physiological benefits.

Together, aerobic exercise and resistance training can promote health, as long as exercise is approached prudently and one's health risks are carefully assessed. Aerobic workouts improve heart and lung function, expend calories, and "burn" fat; resistance exercise builds muscle, bone, and connective tissue. In combination, body composition is regulated as it was throughout human evolution. Exercise is thus a more effective and more physiologically and psychologically sound approach to body maintenance than dieting alone can ever be. Dieting reduces muscle at the same time it reduces body fat; combined aerobic and resistance exercise, even without dieting, typically reduces fat and *increases* lean body mass.

In Western nations, body composition and proportions deteriorate steadily with age, usually beginning in the third decade of life, as lean body mass declines and body fat inexorably increases. Recent hunters and gatherers, however, have been shown to maintain a fairly steady body composition and configuration well into the fifth decade. Even later in life, as total body mass gradually decreases, body composition remains fairly stable. This was probably the original norm, characteristic of human life throughout eons of experience. To emulate this pattern today requires no more than the desire and commitment to foster the very best in ourselves, to put our bodies on the path our biology is best designed to follow.

CHAPTER EIGHT

THE NATURAL CHILD

Compared with some of the topics in earlier chapters of this book—nutrition, exercise, preventive medicine—the subject of child care and development is more elusive and less amenable to definitive statement. Nevertheless the same methods are to some extent applicable. From studies of recent hunters and gatherers, and to a lesser extent of other traditional peoples, much knowledge has accumulated about the range of possibilities of human childhood under preagricultural conditions—without the intervention of centuries of industrial life and dozens of theories from Freud to Montessori. Although childhood under preindustrial conditions, and even among hunters and gatherers, has been variable, certain generalizations are still possible.

Just as human digestion and metabolism were designed by natural selection to accommodate a certain range of dietary conditions, and just as human cardiorespiratory and musculoskeletal physiology were designed by parallel forces to fit certain natural patterns of human activity, so certain aspects of human childhood—its physical and emotional needs, its sequence of stages, and its reaction to environmental influences—were designed by evolution to proceed under conditions that prevailed before the agricultural revolution.

On this foundation, a seemingly infinite number of cultural forms have been built. Nevertheless, the "hard rock" underneath has helped determine the shape of the structure, since the plasticity of human childhood is not limitless.

Some of the early conditions were grim: frequent illness, especially gastrointestinal and respiratory infections; mortality of 10 to 20 percent in the first year of life (often in the first week) and 50 percent before growing up. Obviously and fortunately, Western children are protected from such extreme conditions, so some aspects of the original adaptation to child care may be less important. However, it is difficult to separate those aspects that are tied to such high levels of infection and infant mortality from those aspects that are independent of it and simply related to the fundamental biological nature of growing children. These fundamental features are what we attempt to explore here.

However, as in the cases of nutrition and exercise, we do not rely merely on anthropological data. In no case do we advocate adopting a pattern of infant and child care *merely* because it is common among hunters and gatherers or other traditional peoples. As before, we look for supporting evidence in the modern scientific studies of the same phenomena. Child-development research, and especially child psychology, is somewhat less advanced than is research on nutrition, exercise, and health. Consequently, some of our conclusions must be more tentative. Nevertheless, others can be drawn with some degree of certainty and can point the way to further research.

Finally, even where traditional practices do not provide a direction we *should* follow, they can give us confidence about some practices we might like to try as individuals, but which have not been an accepted part of baby and child care in our culture. (The recent increase in the use of baby carriers, based on African originals, is an obvious example.) Some classic advice of pediatricians and educators can also be seen as offshoots of our Western cultural traditions, and less the unbiased professional or scientific advice we have presumed it to be.

This chapter summarizes what we know about human childhood in hunting and gathering societies and considers whether some or all of its characteristics should be viewed as a paradigm for modern baby and child care.

BREAST-FEEDING

Of all the generalizations that can be made about childhood during the Paleolithic period, the most certain is that infants were breast-fed. Those that were not—as when the mother died giving birth—were in grave danger of dying themselves. Not only every known hunting and gathering society, but virtually every recorded society of any preindustrial type relied heavily if not exclusively on breast-feeding in the first months of life. (Even with social stratification wet-nurses breast-fed infants whose mothers wanted to avoid it.) Many societies continued breast-feeding for years.

One of the best studied examples is the pattern of breast-feeding among !Kung San hunters and gatherers of Botswana in Africa. Their traditional pattern is to breast-feed frequently and intensively for the first three or four years of a child's life. Weaning usually takes place only when the mother becomes pregnant with her next child, and if there is no such pregnancy, nursing may continue, albeit less frequently, for an even longer period. (One active boy who was his mother's last child took occasional sucks until age eight years, when he stopped because his friends were making fun of him!)

The frequency of nursing among the !Kung may be even more impressive than the late age of weaning. The average frequency of nursing is *four times an hour* during the day and several times at night, throughout at least the first *two years* of life. This frequency declines only gradually after that until weaning, at around age three. Infants and young children always sleep with their mothers, and sometimes nurse without the mother waking up—an indication of the casual nature of breast-feeding in this culture. Starting at about six months, however, children are introduced to solid foods and eventually subsist exclusively on them.

The advantages of breast-feeding for children in such a society are numerous. First, there is no adequate substitute—no milk products or formula—and breast-feeding is not merely the ideal infant food (it is in our society, too, as we will see), but there is no runner-up. It is true that mothers in many preindustrial societies give their infants prechewed food—a habit that may seem odd to us—but it does provide the infant with partly digested soft food. (It probably does not transfer many more germs than the infant is already exposed to and it may even transfer some protection against those germs.) But this is by no means an adequate substitute for human milk; at best it is a supplement appropriate only later in the first year of life.

Second, breast milk provides specific protection against many infectious diseases, including some of the most dangerous killers in preindustrial societies. Normal human beings have an immune system that provides at least partial protection against many microbes in the environment. (Those born without such protection for genetic reasons have been kept alive only by being raised in a plastic bubble, cut off from all sources of germs.) However, even in the normal child this self-protective system develops only gradually. The fetus in the womb is incapable of forming antibodies to most microbes, but this is no problem, since the mother's antibodies protect the child she is carrying. However, the capability of forming antibodies does not emerge immediately after birth. Different classes of antibodies develop at different rates. The full protection of a child's own immune system is not in place until around age four.

This potentially deadly gap in protection is bridged in our society by vaccination, which stimulates the infant's rudimentary antibody-forming capacity by introducing the minimal level of microbial challenge at the optimal time. We also reduce the number of dangerous germs the infant is brought into contact with. Neither of these options is open to parents in hunting and gathering and other traditional societies, and their children have only one support for their immature immune systems: breast milk. Breast milk is a powerful protector against microbes in such a medically unbuffered environment. It contains about a million macrophages—germ-eating cells—in each cubic centimeter, as well as high doses of antibodies formed by the mother.

Significantly, these are not just general or random antibodies. They have been produced by the mother to counter the specific germs she herself has been exposed too. Here the hunting and gathering practice of maintaining constant close contact between mother and infant has an advantage beyond physical and psychological warmth. As long as mother and infant are together, the chances are that any microbes the infant encounters are also met by the mother. Therefore the antibodies she produces, and supplies to the infant through her milk, will be specific to the germs that are most threatening to the baby.

Third, peoples such as the !Kung San typically have no effective form of birth control, yet the survival of the baby often depends on adequate birth spacing; twins or infants born too close together have little chance of surviving to adulthood. Unless sex is to be avoided (a choice made in some traditional societies in the form of the postpartum sex taboo), the only effective way to postpone the conception of the next child is by nursing. Physicians in our society caution against relying on breast-feeding as a contraceptive, often ridiculing this connection as an "old wives' tale." But recent evidence has mounted in favor of a marked contraceptive effect for certain patterns of nursing. Moreover, even if the effectiveness of nursing as a contraceptive were rather low, it would still help postpone births in a setting in which no other contraceptives are available.

In reality, the effectiveness of nursing varies with its intensity. Studies have shown that frequent exclusive breast-feeding, including night feeding, is a highly effective contraceptive. That is, it has a failure rate similar to or lower than the rates for barrier and drug methods *as they are used in common practice*. The mechanism is believed to involve the release of the hormone prolactin from the pituitary gland each time the nipple is stimulated by sucking. This hormone in turn suppresses the function of the ovaries. In a setting such as ours, a combination of barrier methods with breast-feeding would probably be ideal. But for our ancestors the role of breast-feeding was critical.

Last but not least, there is the possibility of psychological benefits for the infant. This has been the most difficult of the benefits of nursing to study scientifically. What can be directly observed is that infants and children in hunting and gathering societies obviously enjoy the constant physical closeness they have with their mothers, and it seems likely that this gives them a sense of calm and confidence they might not otherwise have. From another viewpoint, the claim that infants breast-fed for so long would grow up tied to their mothers' apron strings (or carrying-pouch strings, in the case of the !Kung San) is not supported by the data from such societies. And, of course, the psychological bene-fits to the mother should not be ignored. !Kung San women declare that they get physical pleasure from breast-feeding, and many women in a variety of cultures report both physical and spiritual rewards. It is possible, although not proved, that the hormones released in response to the infant's sucking play some role in these psychological effects, and promote greater closeness of the mother and infant to the benefit of both.

Thus it can be seen that prolonged intensive breast-feeding was a central part of the adaptation to life among our ancestors, not only during the Paleolithic but to some extent until the Industrial Age. In a sense it can be said that infants are designed to be breast-fed. But how strong is the case for breast-feeding today?

In 1978 the American Academy of Pediatrics (the main professional association of pediatricians) took an official stand in favor of breast-feeding for all infants. This occurred against the background of many years of neglect of this method of feeding and a wide pendulum swing toward bottle-feeding. In the 1950s, bottle-feeding was considered more convenient, more sanitary, and more modern, and it was thought that scientifically designed formulas could improve on breast milk. By the 1970s, scientific evidence had demonstrated the superiority of breast-feeding in several ways, even in our advanced industrial society.

First, the composition of human milk differs significantly from that of cow's milk or formula. Cow's milk has much more protein, and its protein is entirely casein, while human milk has about equal amounts of casein and whey protein. Whey protein appears to be more readily absorbed in the gastrointestinal tract, and also has larger concentrations of certain sulfur-containing amino acids that may be essential to infants. Human milk also contains twice as much vitamin C.

Second, although cow's milk also has antibodies (immunoglobulins), they are predominantly of the IgG—immunoglobulin G—category, be-cause cows do not transfer IgG to their fetuses via the placenta during gestation. Humans do transfer to their fetuses IgG *in utero*, so this component of immunity against viruses, bacteria, and fungi is less needed in milk. Human milk has much higher concentrations of IgA, which human infants have greater need of, and which acts to protect the lining of the gut against invading microbes. Also, to the extent that the IgA antibodies are specific to germs both the mother and infant have been exposed to, this specificity gives mother's milk a much greater advantage. Finally, the cellular component of immunity—the macrophages that make milk actually a living tissue—are found in human milk only, since those in cow's milk are killed in the process of pasteurization.

Less well understood but also important is the fact that breast-fed infants seem to be less susceptible to food allergies than are bottle-fed infants. Components of the more foreign cow's milk or formula apparently sensitize some infants and promote complex allergic reactions. In any case, breast-fed infants do have fewer allergies.

Is there a role for breast-feeding as a contraceptive in the modern setting? The answer must be a qualified yes—that is, yes in conjunction with other methods of contraception. Since all methods of contraception are imperfect, breast-feeding in addition to some other approaches will increase their overall effectiveness. The physiological role of breast-feeding has been studied in middle-class Western women (in Boston and in Edinburgh, among other places), and there is no doubt that the contraceptive effect of breast-feeding, even in well-nourished modern women, is real. However, a meaningful effect probably depends on a fairly intensive program of breast-feeding: breast-feeding at least once every two hours; continued night feeds; and limited supplementation for the first six months of life. In any case, present knowledge does not permit a firm specification.

The psychological issues surrounding breast-feeding in our society remain controversial. Many studies have been done on the psychological development of infants who are breast-fed and bottle-fed, and they are inconclusive. This may be partly because the frequency and duration of breast-feeding in these studies are so limited when compared to the same occurrence in hunting and gathering societies. But some recent studies of the more intensive nursing practiced by women in La Leche League also failed to show a major psychological impact.

What can be said with some confidence now is that fears of *bad* results of such practices are unfounded, and women should not be discouraged from highly intensive and prolonged breast-feeding if they are inclined in that direction. Many pediatricians recommend supplements of vitamin D, fluoride, and iron, and believe that breast milk should not be the exclusive food for infants after six months of age. Ideally, any infant feeding program, especially an unconventional one, should be carried out in consultation with a pediatrician.

In principle, all mothers should try to breast-feed if they can. But

what about the woman who simply doesn't want to? There is no scientific basis for insisting that she go against her inclinations. In extreme
cases, an unwilling mother can damage her psychological relationship
with her infant instead of enhancing it. Moreover, bottle-feeding can
become the center of a mother-infant relationship that is just as tender
and loving as any centered on breast-feeding. Changes in our culture
with respect to the roles of women and men must be taken into account
as well. The woman who needs to work while her child is young—an
increasingly common and probably now-prevailing pattern—may find
it impossible to breast-feed as she would like. Also, the father may feel
that he too should play a role in infant feeding—an impossibility if the
child is exclusively breast-fed. (Expressing breast milk into a bottle for
his use is an interesting compromise; it gives him his chance for a close
feeding relationship with the baby, while continuing to provide all the
physiological advantages of breast-feeding.)

None of this invalidates the basic recommendation of the American
Academy of Pediatrics that all women should try to breast-feed if possible, nor does it sweep aside its proven advantages as discussed above.
Nevertheless, breast-feeding should not be thought of as primarily a
burden. As more and more mothers who persist in breast-feeding are
discovering, it can be a profoundly rewarding experience for a woman,
both physically and psychologically, especially after the common initial
difficulties are overcome.

CLOSENESS AND DEPENDENCY

A key feature of the care of infants and young children among hunters
and gatherers is already apparent from the discussion of breast-feeding.
Proximity between mother and infant, including close physical contact,
is the rule, and the infant's dependent needs or even mere demands
are routinely indulged. The !Kung San have been more carefully studied
with regard to this pattern than any other hunting and gathering group.
Young infants are in physical contact—contact, not just proximity—with
someone (usually the mother) for at least 90 percent of the time during
the first few months of life, and this declines only gradually to around
25 percent in the middle of the second year. This is direct skin-to-skin
contact with the physical warmth and stimulation that implies. Infants
and young children sleep on a mat beside the mother (the equivalent
of sleeping in the same bed), with the father usually also nearby, at
least until they are weaned at age three or four.

Crying in infancy and early childhood is not considered a symptom
of "spoiling" or any other negative psychological condition, but simply
a condition of infancy. In the words of one !Kung San woman, con-

fronted with Dr. Spock's recommendation that a baby who frequently cries to be picked up must be put through a process of "unspoiling," "Doesn't he realize she's only a baby and that's why she cries? She has no sense yet, so you have to pick her up. Later, when she's older, she'll have sense, and she won't cry any more."

This aptly expresses the !Kung San theory of child development: You can't rush it; they go through stages, and you have to respond promptly to their dependent needs because it would be wrong not to—a form of child abuse or neglect. The common American practice of letting the baby "cry it out" is quite abhorrent to them. Measured objectively, they respond to infant crying within an average of six seconds. They pride themselves on anticipating an infant's needs before crying begins. For example, they are usually successful in anticipating when the baby is about to urinate or defecate, and they take the baby out of its carrying sling for that purpose. Even aggressive acts by the young child are indulged—hitting the mother with a stick, for example—on the grounds that this is just another phase. Of neighboring herding people who are less indulgent and more strict, they say: "They don't like children."

So much for the !Kung San of the Kalahari. But to what extent does this apply to other hunting and gathering groups, or for that matter to other types of preindustrial societies?

The pattern of physical closeness, like the pattern of intensive prolonged breast-feeding, appears to be very general. More or less constant carrying of the infant in a sling or pouch at the mother's side or back is characteristic of hunters and gatherers in widely separated geographic regions, including the Pygmies of Zaire, the Siriono of the Amazon Basin, the Paliyans of the Indian peninsula, the Yahgan of Tierra del Fuego, the sub-Arctic and Arctic Eskimo, and the Australian Aborigines. Among the Aché of Paraguay the pattern of mother-infant contact is even more intense than that of the !Kung. It has been established by cross-cultural analysis that nearly all preindustrial people living in warm climates (whether hunters and gatherers or not) tend to have carrying devices that keep them in direct physical contact with their infants. Since the great majority of human evolution took place in warm climates, this finding increases the likelihood that our ancestors had close mother-infant physical contact. But even cold-climate hunters and gatherers such as the Eskimo and the Yahgan have close contact, suggesting the pattern is characteristic of hunters and gatherers regardless of temperature. Among the Eskimo, for example, the woman's parka was cut larger than the man's so that an infant could fit inside it, and infants rode naked except for their caps most of the time, in a hide sling on the mother's naked back.

What about sleeping proximity? This too has been carefully studied in cross-cultural surveys. Close mother-infant proximity is the rule, not the exception. In a study of ninety preindustrial societies for which information was available in regard to sleeping distance, 46 percent had mother and infant sleeping in the same bed, as with the !Kung San; 33 percent had mother and infant sleeping in the same room, but did not specify whether they were in the same or in separate beds; and 21 percent had mother and infant sleeping in the same room but in separate beds. There was no society in which mother and infant slept in separate rooms, even in societies with multiroom dwellings; this appears to be an innovation of recent European society.

This may in part be related to space availability. But at least one study in the United States found that some working-class families with many rooms still keep infants in the same room with their mothers, while some professional-class families with tiny apartments often keep infants in a crib in the kitchen—just to insure that they have a separate room. Even traditional cultures with one-room houses do not have to keep their infants on the same bed or mat, as half or more of them do. And in any case, whatever the reason for the close sleeping arrangement, the infant's experience is the same. Thus the !Kung San pattern of mother-infant proximity—often even direct physical contact—is a widespread characteristic of hunting and gathering and to a lesser extent other traditional societies, and was consequently almost certainly the pattern followed by our Paleolithic ancestors.

It is not difficult to see why, considering our evolutionary background. Intensive maternal care of the young was not invented by mammals, but it was one of the evolutionary hallmarks of these warm-blooded creatures. By the time our closest relatives, the higher primates, appeared, this pattern had been refined to an exquisite degree. Every known species of monkey or ape without exception has round-the-clock mother-infant physical contact or close proximity, with the time in contact declining only gradually as the infant becomes more independent. This is most likely attributable to the fact that an infant alone in the wild is immediately vulnerable to predation. Scientists studying monkeys in their natural habitats have observed infants taken by hawks and snakes, and this would have been a constant evolutionary force promoting the success of mothers (and, in some species, fathers) and infants who maintained close contact. Against this background, the widespread characteristic parent-infant closeness in the fundamental human adaptation seems easy to understand.

Although the indulgence of dependency (other than breast-feeding) is more difficult to investigate, that too seems to be a pattern widespread among hunters and gatherers. Using a large compendium of cross-cultural data known as Textor's Cross-Cultural Summary, it is possible to show how different types of societies view this issue, according to the descriptions of the ethnographers who have studied them. The results? Simpler societies have more indulgent infant- and child-care practices than do more complex ones. To take the comparison between foraging societies and other nonindustrial societies as an example, the amount of pain inflicted on the infant (through customary scarification, circumcision, and other practices) was found to be less among foragers; the amount of overall indulgence—responsiveness to infant demands— found to be greater; the severity of toilet training less; and the child's anxiety over responsible, obedient, and self-reliant behavior less in each case among foragers.

A more intensive study comparing 10 tropical hunting and gathering societies with 176 other nonindustrial societies was carried out by two pediatricians also interested in what hunting and gathering baby and child care has to tell us about our own practices. Their data confirmed that very close mother-infant contact, late weaning, and indulgent responsiveness to infant crying were more characteristic of hunting and gathering societies than they were of other nonindustrial ones.

The same authors went on to compare the 176 nonindustrial nonforaging societies with ourselves. Despite the fact that these societies were less indulgent of infant dependency and had less close mother-infant contact than did the 10 tropical hunting and gathering societies, they still had more of both than we do. Whether measured by body contact, sleeping distance, response to crying, or weaning age, mother-infant contact and maternal indulgence of infants appeared to be less in the United States than in the broad cross-cultural range. This finding supports the much older finding of anthropologist John Whiting, who in a 1953 study with Irvin Child, reported that patterns of infant and child care in the middle class of Chicago during the 1940s were substantially less indulgent than comparable patterns in a large representative sample of nonindustrial societies (including some hunters and gatherers). Except, that is, in the area of aggressiveness, where the Chicagoans were more permissive. In other words, in the areas of feeding, toilet training, sex and modesty training, and independence training, children were placed under more pressure to conform to pre-set standards in Chicago than in the wide range of nonindustrial societies. Only in the area of children's aggressiveness were the Chicagoans less strict.

Two conclusions seem reasonable. First, that hunters and gatherers are more indulgent of infant needs and demands than are other types of nonindustrial societies, and second, that (although those *other* societies exhibit a great deal of variation) they tend to be less strict with infants and children and more responsive to them than we are. This finding repeats the previous observations regarding the intensity and length of breast-feeding and the amount of mother-infant physical contact and proximity. Overall, then, we can infer that during most of the Paleolithic our early human ancestors extended the patterns of our higher primate ancestors in mother-child relations—patterns that almost certainly go back not only millions but tens of millions of years.

LEARNING AND PLAY

Clearly, learning is one of the hallmarks of our species, and the extensive amount of information transferred from generation to generation in the form of culture provides one of the greatest distinctions between ourselves and other species. Many animals have rudimentary traditions that can be called cultural—for example, the song of the white-crowned sparrow and the termite-fishing of chimpanzees—but these are trivial compared with the vast body of culturally learned behavior and information passed on by humans.

But how does this information transfer take place? In human societies as in other species, there are essentially three methods: observational learning, teaching, and play. Observational learning is technically defined as improvement in the rate of learning as a result of watching members of the same species doing a task to be learned—in plain English, speeding up learning by watching. This kind of learning has been studied in the field and in the laboratory for many mammals. In herbivorous mammals—especially those whose infants follow them or are carried around by them, including most higher primates—observation leads to information about food sources and methods of food extraction. Such information transfer is clearly one of the adaptive functions of the mother-child bond in humans (as well as in other higher primates).

By observing their mothers and imitating them, infants among hunters and gatherers acquire the rudiments of digging for roots, cracking nuts, and grinding with a mortar and pestle by the end of the second year of life. As they grow older, children spend more time observing these and various other subsistence activities. They often go on gathering expeditions with their mothers and gradually absorb the details of distribution and extraction of vegetable foods in a complex environment. Girls usually have more exposure to this than boys, but it is essential information for both sexes; hunters rely on gathered vegetable foods to sustain them while they locate their prey, and often bring bush foods back with them if a hunt is unsuccessful.

Such learning includes little or no formal teaching. Nonhuman primates do very little teaching, but carnivores do quite a lot, especially in relation to hunting. This may have some relevance in understanding the evolution of teaching in human society. For example, lion and tiger mothers must do a substantial amount of teaching in order to transmit hunting skills. These and other feline mothers bring back half-dead prey, which their young then kill and eat; they lead cubs and kittens on expeditions whose main purpose seems to be acquainting the young with stalking; and they partially kill prey on the hunt, leaving the young to finish it off (but intervening when the prey shows signs of escaping).

However, unlike hunting cats, human hunters have an important additional teaching tool: language. Much teaching about hunting occurs in the form of storytelling and answering questions. The kind of teaching engaged in by felines occurs to a limited degree among humans, but usually only during adolescence. Before then, boys have already learned a great deal by watching, asking questions, and playing.

Play—behavior that appears to be enjoyable and has no obvious survival purpose—is very widespread among birds and mammals. Studies by animal behaviorists report that play affords the young creature exercise, helps it acquire information about its environment and about other animals, and sharpens its subsistence and social skills. In some mammals, especially monkeys and apes, it is clear that depriving the young animal can seriously handicap its adult social and reproductive skills. We don't usually think of play as a form of learning, but deprivation studies, such as those done by Harry Harlow and his students on monkeys, show that it is highly essential—especially for basic social skills, sexual behavior, and parenting.

In this connection it cannot be coincidental that the most intelligent mammals—especially primates, carnivores, and whales and dolphins—are also the most playful. If an animal is short-lived, the young do not appear to play very much, probably because there is too little time for them to gain much knowledge or skill from playing. Domesticated Burmese elephants, in contrast, begin to learn lumbering at age five, but may retain their playful natures into their forties. In humans, with our long life span, slow growth, high intelligence, and extensive learning ability, one would expect to find that play serves a critical function during development. This is, of course, the case. In hunting and gathering societies, play is the main activity of children throughout their waking hours, in contrast to other types of societies in which chores and schooling occupy large amounts of children's time after the age of six. Also, for hunting and gathering societies, the period of middle childhood—ages six to twelve or so—is characterized by the encouragement of independence and self-reliance, but not of obedience or responsibility. Quantitative cross-cultural studies have shown that in herding and agricultural societies as well as in our own, obedient and responsible behavior tends to be expected of children during these middle years. (In the realm of training for nurturance, however, hunters and gatherers are comparable to other traditional societies.)

Most aspects of foraging life are served well by this pattern of childhood training. Bands move frequently, there is geographic variability in food availability, and the seasons make dramatically different demands on people. The virtues of self-reliance, initiative, and flexibility are at a premium—less than those of obedience, consistency, and responsibility. It is not difficult to see the relationship between those virtues and play, which encourages them even while it teaches and sharpens social and subsistence skills.

Among the Yahgan of Tierra del Fuego, for example, studied by Martin Gusinde, little formal teaching is done, and adults act as models and advisers to children. Independence usually begins with the arrival of a sibling, when the older child is about three years old. While still remaining close to his mother, he gradually switches over to more active exploratory play—with objects in the environment and with other children. At age four, a boy starts spending time helping his father and uncle, who steadily increase the difficulty of the demands they make on him. His only special toys are imitation weapons and tools. When several families join together, the boys play in groups. Their activities are quite raucous, much more rough and noisy than the girls' play, and they do a lot of exploring. They hunt for birds' nests, beetles, and larvae, catch fish with their hands, dig for clams, wrestle, sling stones at birds, and practice shooting at an old tree trunk with short spears and bows and arrows. From time to time adults will supervise such contests, commenting on each boy's performance.

Girls, meanwhile, from about age four, go gathering with the women, and begin imitating gathering techniques and household activities. They learn to range widely in the bush surrounding their village, and gain great sophistication in the knowledge of edible plants—their classification, desirability, and distribution in space and time. They come to feel at home in the bush even before they are fully grown, learning how to circumvent physical dangers in the environment and to avoid wild predators. Gusinde concludes, "The girl is brought up to do these things almost playfully and becomes so familiar with all of them that after a certain age she can in part replace her mother."

Bronislaw Malinowski, in describing the process in the Australian hunting and gathering tribes, emphasizes the adults' fondness for children and their extreme permissiveness. Fathers make toy weapons and tools and demonstrate their use, and they even delight in the nasty pranks their sons play with these "toys." Sons accompany their fathers on hunting expeditions and rapidly learn the facts about their hunting area. He concludes, "As there was no serious and real training during this time . . . all education, as far as it was given at all by the father, assumed more the form of play, and, during that period great leniency towards the offspring was the chief feature of the father's behavior."

Studies of specific Australian Aborigine groups confirm these generalizations. Among the Murngin, all kinds of imitative play were important in preparation for adulthood, and much of this was group play. Among the Walbiri,

> After the boy is aged five or six, he roams the bush with other lads, and his father sees little of him by day. Men spend much time cutting up damaged boomerangs to make throwing-sticks for their sons to use on these jaunts; and the boys display remarkable accuracy in killing small birds and lizards with the weapons. They now learn which flora and smaller fauna provide the best foods, they develop their tracking skills and acquire an intimate knowledge of the bush for ten miles or so around the camp. During this period, men take little part in educating or disciplining their sons, whose behavior towards them often reflects this lack of control.

Here again, heavy emphasis is laid on the educative function of group play. It is not until the boy approaches puberty that actual teaching begins—teaching of indigenous technology and fighting and hunting techniques.

Among the Eskimo of Nunivak Island (Alaska) studied by Margaret Lantis, a similar pattern prevails, but with less emphasis on group play:

> Nunivak children are conditioned to an aggressive predatory life from the time they can toddle. They desire immensely to kill animals, and they practice by using slingshot, bolas, and darts against birds, foxes, puppies, anything moving.

Among the Kaska Indians of the Yukon:

> There is an absence of authoritarian supervision such as would emphasize the child's humiliation and complete submission to his parents. Native education is also characterized by this lack of authori-

tarianism; little effort is made to specifically direct . . . children are left to work out their own answers to problems.

Among the Mbuti Pygmies,

Beginning at age four children play games, sometimes with adults, in imitation of hunting and gathering activities. They are taught by a youth or adult to make miniature bows and arrows, carrying baskets, etc. By the age of six they are contributing to the economy. Any food they get themselves is cooked and eaten at a "play house."

Finally, of the !Kung San, Lorna Marshall wrote more than twenty years ago,

In their parents' presence the children imitate adult activities in vital, active ways, very exciting to watch, and participate in actual work as they are able. The adults pause to show them how to hold a digging stick, or a toy bow or drill, so that play and learning merge.

Subsequent studies have confirmed and extended this characterization. In a quantitative study of middle childhood among the !Kung San, Patricia Draper tested within one society the hypothesis that had been tested by Barry, Child, and Bacon among different societies. She found that as the !Kung became more settled, kept more goats, and hunted and gathered less, they began to demand more obedience and responsibility from their children, whereas the laissez-faire attitude of the traditional hunting and gathering culture persisted in those groups of !Kung that did not settle down and adopt goatherding as a way of life.

In our own society we require formalized schooling to instill efficiently a large amount of skill and information. But in recent decades there has been increasing realization that learning may be facilitated by a more relaxed rather than a stricter school environment. This trend is certainly consistent with the learning patterns of our ancestors. So is the emphasis on learning social skills through play, especially in the early years; and so is the increasing emphasis on sports for all children, girls as well as boys.

Sexual experimentation is also a hallmark of most hunting and gathering societies. !Kung children become aware of sex because it is almost impossible for adults to be completely secretive about their sexual activities. Children become curious and try things out among themselves during play. Sexual experimentation is done in a playful spirit, long before the age of puberty, and is often part of a larger pattern of "playing house," which involves actual gathering, preparation, and consumption of wild plant foods.

This underscores a general point: The skills that need to be enhanced through play are not just cognitive and physical; they are also social and emotional. The primate studies of Harry Harlow and his students provide a fascinating parallel. Monkeys, deprived during the equivalent of their middle childhood of the opportunity to play with other young monkeys (even though they have normal access to their mothers), grow up with inept sexual behavior (which obviously would be a decisive handicap to reproductive success in the wild). Since the play of young monkeys includes behavior resembling sexual mounting, it is possible that this skill requires such practice. More likely, however, is that the monkeys growing up without free social and physical play with their peers fail to develop the emotional responses that will make them comfortable with the social aspects, as well as the inherent playfulness, of normal sexuality. The suggestion, of course, is that something similar is true in human development—that play with peers, even rudimentary sexual play, is necessary for normal development, not only in monkeys but also in humans.

In our society encouraging early sexual experimentation would certainly be controversial. For centuries, religious prohibitions have banned such behavior, and, in any case, most parents do not want their children to become sexually active too early. The birth of a first child is a watershed in a human life and ideally it should occur after, not before, formal schooling or job training is completed. But even if effective birth control were guaranteed, the rising tide of sexually transmitted diseases—especially the specter of AIDS—will likely reverse our decades-long trend toward leniency in sexual and modesty training. These new concerns may require that we teach our children to be wary of sex, but we shouldn't confuse the pragmatic need for sexual restriction with the underlying psychological reality. A free and playful attitude toward sexuality during childhood is our ancestral heritage and may be most compatible with optimal psychological development.

To summarize, play and learning are almost inseparable concepts in the childhood of hunters and gatherers. Learning by observing plays a critical role in imitative behaviors, but as we will see in the next section, this learning does not usually have to be from observation of adults, especially during the middle-childhood phase of learning. In our own society, some recent encouraging trends in education reflect these Paleolithic principles. We may think of the trends as modern, but actually they are as old as our species, and take us back toward the learning patterns of our hunting and gathering ancestors.

THE STRUCTURE AND FUNCTION
OF CHILDREN'S GROUPS

Most of us think of children's play groups as *peer groups*—groups of children the same age who play together because of common interests. But it can be shown that peer groups in this sense were extremely unlikely among our ancestors because of demographic considerations. Typical band size is thirty members for hunters and gatherers of all types in a wide range of environments. Taking the !Kung San as an example, the proportion of women between first birth (nineteen and a half) and the end of the reproductive period (about forty-five) is 40 percent, or six women in each band of thirty people.

Even with an average birth spacing of four years and infant mortality of 20 percent, the chance of any child's having one same-age peer in the band at a year of age is quite high. However, the chance of having two peers is only about 20 percent, and the chance of having three is only 5 percent. Thus, for purely demographic reasons, same-age peer groups were likely to have been rare in the world of our remote ancestors.

For the !Kung San, multi-age play groups are ubiquitous. Made up mostly of siblings and cousins, the play group may consist of six or eight children of both sexes ranging in age from late infancy to adolescence, or there may be two or three smaller groups of children closer in age. Infants begin to participate from the time they can walk, and the sight of a toddler edging away from his mother to throw himself on a pile of wrestling two- to five-year-olds is not uncommon. Two-year-olds who are better walkers will follow the group around and, if they wander from the camp, will be carried by one of the older children when they tire.

The principal activity of the group is always play, though this may and typically does include (1) observation of adult subsistence activity; (2) play at subsistence, which may produce food; (3) "pretend" subsistence, which does not produce actual food but assumes some semblance of adult subsistence; (4) rough and tumble play; and (5) sex play. It also includes protection and care and teaching of infants and children by older children. There is no child nurse comparable to that found in middle-level agricultural societies—that is, children are not *assigned* to take care of infants—and mothers are always within shouting (or crying) distance, receptive to infant needs. But there is care, protection, and teaching nonetheless, and of course, older children are learning infant and child care. These relations arise from the older children's own volition, partly because they too have few or no peers.

Are the !Kung San representative of hunters and gatherers in general? What happened after hunting and gathering life was replaced by agriculture? Both questions can be approached by referring to the cross-cultural record. One study that attempted to do this analyzed infant and child care in 182 different societies. As expected, a wide range of practices was found. However, two interesting patterns did emerge. First, intermediate-level societies (nonhunting-and-gathering and non-industrial) were more likely to have people other than the mother take care of the young child than were hunters and gatherers. And second, older children were more likely to be assigned the task of caretaker. The child nurse, as this institution is called, is typical of many agricultural societies in which women's work load is heavy. It is, however, quite different from the care offered infants by older children among hunters and gatherers, in that the mother is farther away and the child nurse has more responsibility for longer stretches of time.

The age composition of play groups was less well-documented in the same sample, but it was clear that same-age peer groups only appear in intermediate-level societies. (Significantly, multi-age play groups often continue to exist even in societies in which same-age groups could be formed.) Good data are available only for adolescence, but these show that societies that hunt and gather, that have no social classes, or that have population units smaller than 1,500 are significantly less likely to have peer groups in adolescence than are more complex societies. Formal associations of adolescent males, however, occur more frequently in societies that place a high emphasis on military glory—such as martial prowess, heroism, and death in battle. These peer groups function to separate boys from girls and women, and from their identification with women, the better to make them warriors.

In our culture, same-age peer groups are ubiquitous, both in and out of school and at all ages, including infancy. We seem to believe that it is best for children to be with other children their own age, a belief also held in some agricultural societies. Same-age peer groups probably promote more efficiency in the learning of competition strategies, and may even be indispensable in a society in which competition is so central. Nevertheless, it may be useful to consider how much we may be losing in giving up the special adaptive functions of multi-age child groups.

How does an infant come to have relationships with other children? Several laboratory investigations of human infants and toddlers arrived, by different routes, at the same conclusion: that developmental events that take place during the second year of life make possible a quantum advance in the infant's ability to interact with peers. But this idea of how relations with others develop may be an artificial result of the way modern people structure children's play. !Kung San infants develop the ability to interact with children of various ages (and various degrees of responsiveness) much earlier—throughout the first year. During the second year, they are gradually exposed to increasingly younger children—those less and less like adults in their responsiveness.

Some psychological studies have focused on the effects of varying age composition on the patterns of children's interactions. One study found that, in mixed-age groups, children spend more time with each other and less time in solitary play, that younger children accept instruction more easily from older ones if there is a four-year rather than a two-year age difference, and that the social activity of three-year-old children is more mature when five-year-olds are present. However, five-year-old behavior became less mature in this context, reflecting the concern of many parents that their children may be adversely affected by play with younger children.

Before accepting this hypothesis, let us examine the concept of maturity of social activity more carefully. For example, if a five-year-old is playing with a three-year-old, and in a helping or teaching role, how meaningful is it to suggest that they are playing at the same level of maturity? Most people with experience in nonindustrial societies are struck by the relative aplomb with which young people face parenthood. Surely the greater degree of previous experience in taking care of younger children helps to prepare them. At the same time, this arrangement also benefits the younger child; it may help to explain why, in some African societies, the youngest child in the family ends up performing adult tasks with greater skill than the older—the reverse of the pattern usually found in industrial societies.

In this context we can begin to understand the strange forms of social behavior known in the nursery as "parallel play" and "collective monologue." Infants and toddlers may be inept in relating to each other, in part, because they were rarely called upon to do so during millions of years of evolution; consequently they could not have been selected for an ability to do this. They may, instead, have been selected for dependence (in order to develop normally) on the input from a multi-aged child group. Even at the other end of childhood it works: Adolescents who are in close contact with younger children seem to be less aggressive even as they gain crucial experience that will serve them well in their coming role as parents.

ADOLESCENCE AND SEXUAL MATURATION

Years before the average American parent became alarmed about sexually transmitted diseases, changing sexual mores had led to another serious problem: a rise in teenage, especially school-age, pregnancy and parenthood. Today's adolescents have been exposed to a much more liberal set of standards than was the case for adolescents thirty years ago, whether the measures involve transmission of knowledge, entertainment media, adult models, peer pressure, or rules and restrictions governing their own behavior. It seems logical to account for the increasing proportion of adolescent pregnancies mainly by reference to this cultural change.

But this logic runs aground against at least some anthropological experience, which suggests that liberal premarital sexual mores, however new they may be for us, are not new for a large proportion of the cultures of the ethnological record and that, contrary to what may seem obvious, liberal sexual mores and even active sexual lives among preagricultural adolescents are not necessarily associated with pregnancies. In one study using the Standard Cross-Cultural Sample of the Human Relations Area Files, anthropologists rated twenty sexual practices and attitudes toward sex, including premarital sex, in a wide range of traditional societies. It was possible to rate 107 societies on frequency of premarital sex for males; of these, premarital sex was universal or almost universal in 60 percent, moderate or not uncommon in 18 percent, occasional in 10 percent, and uncommon in 12 percent. For females (rated in 114 societies), the corresponding percentages were 49, 17, 14, and 20.

It was also possible to rate 141 societies on attitudes toward premarital sex, as explicitly expressed in the cultural norms. Premarital sex is rated as "expected, approved—virginity has no value" in 24 percent; "tolerated—accepted if discreet" in 21 percent; and "mildly disapproved—pressure toward chastity but transgressions are not punished and nonvirginity ignored" in 17 percent. The cumulative percentage of these three more lenient categories is 62 percent, with the stricter, more disapproving categories making up the remainder.

Since most of these societies do not place much emphasis on chronological age, many not even keeping track of it, it is not possible to separate premarital sex or attitudes toward it with regard to age. However, it is clear from much of the ethnographic material that teenagers are among the main targets of these strictures, or the lack of them.

It thus appears that our much-discussed liberal shift in mores regarding premarital sex during the past twenty-five years has put the more liberal sector of our population in a category that includes at least 60 percent of the traditional societies in the ethnological record. Yet there is not widespread occurrence of early teenage pregnancies in these societies, as there is in ours.

For example, the cultural atmosphere with regard to sex among the traditional !Kung San was at least as open and liberal as that in the United States during the past few years, yet early teenage pregnancy was unknown and at least half of all women who had children had their first child after age 19. The demographic facts of !Kung life, compiled by Nancy Howell, address this apparent contradiction. She found that !Kung girls menstruate for the first time, on average, at age 16.5, also the average age of first marriage. First birth occurs a few years later, at about age 19. Over a lifetime a !Kung woman will give birth to an average of five children, and will bear her last child in her mid-30s. The situation in other hunting and gathering societies, such as the Agta and the Aché, is similar. (See Table XIX.)

How do these data fit with !Kung cultural practices? Experimentation with sex starts quite early, beginning in early childhood and continuing through middle childhood without the interruption familiar in our society (and in psychoanalytic theory) called the "latency period." Children do not assume responsibility for subsistence until their late teens, and play groups are frequently out of sight of adults; sexual awareness and curiosity flourish in the unrestricted time that comprises most of their day. Adults do not actually approve of sexual play and if it becomes obvious, they make some effort to discourage it. But these efforts are half-hearted—on the order of verbal chastisements with no real or threatened consequences—and do little to ensure that it will not recur. Interviews with adults reveal that they consider sexual experimentation

---

TABLE XIX.

Reproductive Milestones Among Hunting and Gathering Women

	Agta (Philippines)	!Kung (Botswana)	Ache (Paraguay)	Average
Menarche	17.1	16.6	14.3	16
First live birth	20.1	19.9	18.5	19.5
Menarche to first birth	3 yrs.	3.4 yrs.	4.2 yrs.	3.5 yrs.
Birth spacing	3.05 yrs.	4.1 yrs.	3.2 yrs.	3.45 yrs.

in childhood and adolescence to be inevitable, even healthy. Certainly for adults sexual activity is considered essential for mental health, and they often referred to mentally ill people (for example, a woman who ate grass) as having suffered derangement because of sexual deprivation.

For the growing child among the !Kung, as opposed to among ourselves, sex becomes less taboo, less frightening, and less unknown. However, despite childhood sexual experimentation, the transition from the playful sex of childhood to the real sex of adulthood is sometimes difficult, especially for girls. This is probably because girls are married young (half, before first menstruation at age 16.5) to men typically about ten years older than themselves. Thus a teenage girl is confronted with the sexual expectations of an adult man after having had prior experience only with boys. Although in principle sexual advances are delayed until her menarche, the transition from casual sex play with age-mates to adult sex with a husband is stressful for many.

The !Kung present a picture of adolescent sexuality that may be different from conventional assumptions about such societies. Children do have active sexual lives from an early age, and restrictions on sexual relations are few. However, they have a late age of first menstruation, a presumed period of adolescent subfertility, and some contribution from miscarriage that result in a mean age at first live birth of just under 20. Even the kinship system shares responsibility and provides extensive economic and psychological support, diminishing only gradually as the young woman reaches her mid-20s and her family grows.

A broader cross-cultural and historical view presents the spectrum of variation against which we can assess both the modern American and the !Kung San cases. Evidence that the age at first menstruation, or menarche, has been dropping in the United States and Europe for more than a century, has been repeatedly summarized. There is disagreement about the magnitude of this phenomenon, about its cross-national variability, and about whether and where it may be continuing, but there is general agreement that the phenomenon is real. A very conservative estimate would be that the age of menarche has declined two years since the early nineteenth century, and estimates as high as between four and five years have been presented.

This long-term trend in earlier maturation—also called the secular trend—has been well documented not only for age at menarche but for the general rate at which youngsters grow and the height and weight they eventually attain. For example, the age of the girl at the time she reaches five feet in height has decreased at about the same rate as the age that she menstruates for the first time—namely four months per decade. This is of particular significance, since studies of age at menarche are subject to skeptical challenges that do not apply to studies of height.

The long-term trend toward earlier maturation appears to have stopped in some populations, notably Oslo, Norway (where the earliest historical data come from), London, England, and among some Americans at Harvard and eastern women's colleges. The trend is continuing in other populations, however, especially in the underdeveloped world, where menarche may still come later than age 13. In northern Europe, it appears to have stabilized at just about 13 years and in New England at a slightly younger age. For example, girls in Newton, Massachusetts, menstruated for the first time at 12.7 years, no earlier than the menarcheal age of their mothers. In New England families that had been well-to-do the longest, the acceleration of growth apparently ended early in the twentieth century. It now seems possible, despite some exceptions, that the mean age at menarche may not drop much below 12.5 to 13 years anywhere in the world, and that this may be a basic biological lower limit for this milestone in our species. Still, conservatively estimated, there has been a 2- or 3-year decline in northern Europe over a period of 150 years. In our population menarche at age 8 or 9 and pregnancy at age 10 or 11 can no longer be considered to reflect hormonal pathology, as they certainly would have at the turn of the century. More reliable measures of growth, such as height and weight, show a similar acceleration.

The reasons for the growth acceleration are not agreed upon. Demographer Rose Frisch has accumulated evidence that nutritional changes have led to increases in fatness at each age, which in turn lead to earlier menarche through the production of physiologically potent estrogens in fat cells. (The effect of intense and prolonged exercise training in reducing fat ratios has been well demonstrated in studies of young dancers and athletes, who sometimes overtrain to the point where menstruation ceases, possibly because of endocrinological stress.) Other explanations of change in the age at menarche have been advanced, including improved public health and medical care in controlling chronic diseases of childhood, changes in environmental lighting, increased consumption of refined carbohydrates, increased stimulation during infancy, and genetic changes resulting from outbreeding or natural selection. Urban living is definitely associated with earlier maturation, an effect that has been shown throughout the world, but the meaning of this association is difficult to determine, since urbanization is accompanied by changes in most or all of the other, more specific, proposed causes. It is likely that the specification of determinants of the secular trend will await a better understanding of the onset of puberty, a field with many unexpected and puzzling findings.

There is also a period of "adolescent sterility," more properly called adolescent subfertility. The erratic quality of menstrual cycles during the first year or more after menarche has been repeatedly documented. Thus it is not surprising that the first fertile cycle lags behind menarche by a year or more in many populations, and that this lag is longer in underdeveloped countries.

Historical demographers have provided a separate body of evidence on adolescent fertility that also takes into account changing patterns of marriage and mores. Through study of church, family, and other records, the lateness of first childbearing in Europe, England, and the United States during the sixteenth to nineteenth centuries has been shown. The frequently cited case of Shakespeare's Juliet, whose nurse chides her for not marrying and becoming pregnant by age 13 (as Juliet's mother allegedly had done) is carefully considered by social historian Peter Laslett. His discussion shows that the nurse was a poor historical demographer, since such a case would have been exceedingly rare in either Juliet's Italy or Shakespeare's England. (Actually, as Laslett also shows, Juliet's age in Shakespeare's source for the play was 18. The change probably gives the play much of its urgency and poignancy, but it makes the nurse's impatience quite unrealistic.)

For the United States, Philips Cutright has reviewed the history of illegitimacy during the twentieth century. He shows that there have been increases in the rate of teenage childbearing at least since 1940, and attempts to explain these increases in part by reference to the long-range trend toward earlier menarche. He refers specifically to "the myth of an abstinent past," the thrust of this myth being that, because teenagers at the turn of the century had few pregnancies, they must have obeyed their society's much greater strictures against sex. He presents the contrasting view that they were in fact more active sexually than we imagine them to have been, but did not become pregnant because they were reproductively immature.

One hundred fifty years ago, a young woman menstruating at age 15 and becoming a mother by age 18 could take her place as an adult in a relatively uncomplicated society designed to support her in every way through firm institutions of marriage and family. Today, a girl menstruating at age 12 and becoming a mother by age 15, often unmarried and likely to remain so, is only a schoolchild at sea in a grown-up world that is much more complex and unforgiving. Even if all systems of physical maturation have accelerated, so that today's 15-year-old has the body and even the brain of the 18-year-old of the past, there is no way for her to compensate for the three years of lost experience, or to struggle successfully in a complex society in which maturity, education, and experience are increasingly valued. Whatever the causes, it seems reasonable to judge the trend toward earlier physical and sexual maturation to be one of the most profound changes in the biology of the species in recorded history, with what would seem to be important implications for adolescent psychology, education, and law.

Many expect moral restraint from teenagers, reasoning—not illogically—that loose morals explain teenage pregnancy. But seen against the background of the ethnological record, it is clear that most societies traditionally have not had such expectations. Equally important, it must be seen in the context of a different reality, one that is now part of the past—a reality in which late maturation and late fertility combined to prevent teenage pregnancy (and certainly early teenage pregnancy) with or without active moral restraint.

Infancy and adolescence are probably two of the most sensitive periods of human growth. An early teenage pregnancy brought to term thus affects two growing children, one in each of the sensitive periods. Fetuses and infants are resilient, but only within limits, and it is doubtful whether a young teenager can provide the environment necessary for optimal development, even under conditions of optimal support and care for the mother. Young teenage mothers, for their part, are completing the most rapid period of growth they have experienced since their own infancy, and are in hormonal, psychological, and social turmoil that centers on their approach to adulthood. To bring a baby into this turmoil is often to pit two children against each other, children with needs that may be incompatible.

Under the circumstances it is perhaps not too strong to say that to withhold information about contraception from a young teenager who may be sexually active may in itself be a form of child abuse. Added now to the risk of untimely pregnancy there is, in the context of the developing AIDS epidemic, a risk of death. Whatever our opinions of the complex moral issues of contraception and therapeutic abortion, our decisions could be made with a larger measure of compassion for the plight of today's teenager, caught between a precociously mature body and less mature, inexperienced emotions.

Numerous other changes have taken place in the behavior of young teenagers in parallel with the increase in their sexual activity. These include a rise in school-age suicide, school-age alcoholism, and school-age substance abuse. Despite the great complexity of the causes—no doubt mostly cultural—of these trends, they must be understood against the background of the prior long-term change in the rate of maturation. The ultimate and perhaps very general implications of these phenomena—for adolescence specifically and for our society more widely—are only beginning to be explored.

SUMMARY: CHILDHOOD AMONG HUNTERS AND GATHERERS

Generalizations about child-training choices are much more difficult than those about diet and health or even exercise and health. The sciences of child development—whether developmental pediatrics, child psychiatry, developmental psychology, or education—have not reached as exact a state as the "harder" medical and physiological sciences. Nevertheless, it is possible to make valid generalizations about the likely practices of our hunting and gathering ancestors, based on the method of examining hunting and gathering societies, as well as other non-industrial societies, where traditional folkways have survived into the twentieth century. These generalizations can then be held up to the light of modern medical and psychological research, just as we have done for diet and exercise in prior chapters. The following principles emerge.

1. The Paleolithic approach supports the recommendation of the American Academy of Pediatrics that all infants be breast-fed; this was the only method of infant feeding available to our ancestors, and it continues to have advantages for us. It supplies the ideal nutritional components during the early months, provides protection against infection, protects against allergic responses, and offers both physical and psychological warmth that helps promote the relationship between mother and child. Emotional benefits may also result for the mother, and an imperfect but significant added protection against conception can result as well. However, breast-feeding should be supplemented by other foods beginning no later than six months of age. It must not be relied on as the only form of contraception at any time, but should be combined with barrier methods.

Every mother must do her own cost-benefit analysis of how often and how long to breast-feed, taking into account her work life, her other children if any, and her relationship to her husband. Breast-feeding is both the original and the ideal method of infant feeding. It can take time to get it working properly, but when it works, it is very rewarding. Doctrinaire attitudes about it can make it a burden for some women, but others, such as La Leche League members, may want to carry it even to hunting and gathering levels; and as long as they introduce supplementary feeding properly after six months of age, there is no scientific basis for discouraging them.

2. Closeness and dependency in infancy and early childhood are encouraged to a much greater extent among hunters and gatherers than among ourselves. This includes carrying babies in a sling or carrier most of the time, responding immediately to crying without any thought or concept of "spoiling," and sleeping together at night. Some psychological theorists have argued that this kind of treatment results in children being "tied to their mothers' apron strings" while others have claimed that it provides the best foundation for later independence. While it is not possible to support the latter claim with definitive research, the "spoiling" theory has received even less support. Strictness has little place in the care of *infants* at least in most current psychological and pediatric recommendations. Extreme closeness and indulgence of dependency comparable to that of our hunting and gathering ancestors cannot be carried out by all parents in our society, but a general increase in both can be said to be desirable. Finally, those parents who feel inclined to emulate the closeness and indulgence of our past should by no means be discouraged from doing so by health or educational professionals; they are merely returning to a more natural pattern once characteristic of most families.

3. After the end of the phase of early childhood a period of intensified learning takes place in all cultures. This middle-childhood period is heralded in our society by the onset of schooling with all its responsibilities, and in many agricultural and herding societies by the assignment of important chores. But among hunters and gatherers, it is a period in which a large amount of learning takes place *without* a significant increase in responsibility. This paradox is resolved by means of learning through play, a method of proven effectiveness which has increasingly influenced the thinking of educators in our own society.

Obviously not everything we need to transmit to our children in modern American society can be conveyed through loosely structured play sessions. But we should take the learning methods of our hunting and gathering ancestors into account when considering such options as self-paced learning, the "open classroom," extracurricular learning, and fun in learning. In reacting to certain children with special needs, especially hyperactive children, we should consider the fact that hyperactivity would have had a very different meaning, and possibly no meaning at all in the milder cases, in a hunting and gathering society in which learning is constantly and physically active. Furthermore, physical movement of the most strenuous sort was a daily part of the play of our ancestors' children. Although our own games and sports tend to be more organized and have a stronger component of competitiveness, they do emulate the ancestral level of physical activity for children. Whether through sports for both sexes and all ages or through strongly encouraged but less formal exertions on the playground, our children must be set firmly on the course of regular, vigorous exercise, and this cannot be begun too early. Here again, though, play and fun rather than discipline must be the guide.

Finally, the "latency period" described by Freud and still referred to by many psychologists—that is, a period of minimal sexual interest corresponding to middle childhood—does not really seem to exist among hunters and gatherers. Sexual play in childhood carries right through this period, so that the games of middle childhood gradually turn into more mature sexual activity in adolescence. These anthropological observations, as well as studies of laboratory monkeys, indicate that this is a healthy and effective way to learn about sexuality.

4. The groups among which hunting and gathering children play and learn are multi-aged child groups rather than peer groups in the strict sense since substantial numbers of same-aged children would have been a virtual demographic impossibility in small bands. Among the many advantages: a) transfer of information and skill from older to younger children, b) informal surveillance of younger by older children, resulting in experience in child caretaking for the latter as well as relief for adults, c) enhancement of the quality of child–child interactions for very young children, and d) reduction of both competition and physical aggression. For the same demographic reasons, such groups usually include both boys and girls, decreasing the opportunity for rigid gender-specific role learning.

Clearly, in our type of society—where the quintessential social act is comparing oneself to someone else—we value the opportunity for same-age peers to play and work together. It facilitates the process of competition and comparison and allows certain types of age-appropriate play to occur. But it is equally clear that we could find a better balance than we have now. Our usual current prejudice against multi-aged groups, and against pairs of children of different ages playing together, is an unfounded departure from our hunting and gathering past.

5. Finally, the process of sexual and reproductive maturation is now quite different from what it was during most of our past. The trend toward earlier physical maturation—a result of changes in nutrition, disease, exercise, and other factors—has resulted in faster development and earlier attainment of reproductive capability than in the past. The most conservative estimate places the age of first menstruation two years earlier now than it was a little over a century ago, and other

estimates place it four to five years earlier. The historical trend has a parallel in cross-cultural data. For the !Kung San, first menstruation occurred at an average age of sixteen and a half. Many other hunters and gatherers and other nonindustrial peoples had similar late ages of reproductive maturation.

This is the context in which we must understand the fact that hunting and gathering societies had very high levels of premarital sexual freedom compared with other nonindustrial societies or, until very recently, with ourselves. They were able to make a gradual transition from the sexual play of middle childhood to the actual sexual activity of adolescence without fear of pregnancy. Our modern society has introduced two new biological phenomena: the reality of early reproductive capacity resulting in early teenage pregnancy; and, in the last several years, a new and deadly sexually transmitted disease. We must adapt to these realities, but we should not deny that under the conditions of hunting and gathering society premarital sex, like childhood sex play, was ubiquitous. Even in a world whose realities require us to restrict adolescent sexual freedom, the knowledge that such restriction is relatively new may help us to present both sexuality and restrictions on sexuality to young people in a more meaningful and helpful way.

CHAPTER NINE
WOMAN THE GATHERER

As the last rays of sunlight recede from a small village-camp situated on the northernmost fringe of Africa's Kalahari Desert, Naukha appears—a !Kung San woman in her mid-twenties, slight of build. She walks toward an insubstantial-appearing thatched grass hut and drops the firewood she has just collected. After clearing the ashes, she makes a new fire, then begins preparing food for the evening meal. Her younger sister, Chuko, soon appears with her own firewood. Naukha calls to her.

"Hey, Chuko! My stomach will surely rumble tomorrow and my family will complain if all we have to eat are these worthless leftover scraps. Why don't we walk west of the acacia grove to the *tsin* bean flat when the sun first brushes through the grass? That way, we can also see whether the sour plums are ready to be picked."

"Naukha, eh . . . how come my older sister's words always make sense? My mouth watered today when I smelled the roasting *sha* roots. My mother-in-law had brought them back. When she sent little Gau over with some for me, they were so sweet! Those women really did well! Did you see them? The ends of their leather pouches barely tied closed." She pauses, then adds, "What about little Nai? Will she come with us?"

"If she stays behind and plays with the other children, I'll worry that she will cry. If I take her along, it will be harder for me to gather as much food as I want. I suppose I'll ask Mother to tempt her into staying."

Chuko laughs. "Just like last time. Mother tried, and other children even asked her to play. But she wasn't satisfied until you took her along. You had to carry Nai and the baby until we almost reached the flats. Only then was she willing to walk on her own. Eh, children really are something!"

"Just wait until your next baby comes along. Then we'll see who does all the laughing!"

With different names, environmental features, and foods, a conversation such as this could have taken place just as easily 40,000 years ago most anywhere in the world as it might have 10 years ago among the !Kung San of Botswana. In most places and in most times women in hunting and gathering societies have known the importance of their work. Their labor was pivotal in keeping their families healthy and thriving; their efforts as gatherers of wild plant foods—together with the equally necessary contribution of game animals hunted by men—provided the original human diet.

Why has gathering—an activity so central to the lives of our ancestors—never really captured the imagination of most Westerners? Perhaps, because, if we think about it at all, we probably conjure up images of unpleasant, dull, tedious, and backbreaking work. After all, how many of us actually eat foods from the wild, and for those of us who occasionally do, would we not perhaps feel just a little more secure if the foods came wrapped in packages with assurances of edibility? As delicious as uncultivated berries or other wild plants often are, how many of us can imagine that such a diet would keep us satisfied meal after meal after meal? Even in the current vegetables-are-your-friends climate that most of us have been brought up in, we still believe that, while vegetables *are* good for us, they are a distant second to meat, which is far better.

Second to meat. Is this a biological determinant or a cultural construction? Hunting has been, without question, central to human experience throughout time, attractive to the wealthy, to the poor, and to many other groups who have never had to hunt or gather for a living. Hunting, after all, has romance, the lure of the chase; it forges emotional connections between life and death, touching our deepest sensibilities as mortal, vulnerable, and transient beings. No wonder the hunt has been filmed and written about, its techniques—both ancient and modern—exhaustively described, and its importance to early human societies readily acknowledged. The concept of Man the Hunter is so widely held that it seems part of our collective unconscious.

Yet, without the continuing collection of wild plant foods, our species would not have been able to flourish to the extent that we have, settling, ultimately, all habitable regions of the earth. Because, in all but the most northern areas, plant foods have afforded a dietary stability and flexibility that have contrasted with the fluctuating availability of wild game. And in the majority of subtropical locations, plant foods have actually constituted the major dietary resource—a possible model for hunters and gatherers throughout vast stretches of human preagricultural life.

Naukha wakes just before sunrise, but stays in her skin blankets, savoring their warmth and waiting for the morning chill to soften. The baby stirs, expectant. At the taste of Naukha's warm milk, he settles into a familiar rhythm of nursing until, soothed, he goes back to sleep. Four-year-old Nai sleeps undisturbed beside him. As the first shadows are cast by the mounting sun, Naukha sits up. Rubbing the sleep from her eyes, she stokes the fire, takes some water she had carried back from the water hole yesterday, and washes. The rest she leaves for her family.

Daylight brightens, and the first sounds of people talking fill the camp. Her younger sister, Chuko, returns from her morning excursion to the surrounding bush, her skin cloth held snugly around her to protect her two-year-old—Nai's cousin—sleeping in a sling on her side. The sisters exchange greetings and agree to leave before the sun makes much more progress across the sky. Bereft of the warmth and softness of his mother's skin, Naukha's baby wakes again. This time little Nai soothes him, making baby sounds and funny faces until he starts to laugh. Naukha and Nai breakfast on roasted antelope, *sha* roots, and mongongo nuts while the baby nurses again.

Little Nai is called to her grandmother's hut and snuggles close as her grandmother also prepares food for her. Nai has just begun to play when she sees her mother and aunt preparing to leave—slipping infant and toddler into their slings, readying leather carrying pouches, and picking up digging sticks. She runs to them, pleading to go along. Naukha protests. Little Nai protests. There's a moment of hesitation, then, with a shrug and mock sigh of resignation, Naukha gestures to Nai the path they will be taking. Avoiding the amused twinkle sure to be in Chuko's eyes, Naukha starts off. Chuko follows. Little Nai darts ahead, skipping happily, singing softly to herself, triumphant.

Gathering is not for the weak, either of mind or body. It requires sophisticated knowledge of plant life and subtle understanding of the vagaries of the environment. Stamina, strength, visual acuity, memory, willingness to heed the advice of others, and a spirit of cooperation are the requirements for success. For such efforts, the rewards are great. Gatherers in many hunting and gathering societies provide the bulk of their family's food—adequate, varied, and satisfying. Nor is gathering considered drudgery, although, like hunting, it does demand considerable effort to walk the necessary miles and to carry the day's findings back to camp.

In most cases gathering is not a daily occupation. Even in less than ideal environments, women in many contemporary groups gather, on average, only a few days a week. Cuiva women of western Venezuela, for example, working two or at most three days a week, bring in enough food to feed themselves, their families, and other dependents. The rest of their time is spent maintaining their households, preparing food, sewing clothing, visiting nearby villages, or engaging in a variety of leisure activities.

The two women and three children reach the *tsin* bean flats within an hour and a half of leaving the village. They have traveled slowly, digging *sha* roots, collecting the last of the *grewia* berries, and pulling sweet lumps of sap from the bark of certain trees. The oppressive late morning heat permeates the dappled shade of the acacia tree where they sit to rest, so they feel little relief. Still, they light a fire to roast *tsin* beans, which they bury under a thin layer of hot sand beside some glowing coals.

Peeling the coarse, outer skin of a few *sha* roots, they eat the raw, sweet flesh, savoring its moisture. Little Nai drinks water from an ostrich eggshell container her mother has brought along, but is impatient to eat the *tsin* beans. She starts to fret; it seems contagious as her two-year-old cousin soon joins in. The women laugh, then begin a distracting and energetic round of singing, clapping their hands in complex rhythmic counterpoint that starts the two children dancing. By the time the *tsin* beans are cooked, the children stop only reluctantly, and sit down to eat.

The midday sun is ablaze. Little Nai and her cousin now sit beneath a different shade tree, watching their mothers collect *tsin* beans nearby. Naukha has left her powder shell, which dangled from her neck, for Nai to play with. Nai makes a doll—a *tsin* bean stuck on top of a small stick—and pretends it is a person who has just bathed. She takes the piece of tanned animal fur from the emptied tortoiseshell container, dips it deep into the fragrant powder ground from aromatic plants, and applies it to her doll. Another *tsin*-bean doll joins her play, then another and another. Her little cousin, enamored of Nai, holds the dolls dutifully while Nai gives directions.

The scattered piles of gathered beans, roots, and berries show that the two women have collected enough to fill their leather pouches. They join the two children at play, grateful to share the meager shade.

Both women lie down, their little ones nursing; Nai looks wistfully on. Nestling beside her mother, she finds comfort. Holding her close, Naukha says as if to no one, "Maybe it's better Nai did come. If she hadn't, right now we'd be rushing through the heat to get home to her."

Small sounds of the bush surround them—a distant bird calling, flies humming, the dry underbrush crackling ever-so-slightly, a dung beetle moving busily beneath. The intense heat amplifies the stillness of the air, which settles like a dense, monochrome blanket on the broad untainted landscape, mile after mile after mile.

Naukha is the first to awaken. She sits up, looks at the steady progress the sun has made across the sky, then stands to brush off her leather coverings. Adjusting the baby so he can nurse while in the sling, she hums a refrain from the song they were singing earlier. She squats beside the piles she has left, opens her carrying pouch, and loads the food. When she joins the others, Nai and her cousin are already intent in play, tracking a little beetle like a game animal.

Chuko also collects her food, and they start their journey home.

Women are the primary food gatherers. True, men who live in contemporary hunting and gathering cultures have comparable knowledge of plant resources and are capable of gathering enough to feed themselves comfortably. But women are the ones responsible for the daily sustenance of their families. Their contributions include not only plant food, but some animal protein as well, brought back independently of men: small mammals, land turtles, snakes and other reptiles, birds, eggs, insects, some amphibians, and a variety of animals associated with water. Adept observers, women also survey all they see on their crisscross journeys through the environment. They locate honey caches, make note of animal tracks, and mentally mark the position of valuable resources such as succulent water roots or reeds for arrow shafts to be harvested when needed.

Gathering is, ultimately, a satisfying way of earning a living. It is regarded as important and is personally rewarding. Every woman can learn the skills, and all have equal access to the foods available. The schedule and pacing of work is self-determined and flexible. Even though most food is collected primarily for one's family, sharing of food outside the family—while gathering or in the village—is typical: It is a kind of insurance against times of illness or other disability. Gathering is not isolating: Women usually go with others, for protection as much as for companionship. They rely on their own courage and on each other, not on men's weapons, for safety as they traverse environments that are frequently dangerous, scaring off carnivores when necessary—

leopards, lions, cheetahs, hyenas, jackals—and warning each other of poisonous snakes.

Gathering is challenging. It taps a woman's ability to identify, from among what may seem an infinite spectrum, a finite number of edible and seasonally variable plants. Gathering is also efficient. Unlike hunting, which has a variable rate of return, gathering is dependable and predictable. And because it requires only intermittent effort and women alternate their trips, gathering is a job compatible with motherhood; someone is usually in the village-camp, able to supervise children left behind.

Finally, unlike game, gathered foods are a woman's to distribute or to keep. Since success in gathering is universal, all women can provide food for their families and give presents. Personal circumstances and inclination may divide the generous from the selfish, but when obligations are incurred, they can be discharged quickly, if necessary. This is not always true for hunters who, perhaps down on their luck or lacking in skill, may wait weeks or even months before being in a position to return gifts of meat they have received from other men. Therefore, in these essentially egalitarian societies, women's work deflects status differentiation even more effectively than do most of the activities of men.

Sounds are brought by the wind; mere suggestions, at first, that quickly fade away. Yet, as the women walk, the rhythmic pounding of food preparation in the distant village-camp—"mortar-and-pestle talk," as the people call it—becomes clear. The two women quicken their pace and their movements become more energized, determined. Chuko is in the lead; Naukha trails behind, weighted down by both children, the food filling her leather pouch, and pieces of firewood she picks up as she nears the village.

This time the others watch *them*. Naukha and Chuko untie their leather pouches and release their loads. Calls come from across the village-camp, speculating, commenting, teasing:

"Surely two women alone can not have collected so much food. Someone must have helped. Lovers, of course!"

And, "Oooh, I knew it! When just two decide to go off together, they are surely looking for some special food—the sweetest, most wonderful, most delicious food in the world."

And, "Who stays away all day and returns when dark just begins to sit? Without doubt, someone has tasted something as sweet as honey while away from the village-camp today."

Amid the burst of high-spirited laughter, another chides, "Oooh, women are clever!"

Naukha and Chuko shrug off the good-natured banter, accepting the women's barely concealed praise, pleased to be home and at rest. As Naukha separates piles of food to be given as presents—*tsin* beans, sour plums, and *sha* roots—her husband returns. Something small is slung over his shoulder—a guinea fowl caught in one of his traps— and she smiles in anticipation.

But that is all, he explains quietly. He had gone hunting, having left even before Naukha, and had followed what he thought was a promising lead. But although the tracks were quite fresh, he never came within sight of the animal. After a few hours, he finally turned back. Passing the traps he had set late the day before, he found the bird.

As he sits, slightly apart from the others, plucking and preparing the guinea fowl for cooking, Naukha tells him of her day. Little Nai joins her father, leaning against him, and pulls off a few feathers. She gives up, her attention now riveted by the gentle descent of the decorative black, brown, and white feathers she throws into the air. Naukha roasts and cracks some *tsin* beans and pounds them with nut meats and pungent leaves in her mortar. She takes a handful for herself and sets the rest beside them to eat. When the guinea fowl is cooked, others join for a taste, but no one expects much from something so small, and only Naukha and her family have a full share.

Naukha lies down, satisfied, grateful for the warmth of the fire, pleased to rest at last. As night deepens, a group of men sit at one fire, absorbed in the dramatic rendition of a hunting adventure. Chuko is sitting outside her hut, pressing for news of her parents from a woman at another hut who has just returned from their village. A few children burst into song, clapping dance tunes, hoping to entice the adults to join in, perhaps even to precipitate a healing dance. But although their voices are occasionally echoed by the women, enthusiasm is slight. They soon give up, returning to their huts to play and then to sleep.

Amid the intimate circle of soft voices, Naukha drifts toward sleep. She barely notices little Nai slip quietly beside her and the baby, although almost reflexively she draws her near, pulling the leather blanket to cover her. Soon her husband joins them and lies down behind her, also close.

Quiet gradually descends, punctuated only by fires unwilling to give in to the dark—crackling, darting playfully, challenging, defiant—until the battle lost, they are at last subdued and become glowing embers covered by ash. Stillness is broken intermittently as one, then another stirs, filled with sleep, to add wood to the fire: brief bursts of light that seem to anticipate the new day, still hours away.

WOMEN'S LIVES

Imagine an infancy in which most of your needs for love and physical closeness were indulged, a childhood that—if you escaped serious illness—allowed you to flourish and mature at your own rate, absorbing and learning from role models only slightly older than yourself, a reasonably carefree adolescence that promoted individualism and self-confidence, assured you of your physical attractiveness, and didn't expect you to assume full adult responsibilities until you reached your late teens. Imagine, as well, an adulthood that essentially guaranteed marriage (with room for divorce and remarriage if necessary), that made it likely that you would have children, yet would not ostracize you if you couldn't or isolate you if you did, and that had social supports enabling you to balance family obligations with significant contributions to the economy. Although age, accidents, and infectious disease would gradually decrease your physical capabilities, your status within the community, especially within your family group, would be likely to increase. You would be turned to for the knowledge you possess about the past, highly relevant to a world that changes slowly, if at all. You would be the repository of stories told to you by your grandparents, entertaining to young and old alike. You would be vital to the life of your family.

A romantic fantasy of the noble savage? Twentieth-century pie-in-the-sky ideology? Given the unfortunate levels of mortality typical of foragers—and of all societies prior to the last hundred years—in some ways, of course, it is. But a version of life broadly similar to this one has been experienced by more generations of women than has any other. Even though there is and always has been marked diversity among hunting and gathering groups, certain elements affecting the way their lives progress are much more similar to each other than they are to ours today.

What follows, then, is a journey through a number of life stages as they would likely have been experienced by women in hunting and gathering societies.

Girlhood Among the Gatherers

Infancy and early childhood involve few if any distinctive features for girls; both girls and boys experience similarly the nurturance described in Chapter 8. As the toddler grows into a more independent child, play with a multi-age child group takes increasing amounts of time, but at first there is relatively little gender segregation. By age eight or nine, though, girls are more likely than boys to accompany their mothers on gathering expeditions, and so become trained and socialized in the art and science of plant food collecting. Before this age, boys exhibit more fighting behavior than girls, and the child in the play group most likely to be taking care of an infant or toddler is the baby's older sister; this role, however, is much less formal than in some agricultural communities in which young girls, or "child nurses" are responsible for much of the care of younger siblings. Because of demographic conditions (there are relatively few children in any one band so they all tend to play together), foragers have little opportunity for the extreme sex segregation during childhood that occurs routinely in many other societies.

Other features observed among recent hunters and gatherers also presumably characterized multi-age play groups of the past. With few peers, competition is minimized. Winning a game from someone much younger, or trying to beat someone much older is not very satisfying. Cooperation and nurturance is also fostered in children of both sexes. The inclusion of younger children means an expanded group, more diverse, and usually more interesting than solo or limited play.

Girls, as well as boys, spend a great deal of time in this group, which shifts in membership and size according to band composition, from toddlerhood to young adulthood. As described in the previous chapter, much learning of adult skills takes place in this context; older children with more advanced knowledge are powerful role models for younger children. Older girls (and boys) eventually learn from adults as they gradually spend less time in play and more time refining their economic and social skills.

Puberty and Menstruation

The physical transformation from girl to woman is a dramatic occurrence, one that in many traditional societies occasions ritual celebration. First menstruation marks not only physical maturation, but entrance into the adult social world as well. In most societies this is a more important moment than the corresponding herald of male puberty—first seminal emission. The Siriono of eastern Bolivia, for example, celebrate puberty for girls but not for boys. Similarly, among California Indian hunters and gatherers, few groups had formal recognition of male puberty, while strong emphasis was placed on first menstruation.

As young girls in foraging cultures approach adolescence, they spend increasing amounts of time gathering with their mothers. Until puberty, however, their economic contribution is usually minimal. Among the Mbuti Pygmies of Zaire, children participate in all economic activities, including net hunting, where they help adults as "beaters," beating the bushes to drive animals into previously positioned nets. As a group, children also frequently prepare meals for themselves. But it is only after puberty that they actually begin to assume the responsibilities of adults. Among the Tiwi Aborigines of Melville Island in northern Australia, young girls also learn basic economic skills before puberty and are usually betrothed at birth. But only after puberty does a girl experience *ambrinua*, one of the most important rituals in her adult life: She is ceremonially introduced to the man who will become the husband of her yet-unborn daughters, her prospective son-in-law.

First menstruation, as we saw in Chapter 8, generally occurs later in preindustrial societies than it does in our society. The adolescent period is therefore mostly free of the risk of pregnancy even though it is not free of sexual activity; this is especially true of hunting and gathering societies where restrictions on premarital sex tend to be less stringent than in other societies. More important, first birth does not come, on average, until the late-teen years: an average of age 20 for the Agta of the Philippines, 18.5 for the Aché of eastern Paraguay, and 19.5 for the !Kung San of Botswana.

Marriage

Romantic love is as ancient as the human race. The expectation of marrying for romantic love, however, is much more recent, especially in its Western form where it can occur independently of parental sanction. Marriage during the Paleolithic period must have varied widely, much as it does among recent hunters and gatherers, with differing emphasis placed on personal, economic, and political considerations.

Nevertheless Paleolithic marriage would probably have shared some of the features common to recent hunters and gatherers. Early marriage, for example, is virtually universal for women, and remarriage upon divorce or widowhood is fairly assured, especially for women in their reproductive years. Some are betrothed at birth, like Tiwi women of Australia; others, like the Agta of the Philippines, a few years before the onset of menstruation; still others marry sometime around first menstruation, which for the !Kung San of Botswana occurs at an average age of 16.5. !Kung girls who marry before menarche, however, are not expected to have sexual intercourse with their husbands, while premenstrual Tiwi and Agta wives may be introduced to marital sex earlier.

Early marriages are often fragile, however, and divorce is frequent until after the birth of the first child.

While girls marry in their teens, men's marriage rates and ages are more variable. Some groups practice polygyny (the form of polygamy in which a man has more than one wife), enabling older men to monopolize a sometimes significant proportion of women. Other groups are more like the !Kung San. With a 5 percent polygyny rate, most !Kung men marry, although a young man's first marriage may be to an older woman, one recently divorced or widowed. More typically, however, men are older at first marriage than are the women they marry, affording them somewhat more control within the marriage relationship. (Men usually have to prove their worthiness as hunters before becoming eligible, which also helps account for the age difference.) At the other end of the life cycle, however, women often outlive their husbands, and "till death do us part" may translate into only a decade or two. But remarriage after divorce or death of a spouse is commonplace, and both men and women generally have a number of spouses if they live long enough. For the Tlingit of Alaska, for example, the clan of a deceased husband had to provide another spouse, although the woman was not forced to accept.

Where polygyny does occur, it effectively places a premium on young, marriageable girls. A young man may live with the bride's family and hunt for their benefit while waiting for the girl to mature. (The situation appears in Western tradition in the biblical story of Jacob, Rachel, and Leah.) Once the girl matures and if the marriage lasts, the couple will be guided by custom as to whether to stay with her relatives or move to be near his. Among the !Kung San, if the husband has no other wives, a young couple may divide their time between both villages, alternating one with the other until finally settling down with either.

For the Mbuti Pygmies, mutual affection between intended spouses is essential to the promotion of "real" as opposed to "empty" marriages. For the Tlingit of Alaska, a woman had to consent to a proposed marriage. After a formal ceremony, the couple lived together; if the relationship lasted four weeks, the marriage was considered permanent. For the !Kung San, marriages are usually arranged, especially first marriages, but early marriages are fragile and apt not to last. Subsequent marriages take place when a girl may be old enough to voice her own opinion and, depending on her age and the support she gets from other relatives, she may or may not be heeded. For both the Mbuti Pygmies and the !Kung San, however, divorce is accomplished more easily before a child is born than after.

Marriage is not only an affair of the heart, it is an arrangement between two groups of people. For hunters and gatherers, couples are not isolated units, but threads in a net thrown far and wide, connecting people in distant areas, involving them socially, politically, and economically in each other's lives. Marriage expresses interdependence, the mainstay of hunting and gathering existence. This interdependence offers a cushion against times of scarcity. A family or group can visit in-laws living in more bountiful areas for extended periods of time. Even within the village, the presence of relatives translates into having more people to count on in times of personal hardship, such as illness or accident.

The village-camp a couple lives in after marriage determines important aspects of their lives. Each knows the vegetation, terrain, and game-migration patterns in his or her territorial home. It is advantageous for women to live near their own relatives, especially in groups where husbands are more dominant, if only because of age. By living near her parent, a woman's position—both in relation to her husband and to the social life of the camp—is strengthened. Although some foraging groups expect young married couples to reside with the husband's family, others expect them to reside with the wife's family, or have no set pattern at all and allow the couple to live with either family. However, even when the husband's family's residence is preferred, individual couples may be permitted the option of doing otherwise. In any event, the fluid nature of hunting and gathering bands usually translates into extended visits to both groups.

Birth

A woman feels the initial stages of labor and makes no comment, leaves the village quietly when birth seems imminent—taking along, if necessary, a young child—walks a few hundred yards, finds an area in the shade, clears it, arranges a soft bed of leaves, and gives birth while squatting or lying on her side—on her own. Unusual even for other hunters and gatherers, solo birth for !Kung San women is nevertheless an ideal: 35 percent of women attain it by their third birth and the majority do on subsequent births. Showing no fear and not screaming out, they believe, enhances the ease and safety of delivery. Cries of a newborn in the distance alert others, sending them running to the scene. They assist in the delivery of the placenta, cut the umbilical cord, clean the infant, and carry it back to the village. For the most stalwart, however, the first others learn of the birth is when they see the woman sitting near her hut, a small bundle in her arms.

Not all !Kung women attain this ideal, especially not those experiencing their first births. These women welcome the help and support of mothers, sisters, or other female relatives. Nor do most hunters and gatherers share this ideal. For the Siriono of Bolivia, for example, birth was a more public event. It took place in the village, and was attended by women and children; if it occurred at night, the prospective father would also be present. The actual birth, however, was left entirely to the woman to manage, since she received essentially no help throughout labor and delivery. She herself tied a rope above the hammock in which she would give birth, grabbing it when necessary for leverage. As she delivered the infant, it slid onto a pile of softened earth prepared a few inches below the side of the hammock. Birth for women among the Mbuti Pygmies also involves support from other women, not only by their presence but in the offering of help as well.

The experience of pregnancy and birth for Paleolithic women, while certain to have varied widely in cultural expression and meaning, nevertheless must also have been constrained in a number of similar ways— many of which have been observed among recent hunters and gatherers. The rhythm of the menstrual cycle, for example, may have been charted according to lunar cycles. Marked bones that may have served as calendars have been found in European Upper Paleolithic archaeological sites; recording twenty-eight units, they are suggestive of an attempt to establish either the phases of the moon, the menstrual cycle, or both. !Kung San women start anticipating pregnancy when two lunar cycles pass without the onset of menstruation. Additional months confirm this, as do darker nipples, mood swings, and sometimes intense food preferences. Pregnancy doesn't mean coddling, however, either for !Kung women or for other recent hunting and gathering women, who continue their usual work patterns until the very end and may resume them, like the Mbuti Pygmies and the Philippine Agta, within a few days after birth.

Whether with the help of other women or alone, women living in hunting and gathering societies have no choice but to give birth as nature intended. This means an inevitable and unfortunate loss of life, but the pattern is as typical of foragers as of agricultural and even early industrial peoples and continues in many parts of the world today. Attempts are made to prepare young women for the experience, and most girls see childbirth before they experience it themselves. But no amount of preparation can remove the risk. Indeed, our own security in this regard is unprecedented in human experience.

However bravely women may face childbirth, it is a risky affair that until about two generations ago, took a dramatic toll on the lives of women and infants in all societies no matter when or where they lived. (In Europe, for example, from 1500 to 1900, about 25 percent of deaths of women ages fifteen to fifty were related to childbirth.) And, while the !Kung ideal of solitary birth is atypical, beliefs and practices designed to minimize risk are widespread. For the !Kung (and for the Siriono), a solitary or unaided birth may have its positive side; minimizing the number of people present at the birth or who touch the woman throughout labor exposes a woman and her infant to fewer germs. But for the !Kung at least, solitary birth may also mean fewer dissenting voices in the rare cases when infanticide is being considered. Infants with serious deformities jeopardized an entire family's ability to survive, and twins—or children born too closely together—can not both thrive on milk from nursing, the only kind of milk available.

In anthropological usage, "infanticide" refers to the abandonment or killing of an infant at birth or soon after. There is some dispute as to whether it has played (and continues to play), a large or small role in population regulation; either way, it is likely to have been part of our hunting and gathering past. Infanticide has been practiced throughout the world and over a wide span of time. Oedipus, Moses, Romulus, and Remus, like many other heroes in world mythology, were all abandoned; they survived only through extraordinary luck. In addition to its practice by the ancient Greeks and Romans, infanticide has been recorded in other societies both large and small: the Chinese, the Japanese, the high-caste Indians, the Aymara of Bolivia and Peru, the Yaudapu Enga of New Guinea, and the Ibo of Nigeria, as well as the Eskimo and the Australian Aborigines.

Infanticide has not been unknown in Western countries. Anthropologist Susan Scrimshaw writes:

> In London in the 1860's, dead infants were a common sight in parks and ditches. In nineteenth century Florence, children were abandoned or sent to wet nurses who neglected them, while during the same period in France, thousands of infants were sent to wet nurses in the countryside, never to return.

On May 5, 1987, a baby was found in a dumpster in San Francisco— alive and fortunately saved, but a grim reminder of a common practice in our past.

Many studies of infanticide have calculated its incidence among human groups, both in the past and the present. One such study of 112 preindustrial cultures reported that 36 practiced infanticide commonly; an additional 13 practiced it occasionally. John Whiting and associates analyzed the literature on a group of 84 cultures and found similar results: one-third reported infanticide as a means of eliminating defective offspring, and 36 of a group of 72 cultures reported killing infants born too soon after the birth of an older sibling. This was more likely to occur in nomadic hunting, gathering, and fishing societies than in agricultural ones.

The practice of infanticide has had a long history. In trying to understand it, the drastic circumstances many of these people found themselves in have to be considered. Many of these infants would have died later from lack of food or general neglect. If allowed to live, a severely deformed infant could have jeopardized the survival of the entire family. Even normal children born too closely together endangered their siblings. This is not to justify the practice—even many hunters and gatherers do not. !Kung mothers suspected of it are bitterly criticized and their reasons closely scrutinized. As a Jicarilla Apache told anthropologist Morris Opler, "Sometimes unmarried mothers throw their babies away. But there is a strong feeling against it. To kill a child like this is to set yourself against life, and your own life will not be long after that."

Beliefs About Pregnancy and Birth

Birth is an awesome mystery, intense and inexorable, joyful yet dangerous, a moment of transition as the baby enters one world from another. Death of the infant is common, and death of the mother is not rare. It is hardly surprising that hunters and gatherers as well as people living in preindustrial and even industrial societies, have elaborate beliefs about pregnancy and birth, some of which belong in the realm of superstition. We may wonder at the spectrum, but some beliefs seem to have a grain of the truth, if only intuitive. For people who have no better explanations or control over their destiny, myths that calm and comfort are justification enough.

Early in the twentieth century, Elsie Clewes Parsons collected beliefs about birth and sex held by people in all types of society throughout the world, from hunters and gatherers to people living in Western societies. The sheer number and widespread prevalence of pregnancy taboos, for example, are staggering, as are the many common themes. Underlying most of these beliefs, however, seems to be an impulse to protect mothers and infants. Given the insecurity and unpredictability of life for hunters and gatherers, it is probable that our remote ancestors shared analogous conceptions.

The near-universal expression in Parsons's collection is that a woman's mental attitudes, nutrition, and even experiences influence the character, looks, and career of the unborn, with the result that "great circumspection and self-deprivation are required of her." For example, Australian Aborigines believe that congenital deformities are caused by eating forbidden things during pregnancy, and the California Indians, too, imposed many food restrictions. In the Admiralty Islands a woman does not eat yams, lest her child be lanky. Nor does a Thompson River Indian eat hare, lest the baby have a harelip. Among the Dabuis, a pregnant woman may not eat any animal that has died with young. In addition to proscriptions, there are many prescriptions. In the Torres Strait Islands, for example, an expectant mother should eat shellfish that make a hissing sound while roasting to ensure the child a good voice and lusty lungs. Almost all aspects of maternal conduct seem applicable. Many cultures believe women should avoid knots to ensure a safe delivery. In parts of Germany, for instance, a woman shouldn't pass under a clothesline or spin or reel or twist anything.

Similar themes are expressed in a more recent ethnography of maternity and ritual in Bang Chan, Thailand. The author, Jane Richardson Hanks, reports a mother's advice to her pregnant daughter:

> Women are easily upset when pregnant. It is up to you to put yourself in a cheerful mood. Everything you do will affect the infant in your womb. If you see a scarred person, your child will be scarred. Be calm, look only at pleasant things and avoid jerky motions. Do not overeat, lest the child be a glutton. If you sleep during the day and are inactive, you will also have a lazy child.

The list of do's and don'ts throughout the world is virtually endless. Many rituals transmit cultural information and practical advice. But overall, when things go wrong, the woman is considered at fault. In the face of overwhelming insecurity, it is understandable that people should grasp at an illusion of control. The !Kung blame women for any difficulty they have in childbirth, saying that it is caused by their fear or, worse, by an inherent rejection of the infant. A traditional Jicarilla Apache story blames the woman in a way that is even less helpful: "A woman who is kind and good does not suffer when she has a baby, but one who is mean and wicked and always harming others is the one who will have a hard time at childbirth." In labor, Hawaiian women, like the !Kung, were not supposed to cry out in pain, "lest she make herself the talk of the neighborhood."

Motherhood

First motherhood is not often the occasion of special ritual and ceremony, but most cultures recognize it as the true dividing line between childhood and adulthood. The experience of first birth changes a woman. The !Kung San have an expression for the firstborn which applies to no other child, and after the baby comes, the parent is usually given a name derived from that of the baby: Susanna's-father, Adam's-mother (or the equivalents), a tribute to the change in status. Giving birth not only separates the women from the girls but, of course, the women from the men. The words of an Abyssinian woman recorded early in this century express this distinction, as applicable to hunters and gatherers as they are to ourselves:

How can a man know what a woman's life is? A woman's life is quite different from a man's. God has ordered it so. A man is the same from the time of his circumcision to the time of his withering. He is the same before he has sought out a woman for the first time, and afterwards. But the day a woman enjoys her first love cuts her in two. She becomes another woman on that day. The man is the same after his first love as he was before. The man spends a night by a woman and goes away. His life and body are always the same. The woman conceives. As a mother she is another person than the woman without child. She carries the fruit of the night nine months long in her body. Something grows. Something grows into her life that never departs from it. She is a mother. She is and remains a mother even though her child dies, though all her children die. For at one time she carried the child under her heart. And it does not go out of her heart ever again. Not even when it is dead. All this the man does not know; he knows nothing.

Becoming a mother entails a change of status for women in all cultures; among hunters and gatherers, it represents the assumption of full-fledged adult responsibility. The new demands now placed on a woman's time, however, do not contradict her role as economic provider. Mothering in the context of hunting and gathering societies not only provides ample opportunity for "dual careers," it requires them; it is also organized sensibly, and with many more social supports than it is for us. From the moment of birth, the differences are striking.

As described in Chapter 8, infants in hunting and gathering societies, such as the Aché of Paraguay, are likely to be in frequent or even constant physical contact with others throughout the first year or more of life. They are carried wherever their mothers go during the day, often skin to skin in some form of sling, and they sleep beside or near their mothers at night. (North American Indians used cradleboards to comfort infants, but still maintained close physical proximity.) Nursing is "on demand," a pattern of frequency unknown to most mothers in industrial cultures. The !Kung San believe that an infant cries for a reason. Mothers respond to a child's frets immediately—if not before, in anticipation—by putting it to the breast for as often and for as long as it wants—from a few seconds to several minutes. As a child gets older, it nurses whenever it chooses; it simply avails itself of its mother's breasts while being carried in the sling, when sitting near her on the ground, or while sleeping beside her at night. For the first two years or more of life, a !Kung child nurses an average of four times an hour. (One drawback of breast-feeding—that it drains calcium from the mother—is offset by exercise and high calcium intake.)

Few women in our own culture, even those committed to nursing on demand, have adopted a comparable level of frequency or degree of commitment to this mode of feeding. Work schedules and social patterns prohibit it. Breast-feeding in public is available only to the most stalwart, and even then social tension may interfere with it. Frequent breast-feeding also runs counter to the Western ideal of breast-as-sexual-object because of fears that it will hasten the transformation of an adolescent-shaped breast. Among hunters and gatherers, as among many preindustrial peoples, the breast is as much a symbol of nurturance and maternity as of nubility and sexual attractiveness, at least after adolescence.

Another practice common to hunting and gathering societies, sleeping beside the mother at night, seems to pose relatively few problems to the child or to the couple. A concern voiced frequently in the West—that a woman may roll over (also known as overlying) on a child and smother it while both are asleep—was not considered an issue for the !Kung. As far as they knew, no one had ever done that. In fact, infant death caused by smothering or strangling in a crib, away from the mother, is better documented in the medical literature than is overlying. Furthermore, when we consider how most of us sleep—on raised beds several feet above the floor—why don't adults constantly fall out of bed? Because, despite our altered states of consciousness throughout the night, we are capable of making delicate calculations about our body position—the same made by mothers sleeping beside their children.

More problematic, to be sure, are a couple's sexual relations, which are likely to be more restrained in the presence of a sleeping child. Among hunters and gatherers, however, dwellings are often loosely constructed and set close together so that engaging in sex requires extreme discretion whether children are present or not. Sometimes a husband and wife meet like lovers in the bush for a less inhibited encounter. But even for these meetings a small infant would probably not be left behind.

Patterns of child rearing similar to these probably typify the Paleolithic period. Close contact with the mother promotes safety of infants and young children, and frequent nursing assures adequate water, nutrition, and at least some protection against infection. In an environment in which mortality within the first few years of life is high, close physical contact and frequent nursing also help cement a strong bond between a mother and child, maximizing the infant's care and thus its chance of survival.

As the child grows older, experiences unique to this way of life continue to affect its development. During the second year, for example, the child gradually turns its attention from the mother to the world beyond, but the initiation and circumstances of this separation contrast markedly with usual Western practices. As we have seen, because villages consist only of about a dozen families, children of all ages play together. For toddlers, the running, jumping, squealing, dancing, singing, rope jumping, cartwheeling, and all other variety of imaginative games played by multi-age child groups are so appealing that they attract even the youngest. An older sibling, cousin, or friend will pick up little ones eagerly crawling toward them or calling out to play, and include them in their games. When the toddler tires, gets hungry, or just wants more comfort than other children are willing or able to offer, the mother is usually nearby. In this setting it is primarily the child— not the mother—who controls the degree and timing of separation and social growth. The children's play group, therefore, relieves the mother of intensive child care for brief but frequent periods throughout the day.

A common complaint of mothers in the West was voiced by a young American woman caring for her first child. "I love being a mother and I love my son. I also enjoy playing games with him. But when he wants to repeat the same game fifty times the same way each time, I get so bored I can't stand it. I try to change the game, but he insists. Is there something wrong with me that I can't do it his way?"

The answer, from the perspective of our hunting and gathering past, is that nothing is wrong with her; something is wrong with the structure of Western child rearing. Mothers living in hunting and gathering societies are rarely faced with children who are bored, having to devise ever more elaborate strategies to entertain them. Other children are better at that. Other children, working out similar skills, perhaps at a somewhat higher but still immature level, *are* willing to repeat a game endlessly. Other children are also usually more fun. This does not mean that mothers in hunting and gathering societies are not playful with children, for indeed they are, especially with the very young. Their face-to-face and vocal interactions with infants are playful and tender, obviously a source of pleasure to infant and mother alike. But their primary role is to offer what they, and only they, are uniquely qualified to provide: food, nurturance, security, comfort, and, above all, love. Play is what other children do best.

Play also distracts young children from the pain of the ultimate separation from Mother: weaning. This probably took place relatively late among Paleolithic hunters and gatherers, since prolonged nursing provides the only form of milk available for growing children. It also helps maximize birth spacing. A four-year difference between successive children means that a second youngest child is able to walk on its own much of the time. Shorter birth spacing undermines a woman's capacity to work; instead of carrying only the youngest child on routine gathering expeditions (along with heavy loads of food), she has to carry the next oldest as well. The extra weight also severely limits her effectiveness as a provider and so profoundly taxes her energies that the prospects for all members of her family are diminished.

Motherhood is eased not only by the presence of a play group and by long birth spacing, but also by the social context in which it occurs: Other people are always around, adults whom one can rely on to take the baby for a few minutes at least. Fellow band members provide company, companionship, and conversation; they also act as a critical release valve for the tensions that motherhood often produces. All-day isolation of mother and children, so common in middle-class Western societies, is unusual among hunters and gatherers.

Unfortunately, the security and comfort of childhood provided by parents—especially mothers—in preagricultural societies has always been undermined by forces beyond anyone's control: diseases (primarily viral and bacterial infections of the respiratory and gastrointestinal tracts) and other medical problems which we can now control but which they couldn't. These caused high mortality for children of all ages, although the most vulnerable then, as now, must have been infants. Simple infections accompanied by diarrhea can fast become life threatening; dehydration can be swift and lethal in the absence of medical intervention. Having one's siblings, and later, one's children, die was an experience both men and women had to learn to cope with, to endure, and finally, to overcome.

Women and Subsistence

There is some question as to the relative importance of meat and vegetable foods in hunting and gathering diets. The problem arises from the wide variation in subsistence patterns found among contemporary groups, a variation not unexpected considering the diversity of environments in which they live. However, since recent hunters and gatherers occupy marginal areas and since all have been influenced to some degree by outside forces, their diets should not be viewed as direct analogues of the past. Nevertheless, contemporary groups can provide insight into many facets of this way of life, especially those groups living in relatively favorable areas.

To shed some light on what hunters and gatherers do for a living, anthropologists M. Kay Martin and Barbara Voorhies tallied the meat and vegetable content of diets in ninety foraging societies listed in the anthropological record. Their findings suggest that it would be at least as accurate to label these groups "gatherers and hunters" as "hunters and gatherers." In two-thirds of the groups, meat provided only 30 to 40 percent of the diets and gathering was the primary subsistence activity. Of course, these figures probably represent only one set of conditions—not the entire range that existed in the past. But even in environments abundant in game animals, plant foods would not have been ignored. (Whatever the percentage, however, meat is almost always more highly valued.)

The division of labor by sex among hunters and gatherers is ubiquitous but not exclusive, and there is considerable crossover of roles. In most groups men do some gathering, if only for themselves, and women sometimes return from gathering expeditions with animal protein: small mammals, reptiles, aquatic creatures, birds, and insects. Women are occasional participants in the hunt: Mbuti Pygmy women help drive animals into nets where they are killed by men, Cuiva women paddle canoes while their husbands hunt or fish, and family expeditions also occurred among California Indians. Women among the Australian Tiwi sometimes hunted without men—usually with dogs.

But in recent years, a more unusual and dramatic example has been recorded by P. Bion Griffin and Agnes Estioko-Griffin. Among Agta hunters and gatherers of the Philippines, women carry on full careers as hunters—not a handful, but women in general—and are very successful at it. Hunting on a regular basis, women either alone or with other women contribute over 30 percent of all meat brought into camp. (They also hunt jointly with men.) Remarkably, this does not seem to interfere very much with the basic forager pattern of maternal nurtur-

ance—nursing, physical contact, sleeping proximity, and indulgence—
which is roughly the same for the Agta as for the !Kung San.

The extent of Agta women's hunting presents a challenge to traditional anthropological views about the division of labor by sex in hunting
and gathering societies. Although these views derive from data collected
on all other groups in which women rarely if ever hunt, it is nevertheless
intriguing that even one such exception exists. Most theorists have described women as being unsuitable for hunting. Pregnancy, lactation,
and carrying a child—physical realities for women during most of their
reproductive years—appeared incompatible with running long distances, using weapons, and confronting dangerous situations. Yet, Agta
women confound this theory. They hunt (usually with the aid of dogs)
with other women, with men, or alone. When hunting in mixed groups,
they are just as likely as men to kill an animal, using knives or bows
and arrows. Even more dramatic—and probably tied to their success
in using dogs—women hunters, alone or in all-female groups, are almost
twice as successful in the hunt as are male hunters. Not all Agta women
want to hunt, and some choose not to. But for those who do, pregnancy
doesn't prevent participation; most women continue until the time of
delivery. Even women carrying infants (over six months old) hunt, but
because of the difficulty of transporting both child and meat, they are
not among the 9.5 percent who occasionally hunt alone. As a group,
however, women who are lactating are less active as hunters than are
nonlactating women.

Given the exceptional nature of Agta women hunters, it would be
inappropriate to suggest that they typify our remote female ancestors.
Still, their experiences are provocative. Few scientists previously con-
templated, with any seriousness, the possibility that women in these
kinds of societies (either remote or recent) might have been capable of
hunting. Yet, the incentive for procuring meat has always been great
and this one example—even with meat being used in trade—opens the
door to the possibility that other examples, in different times and places,
may have occasionally existed.

Remote and rare though that possibility may be, the experience of
the Agta has other lessons to teach. First, it vividly illustrates the physical strength and stamina typical of women in the foraging setting. Second, Agta women exhibit an assertive independence associated with
males more often than females. Agta women stand beside men as equals,
fully participant, with comparable access to activities that promote influence and prestige, even hunting.

There is no reason to believe that women of the past were more
passive players. They may not have been hunters, but there is little

doubt that they were aggressively involved in a broad range of band activities, made important economic contributions, and participated actively in decisions affecting their families and the band. As we will see, it is among recent hunters and gatherers, more than for most societies of other types, that equal opportunities exist for men and women to share in all spheres of life, whether productive or reproductive.

Women and Physical Fitness

The nature of women's physical work in hunting and gathering societies has been well characterized. They collect fruits, vegetables, seeds and nuts, and dig roots and tubers, frequently from drought-hardened ground; they haul heavy loads of water, food, or firewood, often while carrying a young child; they walk long distances across hard-baked semi-desert, through fields of high grass, or in the forest—while gathering, moving, or visiting; and, for recreation, they often dance vigorously, sometimes for hours. Women foragers have the strength and stamina to cope with these demands—without obvious discomfort or harm—as a natural consequence of their way of living. Like men, they maintain both cardiovascular and musculoskeletal fitness throughout life.

The beneficial effects of these activities (combined, of course, with diet) generally parallel those for men; for example, women over fifty in hunting and gathering societies rarely experience the strokes and heart attacks so common among postmenopausal women in industrialized societies. But in other respects, hunting and gathering life has special relevance for women. Since exercise, particularly resistance exercise, promotes bone growth, the peak bone mass achieved by women foragers is likely to exceed that of women in our own society, especially since their calcium intake is generally greater than is ours. During later life, their continuing physical activity, also in contrast with the sedentary existence of older women in affluent nations, helps to forestall bone loss. These factors tend to offset the calcium loss associated with prolonged lactation and help women foragers avoid osteoporosis, the bone loss that afflicts so many Western women.

Aerobic exercise also affects women's physiology—especially the reproductive system. Rose Frisch and others have shown that young girls training intensively for athletic competition or ballet experience menarche substantially later than more sedentary girls. Further studies have shown that vigorous exercise, such as that involved in marathon running or long-distance swimming, can induce menstrual irregularity in women whose menses previously occurred with great regularity. In both cases, increased physical activity, coupled with a reduction in body fat, seems to be the causal factor.

These findings have broad significance for women in hunting and gathering societies. Their patterns of lifelong exercise almost certainly influence their fertility. First birth occurs at an age—twenty years among the Agta—when the young woman is mature enough to make the transition to motherhood, thus avoiding the tragedy of early-teenage pregnancy that afflicts our population. Throughout the reproductive years, Agta women who are fertile maintain a birth spacing of about three years, and while lactation plays a role in this, physical activity helps as well. Without long birth spacing, infants would be born too closely together, jeopardizing each other's already precarious chances for survival.

The Older Woman

Whatever one's level of nutrition and exercise, fitness comes to an end eventually. Life expectancy among hunters and gatherers is, of course, abbreviated compared to contemporary Western standards, but it is similar to what was experienced by most human societies until the nineteenth century. Today's impressive average longevity—of well over seventy years—is new, achieved in the United States only in the most recent generations.

But even among modern hunters and gatherers, once the vulnerable period of childhood is successfully negotiated, survival to age sixty is not unusual. That means there are enough older people around to ensure continuity of traditions and ritual. In most groups, the people who survive to old age are recognized with a name category, an equivalent to "senior citizens." (Usually another distinction is made between those who can attend to their own needs and those who can't.) Older people typically gain in prestige and influence and become privileged in ways that younger people are not. Food taboos may be lifted and participation in ritual matters increased. Old people are often respected, turned to for advice in times of conflict, expected to transmit skills and lore to younger people, and counted on to help with child care (while forming intense bonds with their grandchildren). Because of the lack of medical care, however, many suffer from old injuries and chronic infections that make them dependent on others, although they are likely to be free of most of the degenerative diseases of civilization common to older people in the West.

Older people among the Mbuti Pygmies, for example, do not participate in communal hunts, but no stigma results. They look after children left in camp, make twine used in hunting nets, prepare food, and perform other essential functions. They are fed by others. They do some hunting and gathering on their own, but they are not expected to fend for themselves. The !Kung San are reasonably similar. Among the Tiwi, older women assume positions of influence within the domestic group, directing the activities of younger cowives, and attain considerable prestige. Older people among the Siriono of Bolivia, however, living under more stressful nutritional conditions, were considered a burden and were afforded little care.

In many ways women among hunters and gatherers come into their own after menopause. Freed from the heavy physical and physiological burdens of pregnancy and lactation, from the psychological burdens of small children, and usually from the necessity to provide for others, they often take a more active role in group discussions—the de facto equivalent of leadership in such small-scale societies. If they have been successful in reproduction, they can also reap the benefits of that success, gaining prestige from the presence of their growing and grown offspring and, later, of those children's spouses and children. New bands are frequently formed because a single couple's children produce enough offspring to make up the core of a group and bring in other relatives through marriage.

However, the care of older people in the hunting and gathering setting is not uniform and should not be romanticized. Their experience depends in large measure on the availability of family and kin. Under extreme and stressful conditions, the cost of maintaining older people can be greater than the contribution they make, and then geronticide—the counterpart of infanticide, at the other end of the life cycle—may occur. Very old, frail, and sick people—among the Siriono of Bolivia and the Chipewyan of Canada, for example—were abandoned when the group had to move due to severe food shortage and when continuing to support them endangered the survival of all. Such abandonment probably occurred in many hunting and gathering groups, frequently with the concurrence of the elderly people involved and often, although not inevitably, resulted in their death.

THE QUESTION OF EQUALITY

The battle between the sexes rages not only in our lives, but in the literature interpreting our lives. Not surprisingly, our hunting and gathering past is invoked by many as holding essential keys to the meaning of "male" and "female" as well as the possibilities and limitations of the two together. But, in contrast to diet and exercise, or even certain aspects of infant and child care, the relationship between men and women in hunting and gathering societies is more elusive; humans are forever innovative, and their social arrangements infinitely complex.

Disentangling the threads of the hunting and gathering adaptation from the fabric of culture may be difficult, but tracing a few common themes can provide useful insights and establish a range of possibilities and limitations that may have characterized our ancient past.

Perhaps the most intriguing finding, true in varying degrees of most hunters and gatherers, is one that defies the common "caveman" stereotype of our Stone Age past. Instead of being subservient and dependent, women are central to the economy, autonomous in their actions, and in positions of influence quite comparable to those of males. Relations between the sexes, instead of resembling a battle, are usually more like a skirmish; and in at least one group, the Agta of the Philippines, the conflict may be almost nonexistent. If human societies were ranked along a continuum according to the status of women, most foragers would be positioned near the end closest to full equality.

Another striking finding is that little in the structure of the foraging life-style requires male privilege. Instead, many features encourage an egalitarian system and a position of overall strength for women, along with men: (1) the importance of gathered food and the economic independence of women; (2) comparable mobility for men and women; (3) the absence of social or economic class structure; (4) leadership that is informal, nonheritable, and antiauthoritarian; (5) problem resolution that maximizes individuals' participation in group decisions; (6) an emphasis on cooperation, sharing, and generalized reciprocity; (7) minimal property ownership with little value placed on accumulation; (8) fluid band composition; (9) small living groups in which men and women mix freely; and, at least among recent groups, (10) a low frequency of war and of elaborate preparations for war.

Women's economic role is overwhelmingly as providers of gathered food. Depending on environmental factors, wild plants in the diet range from insignificant (for people such as the Eskimos, who live in extreme northern climates with little vegetation) to the vast majority (for people such as the Aborigines of the Central Australian desert, where game is scarce). Since foragers of the past lived in the most advantageous areas, it is possible that women's contribution of plant foods was less significant. However, contemporary hunters and gatherers such as the Hadza of Tanzania and the Tiwi of Australia live in environments rich with game, yet gathered foods still comprise at least 50 percent of their diets.

What about societies in which game *is* more prominent than plant foods? This probably typified some groups during the Late Paleolithic, especially those living near the receding glaciers, where game was abundant but plant growth was limited. High meat consumption also characterizes many contemporary groups living in northern latitudes, as well as some tropical forest dwellers such as the Aché of Paraguay. The status of women among the noncoastal, traditional "Caribou-Eater" Chipewyan Indians of Canada—whose diet consisted of more than 90 percent meat—has been described as being one of the lowest for any North American Indian tribe. Women participated only in food processing, not in food getting, which was almost entirely the responsibility of men.

A different picture emerges, however, among more recent tropical forest hunters and gatherers. Contrary to expectation, edible plant food is widely scattered and less available in the tropical forest than it is in mixed or open environments; the deep shade and high tree cover nevertheless provide ideal conditions for a wide range of game (as well as honeybees). For the Aché of Paraguay, the Maku Indians of northwestern Amazonia, the Efe Pygmies of Zaire, and the Agta of the Philippines, meat and honey constitute more of their diets than does plant food. Among these groups, women's contribution to the economy is still significant, not only as gatherers, but also as hunters. Among Efe Pygmy net hunters, women participate in the hunt, driving animals into nets; among the Agta, women hunt as do men. Perhaps it is not coincidental that the relations between the sexes in these two groups are portrayed as being essentially equal.

Women hunters have also been described among the Tiwi of Australia, for whom the division of labor seems not so strictly dichotomized along sexual lines—at least in the economic sphere. Tiwi men and women both hunt and gather; their resources, not activities, are categorized into male domains (those of the sea and air) and female domains (those of the land). Men typically fish and hunt birds, aquatic reptiles, and mammals; women collect wild foods, shellfish, and hunt land animals with the aid of dogs. (The largest, strongest, and most-difficult-to-obtain land animals, however, are usually hunted by men.)

But in the social sphere, relationships seem less equitable, especially within marriage: Tiwi women are betrothed before birth into polygynous households (helping to establish their husbands as "big men" who command considerable power within the community) and they have little opportunity for divorce. As wives, they are "inherited" by other males when their husbands, who are much older, die. A woman eventually gains influence in this realm by the establishment of a formal relationship with a prospective son-in-law (the husband-to-be for all her female children) arranged even before she becomes pregnant. Age also brings increased status as she moves into the position of senior wife.

Work that equals or even exceeds that of men in practical value does not automatically lead to equality. Women in many small-scale agricultural societies also make significant contributions to subsistence, working hard in the fields, often much harder than men, yet their status usually remains quite low. Perhaps the most significant difference is that for most foragers, food is gathered for use—not for exchange or for translation into forms of currency or prestige items. Women foragers control the conditions of their work, and the foods they gather are theirs to distribute. By being major participants in the food-procuring (as well as processing) part of the economy and by disposing of the fruits (literally) of their labor according to their will, women build strong social networks that lead to influence within the group.

The hunting and gathering economy also entails considerable time spent away from home base, with comparable mobility for men and women. Women leave camp often, usually with other women, and spend anywhere from a few hours to a full day away. (Men, who also leave camp frequently, are more likely to stay overnight in the pursuit of game.) The decision when and where to gather is a woman's to make, although when hunting strategies are considered, men become involved. Cohesion and cooperation among women are fostered in this setting, together with autonomy and mobility. Child care—the near-exclusive domain of women—takes place in the context of this economic contribution, not to the exclusion of it.

The absence of social classes and other forms of status hierarchies are additional features of the foraging life-style, ones that limit authority which might otherwise reside with males. Within a camp, just about everything enters the sharing network, be it food or material goods. Leadership itself is usually informal. With thirty or fewer people living together, always having the option to leave one camp for another, it is difficult to develop or maintain arbitrary leadership. Leaders do emerge, more often men than women, but their influence is informal at best; they listen, they suggest, and they argue. Their role is to reflect group consensus, not create it. People participate in the decision-making and conflict-resolution process freely, expressing their opinions and having their views considered.

Even ownership of resources is egalitarian. The land and its food are usually owned collectively, with all people in the group having equal rights of access, although "ownership" by one or more individuals is sometimes designated. !Kung visitors, for example, ask permission to exploit local resources and this permission will not be denied; granting use assures reciprocal access to the visitors' resources another time— an "insurance" policy against periods of local hardship or scarcity. Material goods owned by individuals are not hoarded since most items can be produced by individual families. More exotic ones invariably become part of an exchange network, so that there is no institutional separation of haves from have-nots. After all, when mobility and adaptability are at a premium, accumulation of goods becomes a liability. It is better to translate material advantage into obligations that can be "harvested" in times of stress than to be overburdened with coveted items during times of abundance.

Another feature that affects women's status is the site of residence after marriage. Many hunters and gatherers prefer a couple to live with the husband's group after marriage. The experience of living in the husband's village, quite common among agriculturalists, has been eloquently described by anthropologist Naomi Quinn:

> Such a bride suffers the loneliness and the scrutiny of her affines [in-laws] which typifies the lot of all virilocally married women . . . , in addition she may find herself under the authority of a hostile mother-in-law, whose interests are opposed to hers in competition for the affection and loyalty of her husband. Her only claim to status rests on her success in bearing and raising sons and her eventual position as mother-in-law herself. Typically, women can only gain power in such households indirectly, through men, and their strategies for so doing may be characterized by gossip, persuasion, indirection and guile.

In Martin and Voorhies' sample of ninety foraging societies, nearly 65 percent either favor living with the woman's family or at least allow the option of living with them. By being based for at least some time with her family, a young woman has support for decisions that affect her life, and has the protection of family members in times of stress— physical, social, and even marital. Because there is a reasonable chance a girl may live with her parents' group after marriage, her value, even at birth, is not diminished. Just as a son may enhance his family's standing in the community by bringing in his bride, so can a daughter, by bringing in her husband. Among some Native American hunters, ownership of the home was seen as residing in the hands of the woman who built it; her husband was viewed as a long-term guest.

Within the family, women's standing is also enhanced by long birth spacing (only one small child to care for at a time), permissive child-rearing attitudes, and nonauthoritarian family structure. Together, these factors point to the hunting and gathering mode as one that maximizes mutual respect and easy dependence between the sexes—a lesson for our own times.

Yet a number of issues need further consideration. First, equality between the sexes is not universal among hunters and gatherers. Substantial diversity exists, ranging from groups in which women attain considerable influence and recognition (as among the !Kung San or the Philippine Agta) to those which are "less equitable" (as among some Eskimos and many Australian Aborigine groups). Second, among groups that *are,* for most practical considerations, egalitarian, men still invariably seem to have an edge. They are more likely to become leaders, both political and spiritual, more likely to use aggressive force against women (as well as against men), and, being generally older than their wives, are likely to be dominant in the marriage relationship, including exercising the option to have more than one wife. Men are also more likely to be *considered* dominant—by men and women alike.

Contemporary forces have been accused of being partly responsible for distorting what otherwise might be a more symmetrical male-female relationship. Some anthropologists condemn the colonial presence as having tipped the scales in favor of men. They argue that when hunters and gatherers were asked to present their "chief" to colonialists, it was made clear that a high-status male was to step forward. (For groups that downplayed "high status" anything, this was considered an affront to good manners.) Missionary influences often produced similar results— not only on foragers, but also on neighboring people with whom foragers had economic and cultural contact. Others criticize male observers (and most early observers were male) for concentrating primarily on male activities and for projecting their own sex-stereotyped images. This imbalance created an "androcentric," or male-oriented, view of hunting and gathering life.

Other influences have also inevitably clouded the picture. Recent hunters and gatherers live in a contemporary world; all have had contact with outside forces, some for hundreds of years. The Pygmies of Zaire, for example, only speak the language of their agricultural neighbors, having lost their original tongue. Others, like the Mashco-Piro of Peru, have remained more isolated, but none has been "untouched." In light of these circumstances, then, it seems all the more intriguing that a general pattern of high status for women characterizes most contemporary hunting and gathering groups—especially when they are compared to many agricultural and industrial societies in which extreme forms of female subordination often exist. Indeed, although not all agricultural societies should be implicated, the shift to agriculture generally heralded a decline in the overall status of women. This was probably due in part to an increase in the importance of war.

Archaeological evidence suggests that just before agriculture was introduced, areas with rich, abundant resources started supporting larger, more sedentary, and socially stratified settlements somewhat more oriented to war. A number of contemporary examples of this late hunting and gathering adaptation have been recorded, especially among various Native American groups living on the northwest Pacific coast. For the Tlingit of Alaska, in a good year the three-month salmon run could provide enough fish to last (when preserved) until the next season, twelve months later. Known for their rigid social classes, including slaves, and elaborate storage techniques, the Tlingit held widely publicized potlatches—or social gatherings—during which large quantities of food and wealth were given away.

Yet anthropologist Laura Klein found that, historically, women's status was quite high in this stratified society. A report from 1874 reads, ". . . there are few savage nations in which the [female] sex have greater influence or command greater respect . . . the truth is that not only old men, but old women, are respected." And, "The women possess a predominant influence, and acknowledge superiority over the other sex." Indeed, she comments that in this society in which status was so important, "Women and men held similar positions in the ranking system." Not all stratified groups reflect this high degree of equality, but the Tlingit case makes clear that more complex societal organization didn't necessarily preclude women from enjoying privilege along with men.

That "true" equality between the sexes may have existed during the Paleolithic is clearly a theoretical possibility; many contemporary groups exhibit something quite close to it. Yet, contemporary analogues suggest that a balance of power favoring men also may have prevailed in many societies. What is least likely, however, is that the extremes of oppression experienced by women in many parts of the world today existed before the introduction of agriculture. Too many features of the hunting and gathering life-style guard against such conditions.

Contrary to popular belief, then, our remote past provides no precedent for extreme sexual or social inequality: It is not ubiquitous or inevitable. To survive during the long course of the Paleolithic period, humans had to be flexible more than anything else, so that they could freely adapt to diverse and variable conditions. Rigid social categorization would have undermined and limited their ability to fine-tune their social worlds to a wide range of environmental challenges. Gender roles were surely well elaborated, but must have existed in a variety of guises, responsive to the specific demands of a wide range of circumstances. Yet, the potential for human inequity—social classes, war, and the oppression of women—does seem part of the human makeup, never far below the surface. When the checks and balances against the extremes of its expression erode, inequality is only too quick to blossom.

But humans can clearly function quite successfully in an egalitarian framework. Recent hunters and gatherers are living proof: They discourage self-aggrandizement and encourage social equality. Thus the goal of an equitable and decent world order is not inconsistent with the original human condition.

WOMEN IN HUMAN EVOLUTION

We are bombarded by sexist images about our "caveman" past: Alley-Oop drags Betty-Boop (or whomever) along by the hair; he is rudely masculine, she is demurely accepting. Only slightly more sophisticated are images of hunters protecting and providing for their dependent wives and children, valiantly braving carnivore-infested wilds, stalking dangerous animals, and risking their lives to bring home "the bacon" (or wild boar, as the case may be). These images depict women as passive actors in the grand sweep of human evolution and men's hunting and warring activities as the dynamic forces shaping human existence. Not mere cartoon and movie conventions, these images also reflect the legacy of nineteenth- and early-twentieth-century beliefs—both scientific and popular—about the fundamental nature of the sexes and their roles in the development of early human society.

The most popular nineteenth-century theories described "the beginning" as a time of human promiscuity and group marriage. Women were not seen as sharing comparable sexual appetites with males and were portrayed as asexual "victims" of male sexual drive, dependent, and nonproductive. All that changed when women took charge; promiscuity ended as women redirected male sexuality into monogamy, marriage, and the family. In this stage, called matriliny, males continued to be sexually driven, competitive, and aggressive, but females were able to keep them in check. By some accounts, these females were amazons, political and religious leaders—aggressive in nature—and in control of power, property, and the family.

Eventually, so the scenario goes, males "rightfully" wrested power back from females and reasserted their dominance in all areas of cultural life—social, political, economic, and intellectual—but without a return to promiscuity. During this last and final stage, called patriliny, marriage came under the control of men and women again became subservient. Not coincidentally, Victorian Europe was viewed as having reached this ultimate stage, the pinnacle of human potential and possibility.

With time, these unscientific speculations were challenged: New data from "primitive" cultures did not support the theory of universal stages in societal development. All societies had some form of marriage and family structure; and matriarchy, or rule by women—with or without general promiscuity—was unknown. Also, the view of females as weak and dependent and males as virile and aggressive was so parallel to nineteenth-century stereotypes of the sexes that they were eventually seen for the thinly veiled, ethnocentric projections that they were.

Nevertheless, this intellectual tradition did not die out completely. Some twentieth-century theorists continued to stress a male-oriented view of human beginnings. Hunting was seen as the driving force behind human evolution. Pressure on men to cooperate during the hunt, they argued—locating, approaching, and killing big game animals—was the central impetus for brain enlargement and cultural progress. Man the Hunter was synonymous with the evolution of human biological and social complexity.

But in the last two decades, a more balanced theory has become increasingly accepted. This view stresses the use of implements—of stone, wood, and leather—for hunting *and* gathering. Wooden spears and stone knives increased the variety of accessible game and the yield per kill. Wooden digging sticks provided access to underground roots and tubers while stone processing tools expanded the spectrum of edible vegetable foods. Such implements permitted the development of increasingly sophisticated techniques for both activities—and favored the survival of males and females intelligent enough to devise and employ such techniques.

Tool use, together with the need to care for an increasingly dependent child, promoted a two-level approach to food getting, resulting in a sexual division of labor exceptional among mammals. *But,* neither hunting nor gathering was necessarily more important; both animal and vegetable foods make vital contributions to human nutrition. Moreover, the ability to simultaneously harvest foods from two different environmental levels gave early humans a unique advantage over their competition, while favoring further evolution toward intelligence and communications.

Brain enlargement may also have been fostered by baby and child care. During human evolution, infants were born at an increasingly helpless stage (compared with the offspring of apes and other primates). The proper care of such infants must have necessitated corresponding increases in the intelligence of protohuman females. Even upright posture may have been the result of the early human female's need to carry an infant with one hand while carrying fruit or vegetables with the other. Some have postulated that the earliest human tool may have been an infant carrying device. Furthermore, anthropologist Jane Lancaster has argued that provisioning young children with food after weaning—something only humans do among the higher primates—may explain why we have lower mortality rates after weaning than do monkeys and apes.

The view of early females as being weak and dependent has also been challenged by the realities of contemporary hunting and gathering life. Recent foraging economies reflect women's contributions as being vital to the life of the community. Because of the importance of gathered foods, some anthropologists say that "Woman the Gatherer" is at least as apt a description of these societies as "Man the Hunter."

This is not to suggest that a universal stage of woman rule, or matriarchy, ever actually existed. Yet, a sizable minority (15 percent) of societies are arranged along matrilineal lines. In these groups, inheritance passes on through women, children are identified through female relatives, and about 50 percent of couples live with the woman's family. But even in these societies, men tend to dominate politically—a far cry from women's rule.

Perhaps the most appealing aspect of a theory of matriarchy, however, is its depiction of women as a dynamic force in human evolution—with political savvy and sexual drive. Anthropologist and primatologist Sarah Blaffer Hrdy, in a book reviewing recent research on the social role of females in primate groups, has shown that females always play an active role in initiating sexual relations (usually with a variety of partners), in fighting to protect their offspring, and in struggling actively with each other for precedence in the social hierarchy—a major determinant of the social rank of both their sons and daughters. Other studies have also shown that, in several monkey species, females determine which males will succeed in reproducing, by choosing those who are capable of forming long-term friendships with females. And, in looking at the ability to form cooperative social groups and "bonds" among our closest primate relatives, the apes—females and their offspring—are at center stage while males generally remain in the wings. With the exception of defending offspring, these findings overturn smug convictions that have long been held by a male-centered approach to primate evolution.

These new ideas may be speculative, but they are transforming the way anthropologists and paleontologists think about human evolution. Women are finally emerging as members of the team: selectively choosing males, forming cooperative groups with offspring and other females, competing with females and with males, maintaining a major role in subsistence, and performing the vast majority of baby and child care— essentially grappling with all human issues side by side with males. As Sarah Blaffer Hrdy writes,

> If it is shown—as I believe it will be—that there are no important differences between males and females in intelligence, initiative, or administrative and political capabilities, that women are no less qualified in these areas than men are, one has to accept that these potentials did not appear gratuitously as a gift from Nature. Competition was the trial by fire from which these capacities emerged. The feminist ideal of a [female] sex less egotistical, less competitive by nature, less interested in dominance . . . is a dream that may not be well founded.

The lesson from the past, then, is one of complementary roles, not dominance. Males and females both played hard, won and lost, and together contributed to the dynamic and complex patterns of human culture as we know them today. Yet our society's opportunities for women who want to contribute both productively and reproductively are limited. Young children can rarely be brought to the workplace, and most women cannot (and might not want to) bring their work home. Supports for child care are often inadequate, and women's pay sometimes barely covers the expense. Western women are forced to choose between career and motherhood, a dilemma "working women" foragers never had to face. Their system valued women's contributions to the economy and to the family and was set up to support both.

Women have always had the propensity and talent for contributing to society, both within and outside the family. Sigmund Freud recognized how important both aspects were for mental health as reflected in his motto "love and work." Erik Erikson also defined the fulfilled life as one which included both. Yet, many women in our society have to give up one in order to have the other. Or else they try both, stretching themselves beyond comfort, worried that neither job is being done well. If our ancient female forebears were to contemplate the life of today's superwomen—with minimal supports and maximal demands—they would no doubt wonder at the "primitive" conditions under which these women are forced to live.

Our female legacy from the past, then, is not only one to be proud of, it can also serve as a guide for the future. Women *can* and *should* have it all—they were meant to, and did so for most of the time people have been on earth. In order for women today to match the contributions made in the past, changes are necessary in the workplace to accommodate parenting. Nurseries have to be set up in buildings where parents work. Flexible and part-time hours have to be options available for parents involved with school-age or younger children.

Another way to ease the demands of parenting (so often exclusive and isolating) is to design apartment buildings with safe spaces where children can play—a re-creation of a hunting and gathering village. Communal playrooms, perhaps on every floor, with only inside access from each apartment, would be a haven for children of all ages and a compelling alternative to television. It would also help break the isolation of parenting within one's own four walls, an "unnatural" consequence of civilization.

To move forward—to regain the Stone Age standard—women have to shape their futures, a task well within reach. After all, there was a time when scientists failed to recognize women as one of the dynamic forces behind evolutionary change. Not so long ago women were also expected to stay at home to raise their families—and to feel fulfilled; those with other ambitions were seen as somehow lacking. Yet, when women entered the previously male-dominated intellectual arenas of paleontology and anthropology, they changed views of human origins just as the massive flow of women into the workforce changed women's relationship to the economy. These changes are praiseworthy, but from a Paleolithic perspective, it is no more natural to expect women to devote themselves exclusively to work and to be fulfilled than it once was to expect complete devotion to family.

One additional step is now needed to integrate "love and work": a modern restatement of an ancient principle. As women's contributions to the economy become more widely valued, there is no doubt that they will eventually gain the confidence to recreate conditions that better serve their, and perhaps even men's, needs.

CHAPTER TEN

THE PALEOLITHIC PRESCRIPTION: OLD WAYS, NEW PROSPECTS

DISCORDANCE RESTATED

For poker players, a "bust hand" is one with no realistic possibilities for improvement: no high cards, no partial straights or flushes, no wild cards, no potential toward which to draw new cards. Good poker players sometimes bluff with such hands, but more often they throw them in, abandon their ante, and await the next deal. The opposite is a "pat hand." Here, a player is dealt such exceptional cards that it is possible to "stand pat"—play without drawing any new cards—and, in most cases, win.

The genetic constitution of each of us can be likened to an enormous poker hand—with tens of thousands of cards, not just five. Some people have the equivalent of a "pat hand," genes so favorable that they can avoid the diseases of civilization despite shockingly unhealthful lifestyles. Winston Churchill was an example of this fortunate constitution: He was obese, known for his love of brandy and cigars, and—despite his well-publicized bricklaying—almost never exercised. Nevertheless, he lived to the ripe age of ninety and enjoyed excellent health throughout nearly all his life.

The corollary, of course, is that some of us have drawn very bad genetic "hands." Individuals with inherited diseases ranging from retinoblastoma (an eye cancer that strikes in early childhood) to phenylketonuria—PKU (an inherited defect in amino acid metabolism that can produce irreversible mental deficiency during the first year of life)—are special cases. Fortunately most of us face genetic odds that are not quite so extreme. But we never really know for sure. Take tennis star Arthur Ashe, for example. A superb athlete, Ashe maintained excellent physical condition and lived moderately (by affluent Western standards

265

at least), but nevertheless suffered through two separate heart attacks during his early and mid-thirties.

For people with a genetic inheritance like Churchill, it would seem to make little difference how they play their genetic hands—their medical fates are predetermined by heredity. If we could only be certain that we, individually, had genes that put us in the "pat hand" category, we could live as hedonistically as we wish, secure in the knowledge that "it wouldn't make any difference." But unfortunately, at present, we don't have a way of knowing precisely what genetic constitution each of us actually has. And, of course, few of us possess genes that place us at the very fortunate end of the health spectrum. Rather, we fall into the great, poorly defined midrange of disease susceptibility, while an unfortunate few are especially vulnerable. For nearly all of us, therefore, how we play our hand makes a great deal of difference.

Evolution has been shuffling and redealing our genetic cards for over a billion years, and as a result, the hands we are likely to have drawn at conception are well-suited for the game of life. However, the game we're genetically suited for has rules established geological eras ago and fine-tuned during the Stone Age. If we still played by such rules, nearly all of us would hold a winning hand. But we now play a new game—one with rules much different from those by which our ancestors played. In the new game many of us have losing hands—cards that will insure the development of degenerative disease and, in many cases, premature death.

Genetic predisposition to familial hypercholesterolemia is an example of such a losing hand. In 1985 American investigators Joseph Goldstein and Michael Brown were awarded the Nobel Prize for their work on this inherited condition. Homozygous individuals (those with two genes for the disorder) typically have serum cholesterol levels of 600 mg/dl or even higher and not uncommonly develop coronary atherosclerosis (and, in some cases, heart attack and death) during their teen years. Heterozygotes (people with just one gene for this condition) usually have serum cholesterol levels of 300 or more and generally experience the onset of coronary disease in their thirties and forties.

In Salt Lake City, the Church of Jesus Christ of Latter Day Saints (the Mormons) maintains the most extensive collection of genealogical records to be found anywhere in the world. Working from these records, medical geneticists recently traced the pedigrees of people afflicted with familial hypercholesterolemia. For these families, males in recent generations had serum cholesterol levels averaging 352 mg/dl, experienced their first heart attack at an average age of forty-two years, and died of coronary disease at average age forty-five. For prior generations the ancestors' positions in the pedigree allowed determination of whether they also carried the gene, much in the way we know that Queen Victoria carried hemophilia. To their great surprise, the geneticists identified several male ancestors, born between 1815 and 1870, who without question were heterozygous for familial hypercholesterolemia, but who nevertheless lived to ages of sixty, seventy, and even eighty years.

The Utah researchers concluded that these nineteenth-century males were able to achieve normal life spans—averaging thirty years longer than those of their afflicted great grandsons—because their healthier life-style (all the nineteenth-century males were nonsmokers and had physically active occupations) protected them against coronary heart disease despite their genes—the same genes which prove lethal in the twentieth century.

Genetic determinism is far from absolute. How we play our cards makes a difference for nearly all of us. And the difference affects not only the diseases we are likely to develop, but also the quality of our lives from beginning to end.

HUMAN PLASTICITY—WHAT'S A NORMAL HUMAN?

Americans, including many physicians and scientists, base their definition of "normal" on what is common within local populations. People with normal body configuration or normal endurance, for example, do not stand out from their contemporaries. We intuitively reason that what is average for us is average for all humans and therefore acceptable. Yet, researchers who have broadened their scope to include cross-cultural or multinational comparisons, have raised some intriguing questions. Why, for example, are average serum cholesterol levels in Finland so much higher than they are in Japan; and why do Japanese-Americans manifest average serum cholesterol levels 20 mg/dl higher than Japanese living in Japan? If it is normal for blood pressure to increase with age in Western society, why does it not do so among recent hunters and gatherers?

Other findings also cross geographic and temporal boundaries. In the 1850s, for example, European and American girls experienced their first menstrual period at an average age of 15 or later. This age, much like that of !Kung girls (who undergo menarche at an average age of 16.5), contrasts dramatically with the experience of most girls in Western society today who typically begin menstruating at about age 12.5.

Average heights have also varied. During the Revolutionary War, American soldiers averaged 5′ 5½″ in height; now American men of similar age average about 5' 9". This pattern parallels that of Japanese immigrants to the United States whose Americanized grandchildren average nearly 6 inches taller than their immigrant grandparents. And, of course, most current European men are too tall to fit into the armor made for medieval knights. As recently as 1959 the American life insurance industry established a table of normal weight ranges for people of differing stature. Just twenty-four years later, in 1983, these tables were updated—the new "normal" weights were, in each case, several pounds greater for any given height.

Were the people in 1776 "normal"? In 1959? Or is it we in the late twentieth century who deserve to be so-called? Certainly our genes haven't changed over this relatively brief period, so what is the truly normal human pattern?

Our disease patterns have also changed. In the early decades of this century, gastric cancer was the leading cause of death from cancer, but since about 1950 its incidence has declined dramatically. Over the same time interval, lung cancer, which in the early 1900s was called "one of the rarest forms of human malignancy," became the most common cancer killer. And consider coronary atherosclerosis: In 1910, Sir William Osler, considered by many the greatest physician of his time, was asked to lecture on heart disease. He described angina pectoris (a painful, but nonfatal condition caused by coronary atherosclerosis) as a relative rarity and failed to mention heart attack altogether.

Unlikely as it seems, heart attack was not described as a clinical entity until 1912, but soon after, physicians everywhere became aware of its existence. When reflecting on his early years in practice, Paul Dudley White, an outstanding cardiologist of the midcentury, noted that before 1920, heart attacks and other symptoms of coronary atherosclerosis were relatively uncommon. His statement was not based solely on his memory; rather, in reviewing his earliest office records for telltale signs of heart disease, he just did not see them occurring with any frequency.

What accounts for these changes in height, weight, sexual maturation, and patterns of disease within a time frame far too short to reflect genetic alterations? The answer is relatively straightforward: We do not inherit specific attributes such as adult height—we inherit genes which establish a range of genetic potential. Extremely short parents are not likely to have a son who will play center in the National Basketball Association, but, like Japanese immigrants to America, their children and grandchildren may become significantly taller because of nutritional and environmental factors. Similarly, our genes do not doom us to hypertension or diabetes; rather, they establish our innate susceptibility to these chronic degenerative diseases. Each of us inherits a greater or lesser predisposition for developing such illnesses. Whether we actually contract any of them depends not on genetic factors alone, but on the interaction between our genes and our lives.

Anthropologists use the term "plasticity" to describe this concept. For most biologically based characteristics, our genes set the limits, but within these limits our life-style determines whether we incline toward the maximum or the minimum end of our inherited range. The arguments about environment versus heredity in human intelligence can be seen in this light. An individual with the genetic potential to rival Albert Einstein can become an illiterate high school dropout given an overwhelmingly unfavorable upbringing, while with hard work and unceasing dedication, a person with ordinary genetic endowment can make outstanding contributions.

But plasticity still does not answer the question "What is normal for humans?" Is it the pattern that exists in our lives today—where blood pressure, serum cholesterol, and body fat all increase with age and lean body mass decreases? Or is it the pattern experienced by recent hunters and gatherers in whom none of these trends occur?

The "normal" human pattern is, ultimately, whatever encourages the optimal functioning of our biochemical and physiological endowment— an endowment refined in the context of Late Paleolithic experience. By looking at life as it was probably experienced by our Stone Age ancestors, we can form a concept of what is normal for humans. At present, the disparity between our genes and our lives promotes chronic degenerative disorders at the same time it creates false biological "norms." We have come to accept gradually rising blood pressure, slow deterioration of body composition, and high serum cholesterol levels as the natural human pattern. Yet, they are, in reality, deviations from the true human norm as much as they are harbingers of impending symptomatic illness.

Our genes cannot (at present, anyway) be changed, but our diet, exercise habits, use of tobacco and alcohol, child care patterns, social relations, and other aspects of our life-styles can. They can be selectively aligned to fit more closely with our basic human design. Twentieth-century life has, in many ways, led us in the opposite direction, creating new ills—from heart attack to early teenage pregnancy. Yet, with essentially the same genetic constitution, these and other "modern" conditions were uncommon, rare, or nonexistent for our Late Paleolithic ancestors.

THE PALEOLITHIC PARADIGM

The life-styles of our Stone Age ancestors can be seen as paradigms for human life today. We share their genes and, despite the millennia which separate us, we can mold many aspects of our lives so as to recreate, selectively, some of the biological conditions under which they lived—conditions which remain appropriate and "natural" for humans today. Their experience can also help us assess the endless stream of health promotion and disease prevention recommendations which issue forth from friends, doctors, popular health books, the media, academic institutions, medical organizations, and the government. More often than not, these sources differ in detail and give contradictory advice; some are so extreme they seem preposterous. Our Paleolithic ancestors' 2 million year experience, however, provides a guide to optimal human functioning—a benchmark against which these recommendations can be sorted, judged, and selected.

Indicators of Paleolithic Health

Numerous biochemical and physiological markers reflect our health status, but the truly significant ones are few in number, and relatively inexpensive to determine. In most cases they can accurately assess individual health profiles; they are therefore useful in measuring the success of efforts to recreate key features of our ancestral physiology.

Body Composition

The relative proportion of fat and lean tissue is more indicative of health status than is total body weight. As measured by differences in skinfold thicknesses, people living in affluent countries are typically encased in unnecessary fat "envelopes" when compared to people who live by hunting and gathering. This excess tissue encumbers and burdens the musculoskeletal, cardiorespiratory, and glandular systems of our bodies. As Kenneth Cooper's aerobic studies have shown, superior physical fitness is correlated with a body composition which includes no more than 15 percent of body weight as fat for men and 25 percent for women. Lower limits are addressed by other studies, which correlate body composition and ovulatory function in women and libido in men. These findings suggest that body fat should range between 5 and 15 percent in men and between 20 and 25 percent in women regardless of age.

Blood Pressure and Blood Sugar

Among hunters and gatherers (as well as most traditional people) these values almost invariably fall within the lower range of the normal spectrum observed in young adult Americans. Furthermore, these parameters do not increase with age. The typical Western age-related increases in blood pressure and blood sugar levels should therefore be considered as warnings of incipient disease.

Serum Cholesterol

Levels in recent foragers and most preindustrial people rarely exceed 150 mg/dl, and this figure should be the goal for healthy Americans. Furthermore, like blood sugar and blood pressure, serum cholesterol levels should remain constant throughout life. Those unable to achieve and maintain a level of less than 175 mg/dl should adopt more stringent dietary guidelines than those advocated for general use in Chapter 6.

Populations in whom total serum cholesterol levels average below 150 mg/dl have little or no atherosclerotic heart disease, regardless of what percentage of their cholesterol is associated with high density lipoprotein (HDL). For example, the Tarahumaras, whose serum cholesterol levels average about 133 mg/dl, have no coronary atherosclerosis even though their average HDL-cholesterol levels are only 25 mg/dl—that is, HDL cholesterol makes up only 19 percent of their total serum cholesterol. On the other hand, in Western populations, where high serum cholesterol values are common, the proportion of total cholesterol associated with HDL is more significant, because a high proportion of HDL cholesterol tends to protect against development of coronary atherosclerosis. Data from the prestigious Framingham Study suggests that the proportion of total serum cholesterol associated with HDL is more important than the absolute concentration of HDL and that individuals whose HDL cholesterol comprises more than 29 percent of their total serum cholesterol have a significantly lower risk of developing coronary heart disease than are otherwise similar people with a lower proportion of HDL cholesterol. High proportions of HDL cholesterol are common among rural agriculturalists whose total cholesterol values exceed 150 mg/dl (for example, 46 percent for the Tswana of South Africa) and, more importantly, for partially Westernized Eskimos, who remain remarkably free from coronary disease despite total serum cholesterol levels similar to those of Western Europeans (for example, 44 percent for Greenland Eskimos and 43 percent for those in Alaska). The Japanese, who have little coronary atherosclerosis despite their heavily industrialized culture, generally maintain HDL cholesterol values exceeding 29 percent of their total serum cholesterol levels, and this figure seems a reasonable physiological marker for individuals who seek to achieve Paleolithic health while living in Western society.

Maximum Oxygen Uptake Capacity (VO$_2$ max)

This parameter best characterizes endurance fitness and can be estimated by treadmill testing. Data on hunters and gatherers and other preindustrial populations together with studies of Americans conducted by Dr. Cooper suggest that VO$_2$ max should be at least 40–50 ml/kg/min for men and 30–40 ml/kg/min for women who wish to approximate the endurance of Paleolithic humans.

Strength Fitness

While the skeletal remains of early *Homo sapiens sapiens* indicate that they were extremely powerful, we have no way of knowing just how strong they actually were. And, although many anecdotes attest to the physical strength of today's hunters and gatherers, little systematic testing of their muscular power has been carried out. The strength fitness standards recommended here, therefore, are based on data provided by sports physiologists. These findings suggest that males of all ages should—*under appropriate medical supervision*—pursue a program with the *ultimate* goal of bench pressing a minimum of their body weight and leg pressing 1.5 times their weight; women should aim at bench pressing two-thirds of their body weight and leg pressing 100 percent of their body weight.

These goals—for both endurance and strength—must be pursued gradually and carefully; people over forty, and those having trouble attaining the fitness standards outlined in this book, should approach fitness training with special caution because these activities can be hazardous (as described in Chapter 7). In such cases the advice of physicians and exercise specialists can be invaluable and is recommended. And remember: Even modest gains in overall fitness can be a great boon to health.

People living in today's world cannot, and would certainly not wish to, reestablish all elements of the Paleolithic world. However, it is possible to recreate those most beneficial biological conditions which influenced the biochemistry and physiology of people living before the beginnings of agriculture. Since our genes are basically similar to theirs, we can—by adjusting our habits, nutritional practices, and exercise patterns—achieve the basic vigor inherent in our human design. Success can be measured by comparison with the criteria described here. If all Americans were to maintain these standards throughout their lives, the prevalence of chronic diseases in this country should parallel that which probably characterized the Late Paleolithic; that is, such diseases should be minimized, postponed, or reduced to negligible importance.

The Paleolithic Standard: A Light From the Past

It is often difficult to feel confident about which health advice to follow. "Orthomolecular" enthusiasts, for example, recommend vitamin C and other vitamins in doses far greater than those suggested by the government, nutritionists, and most physicians. The debate that results is often acrimonious, pitting, as it does, traditional medical physicians against "alternative" practitioners. This may confuse us, but it pales beside the confusion wrought when respected authorities within mainstream medicine disagree among themselves. Conflicting advice about human requirements for calcium and its role in preventing and treating osteoporosis, for example, is championed by physicians of impeccable credentials—to the dismay of most people, but especially women, who are more vulnerable to the condition and impatient for consensus. The official stand regarding issues such as breast-feeding, permissive child rearing, and even the "natural" role of women has also changed over the decades, often fluctuating between extremes. Exercise too has been promoted and derided. And, of course, new research "breakthroughs" are announced regularly in the media—water-soluble fiber, monounsaturated fat, selenium, fish oil—each purportedly the answer to one or more health problems.

Amid the welter of continuing argument, the Paleolithic paradigm is a standard to be turned to—the very foundation of the human condition. As each new recommendation, research finding, and health promotion claim arises, the past can be evoked to help evaluate it—a past in harmony with the genetic heritage of which we are heirs. Often our ancestors' experience supports a middle ground. For example, their diets contained levels of vitamin C intermediate between the current RDA and the megadoses advocated by orthomolecular proponents. Sometimes the past suggests a more extreme position. For example, their calcium intake approximated the highest current recommendations. But whatever the issue, the past provides much needed time depth; it can illuminate our discussion of infant and child care and male-female relationships just as it can indicate why extensive and lifelong physical exertion, having once been the rule, should not now be the exception.

Take, for example, the debate about serum cholesterol levels. In 1984 a National Institutes of Health (NIH) Consensus Conference concluded that "elevation of blood cholesterol is a major cause of coronary artery disease" and that lowering blood cholesterol levels would reduce the risk of heart attacks caused by coronary heart disease. But in 1987 heart surgeon Michael De Bakey was quoted as saying that cholesterol is *not* the main cause of coronary atherosclerosis, that cholesterol levels do *not* appear related to the rates of the disease's progression, and that some people with *low* cholesterol levels were as likely as people with higher levels to develop atherosclerotic plaques. Dr. De Bakey also claimed that about a third of patients with heart attacks had "perfectly normal" cholesterol levels.

How can we determine which one is right? After all, the NIH panel was composed of leading national authorities while Dr. De Bakey is commonly recognized as one of America's premier heart surgeons. The answer can readily be found in the "small print" of the respective articles. The NIH panel was primarily concerned with people whose serum cholesterol levels were above the 75th percentile (which, for Americans over age forty, is about 240 mg/dl) while Dr. De Bakey defined "low" cholesterol levels as those below 200 mg/dl. However, while Dr. De Bakey's levels are "low" by contemporary American standards, they are still very high when judged against the Paleolithic benchmark of 150 mg/dl. The differences between the NIH and De Bakey are therefore somewhat academic—akin to arguing about whether you are more likely to cause a fatal accident while driving through town at 50 as opposed to 70 miles per hour when the real speed limit is 25.

This same perspective will continue to clarify a wide range of claims and recommendations into the future. It is a Stone Age standard against which to view the outcome of Computer Age research.

THE PALEOLITHIC PRESCRIPTION

The following life-style recommendations are based on our current understanding of what life must have been like during the Late Paleolithic (generally between 35,000 and 20,000 years ago). They are also balanced as closely as possible with the consensus views of mainstream scientists and physicians concerned with health promotion and disease prevention. They have been modified still further to accommodate the realities of life as most of us experience it today. They are intended to be practicable, not ideal and unattainable.

Their implementation will require alterations in both habit and taste, changes some may deride as being unlikely. Such critics might do well to remember the movie *Loneliness of the Long Distance Runner*, a title reasonable in the early 1960s when the movie was made, but implausible in the 1980s when the roads are clogged with joggers. Culinary taste is similarly influenced by custom and learning. One has only to consider that the snails and raw oysters Americans regard as delicacies are no more (or less) intrinsically appealing than are the sheep's eyes of the Arabs, the moth larvae of the Australian Aborigines, or the whole calves brains of the culinarily prestigious French. And the ancient Romans enthusiastically consumed great quantities of a flavorful sauce made from rotten fish.

The dietary modifications necessitated by Paleolithic recommendations are far less extreme. Their acceptance is no less likely than a nation of joggers would have seemed to a skeptic of the early 1960s; the dramatic increase in fitness consciousness since then proves how receptive we are to change—and how willing we are to implement new ideas.

Nutrition

Our nutritional protocol attempts to balance the dietary patterns of our ancestors with twentieth-century food availability.

Carbohydrates should provide about 60 percent of an average day's calories; sugar and refined flour should be minimized while fruits, vegetables, and whole grains—sources of complex carbohydrates—should be emphasized.

Protein should constitute about 20 percent of average daily calories and should come from low-fat sources.

Fat should constitute the remaining 20 percent of each day's calories. More should be polyunsaturated than saturated; avoid butter and lard as well as the highly saturated coconut, palm, and palm kernel vegetable oils.

Dietary cholesterol is less critical than total fat intake and can be as much as 600 mg/day *providing*, first, that total fat intake provides no more than 20 percent of overall food energy, and, second, that polyunsaturated fat exceeds saturated fat in the diet. These qualifications are absolutely essential; otherwise dietary cholesterol should be restricted to 300 mg/day or less.

Dietary fiber should come from fruits, vegetables, and whole grain breads and cereals, but a tablespoon each of wheat and oat bran at breakfast can help ensure a sufficiency of both soluble and insoluble fiber.

Dietary supplementation with RDA (not megadose) levels of the water soluble vitamins, beta-carotene, and vitamin E provides reasonable assurance of adequate intake, as does taking a multimineral tablet (including iron, iodine, magnesium, chromium, selenium, zinc, and copper). Supplemental essential fatty acids such as eicosapentaenoic acid (EPA) may ultimately prove beneficial, but at present their benefits are uncertain.

Calcium should probably be supplemented in amounts necessary to bring total daily intake up to a 1,500 mg level (providing there is no medical history of kidney stones).

Sodium intake needs to be minimized as much as possible. Restricting dietary sodium to Late Paleolithic levels is one of the most difficult and, to many people, most important current nutritional challenges.

Our foods can be chosen from the four contemporary food groups, even though our ancestors' nutrition was derived from just two of these. Our meals should emphasize whole-grain bread, rolls, pancakes, and cereals, fresh fruits and vegetables, fish, poultry (without skin), and shellfish, and low-fat dairy products. When processed foods are included, select those with the least possible fat (especially saturated fat), sodium, cholesterol, refined flour, and sugar. Those made with complex carbohydrates, nonnutrient fiber, protein, and calcium are good choices. Where possible, caloric contribution from protein should exceed that from fat, and polyunsaturated fat should exceed saturated fat.

Tobacco and Alcohol

Our recommendations regarding drinking and smoking (or other tobacco use) are based as much, or more, on the results of current scientific and medical investigation as on anthropological observation.

Wild tobacco is known to have been used by hunters and gatherers only in Australia, which was first reached by the ancestors of the Aborigines only about 40,000 years ago. In the Americas, its use postdates the appearance of agriculture (about 5,000 years ago), while Africans, Asians, and Europeans had no exposure to it until the voyages of discovery five hundred years ago. Tobacco use, therefore, is essentially foreign to our genetic heritage and, given its disastrous medical consequences, should be eliminated from our lives. Its detrimental effects on health are disputed only by tobacco company apologists and by some legislators from tobacco-producing states, people unlikely to be favorably treated by future historians.

Alcohol use by Stone Age hunters and gatherers must have been limited. But since honey and fruits with sufficient sugar content can undergo spontaneous fermentation, it is possible that some groups made seasonal drinks containing alcohol. However, widespread manufacture and consumption of alcoholic beverages is likely to have begun only after the appearance of agriculture, an assumption supported by its absence in preagricultural populations around the world even well into the twentieth century. In traditional groups where alcohol does exist, it is naturally fermented (that is, beer, wine, or mead, not distilled liquor) and its consumption is socially integrated, usually in a well-defined, often ritual, context. Solitary, addictive, pathological drinking is highly unusual among preliterate peoples living under traditional conditions. Abstinence or at least scrupulous restraint in the use of alcohol is therefore most in keeping with our basic biology. Modern medical experience clearly shows that excessive intake over extended periods is extremely damaging to health. Even one episode of intoxication, if it results in a serious accident, can destroy a life.

Exercise

Skeletal remains from throughout the Paleolithic indicate that humans were heavily muscled and physically powerful. In addition, our unique physiological mechanisms for heat loss (the lack of functional body hair and the ability to sweat) show that strenuous aerobic exercise—the activity most likely to generate heat—must have been central to our ancestors' lives following their divergence from our apelike forebears 5 to 10 million years ago. An ongoing program of physical exercise should therefore become integral to each person's daily schedule, a conclusion also widely recommended by cardiologists, diabetologists, orthopedists, and a variety of other physicians.

Exercise physiologists have shown how we can efficiently duplicate the positive physiological effects of our ancestors' strenuous existence:

Exercise Modes
Both aerobic (endurance) and resistance (strength) exercise are necessary. Emphasize different forms of activity on alternate days of the week.

Periodic Variation
Vary the specific type of exercise on a monthly, seasonal, semiannual, or even yearly basis to forestall burnout and to maximize enjoyment.

Aerobic Training

This can include jogging, rowing, bicycling, swimming, aerobics, walking, and like activities; these should be varied within the context of a lifelong program.

Resistance Training

Variation can be built into the specific exercises, sets, repetitions, and weights and used according to the principles of periodization, as described in Chapter 7. Alternating between free weights and resistance machines is another approach to the same end.

Warming-up

This is mandatory and should last from 5 to 15 minutes (the shorter period in warm weather, the longer period in cool or cold weather). Exercises should consist of easy, simple repetitive movements (very slow jogging in place, jumping jacks, sit-ups, etc.). If stretching is included in the warm-up, it should come at the end—after the muscles and joints have become "loose."

Cooling Down

This, too, is mandatory and should begin with walking—vigorously at first, then more slowly. A flexibility routine is an excellent way of finishing, since the body is in optimal condition for stretching at this point.

An ideal exercise program expends about 2,000 calories a week. Most of this should be contributed by aerobic activities, but the resistance and flexibility components are also important, since each makes significant and unique contributions to overall health. This level of activity does not require an inordinate commitment of time; the entire fitness program need involve no more than 30 to 90 minutes a day.

THE PALEOLITHIC PRESCRIPTION VERSUS CURRENT MEDICAL RECOMMENDATIONS: A GUIDE TO RESEARCH CONSENSUS

The Paleolithic Prescription consists of proposals for contemporary life drawn from anthropological and paleontological principles. *In most respects,* our recommendations are consistent with the advice given by physicians, nutritionists, and sports physiologists concerned with health promotion and disease prevention, as well as with that of pediatricians, psychologists, and educators concerned with a broad range of social issues. There are, however, different levels of research agreement regarding these proposals; some are even contrary to generally accepted views of more conventional authorities.

Table XX lists our major recommendations and assigns for each a rating of the degree of medical or behavioral research consensus regarding them. The scale is as follows:

1. Noncontroversial—almost uniformly accepted
2. Widely, but not invariably, accepted
3. Controversial—much debate, or no consensus
4. Would be generally rejected
5. Not commonly addressed by authorities

TABLE XX.

The Paleolithic Prescription: Research Consensus

Paleolithic Prescription	Research Consensus	Comments*
Nutrition		
1. High protein, approx. 20% of calories	3 or 4	Nephrologists raise possibility of accelerated kidney degeneration
2. Low-fat, approx. 20% of calories	1	SSCN: 30%; AHA: 20–30%
3. Polyunsaturates greater than saturates	2 or 3	AHA and SSCN both recommend P = S
4. Dietary cholesterol less important than fat intake; up to 600 mg/day acceptable *if* fat is less than 20% of total calories and if polyunsaturates are greater than saturates	3 or 4	SSCN and AHA both recommend 300 mg/day or less
5. High carbohydrate, approx. 60% of calories	2	SSCN: 55–60%; ADA: 50–60%; AHA: 50–60%
6. Majority from complex carbohydrate; marked reduction in sugar and refined flour intake	1	Recommended by SSCN

(Continued on next page)

TABLE XX.   *(Continued)*

The Paleolithic Prescription: Research Consensus

Paleolithic Prescription	Research Consensus	Comments*
Nutrition		
7. High fiber intake approx. 50–100 gms/day (includes both soluble and insoluble fiber)	3	Most authorities recommend increase over current intake; recommendations range from 25 to over 100 gms/day
8. Majority of fiber from fruits and vegetables rather than cereal grains	3 or 5	Insures sufficient soluble fiber
9. Supplementation with beta-carotene, vitamin E, and water soluble vitamins—to RDA, *not* to megadose, levels	3	One of the most contentious areas in medicine today
10. Marked reduction in sodium intake	2	Recommended by AHA and SSCN
11. Dietary potassium to exceed sodium	2 or 5	Generally accepted, but not often specifically addressed
12. Calcium intake approx. 1500 mg/day (except in people with kidney stones)	3	Recommendations range from 400 to 1600 mg/day
Tobacco and Alcohol		
13. No tobacco use	1	Essentially universal agreement—more than for any other recommendation
14. No alcohol or very moderate drinking	1 or 2	ACS: drink alcohol only in moderation if at all. None for women who are or may be pregnant
Exercise		
15. Aerobic exercise 30–90 minutes, 3 times weekly	2	AHA: 15–30 min, at least every other day; ACSM: 15–60 min, 3–5 days/week

(Continued on next page)

TABLE XX. *(Continued)*

The Paleolithic Prescription: Research Consensus

Paleolithic Prescription	Research Consensus	Comments*
Exercise		
16. Resistance exercise 30–90 minutes, 3 times weekly	3 or 5	Major advocates are athletic trainers
17. Warm-up period: 5–15 min	1	Reduces likelihood of injury and decreases risk of cardiac arrhythmia
18. Cool-down period: 5–15 min	1	
19. Stretching as last part of cool-down	1	Reduces likelihood of injury—most effective after body is warmed up, especially at end of workout
20. Stretching at end of warm-up	2	
21. Cyclical variation in form of specific exercise—"periodization"	5	Increasingly advocated by sports physiologists and athletic trainers
Baby and Child Care		
22. Breast-feeding at least one year	1	Should not be pressed on very reluctant mothers. AAP recommends through the first year
23. Early indulgence	2	Some authorities believe "spoiling" of infants is possible
24. Close physical contact with parents	3	Day-care in the workplace and "flextime" will help
25. Sleeping with infant	4 or 5	Extremely widespread in nonindustrial societies
26. Avoidance of physical punishment	2	Extremes of physical punishment must be reported as child abuse

(Continued on next page)

TABLE XX.   *(Continued)*

The Paleolithic Prescription: Research Consensus

Paleolithic Prescription	Research Consensus	Comments*
Baby and Child Care		
27. Multi-age playgroups	5	Reduce competition, take pressure off adults
28. Learning through play	2	Classrooms can promote individual pacing, enjoyment
29. Sexual restrictions liberal	4	Dangers of disease and pregnancy must be considered
30. No early teenage pregnancy	1	Menarche now much earlier than for our ancestors
Women's Roles		
31. Equal participation with men in social, political, and economic spheres	3	Approximated among recent hunters and gatherers
32. Women's economic (other than housework) contribution valued	2	Universal among recent hunters and gatherers
33. Fitness and exercise high priorities for women (as well as for men) from childhood on	1	Universal among recent hunters and gatherers
34. Close and frequent physical contact with children	3	Universal among recent hunters and gatherers. Day-care in the workplace and "flextime" will help
35. Cooperation among women in child care and in the workplace	2 or 3	Universal among recent hunters and gatherers
36. Safe play groups for children with access to parents	2	Protected play areas in apartment houses and neighborhoods; day-care facilities

(Continued on next page)

TABLE XX. *(Continued)*

The Paleolithic Prescription: Research Consensus

Paleolithic Prescription	Research Consensus	Comments*
Women's Roles		
37. No sex segregation in childhood activities	3 or 4	Competitive contact sports probably require grouping by sex
38. Grandmothers active in care of children	2	Typical of all traditional cultures
39. Women as assertive achievers	2	The passive female is an evolutionary myth

*AHA = American Heart Association
ACS = American Cancer Society
SSCN = U.S. Senate Select Committee on Nutrition
ADA = American Diabetes Association
ACSM = American College of Sports Medicine
AAP = American Academy of Pediatrics

A CHOICE—NOT AN ECHO

It is easy to become overenthusiastic about the remote past, to become an apologist for a way of life that—through the romantic mists of time—can seem more nearly ideal than it was. The Late Paleolithic *was* a period when human existence was in accord with nature and when our life-styles and our biology were generally in harmony. But, of course, such a view is skewed, an undeserved glorification of a time when half of all children died before reaching adulthood, when posttraumatic disfigurement and disability were distressingly common, and when the comfort and basic security of life were orders of magnitude less than they are at present.

If it were possible to make an informed choice, few today would volunteer for Stone Age existence, especially if there were a trial year or two during which to combat the rain, heat, microbes, insects, and dirt our ancestors encountered each day. On the other hand, the safety, convenience, and unprecedented security of modern life would have tempted Cro-Magnons sorely—just as they have caused recent foragers and members of other traditional societies to abandon their long-standing folkways for a Western life-style.

Of course, people living in the Stone Age could not incorporate elements from our time into theirs. But we are more fortunate. We can pick and choose the best from both worlds. After all, the benefits of life today are incontestable. Our health is buttressed by sanitation, periodic health evaluations, immunizations, antibiotics, anesthesia, supportive care, screening examinations, specialized surgery, and a host of other modern medical miracles. But there are other, less immediate advantages to contemporary life as well.

For them, exercise was obligatory. Preagricultural people traveled long distances on foot, often while carrying heavy loads. Although this imparted important health benefits, the extent of their exercise also created problems. The prevalence of degenerative arthritis in Stone Age skeletal remains, for example, is phenomenal—far in excess of that found among contemporary humans. This finding reflects the complex relationship between the intensity of physical exercise and the effect on health. Almost all parameters (such as endurance, blood lipid profile, and strength) improve with increasing exercise intensity at first, but above a certain level the rate of improvement decreases. In many cases, exercise stress can become so severe that it actually causes harm. Our ancestors had to do what was necessary, not necessarily what was physically ideal; we, however, can choose routines that produce optimal results.

For most of us access to food is essentially constant. We are assured that, once we achieve satisfactory body composition (*not* just body weight), the regular and predictable nature of our food supply will allow us to maintain this composition indefinitely. For recent hunters and gatherers (and presumably for people living in the Stone Age as well) seasonable periods of food shortage and abundance produce regular weight fluctuations. For them, gains and losses of 3 to 5 percent are common over the course of a year, while once a decade or so the percent of weight variation is considerably greater because of near-famine conditions. *We* can voluntarily impose artificial "shortages" when we become obese; for them, shortages occurred without regard to their physical condition.

Nevertheless, we have also seen how the present undermines human health in ways that would have been rare during the Late Paleolithic. To play our cards right, then, we have to adopt the positive necessities of the past and make them a part of our lives today. Fortunately, our bodies are highly tolerant; without built-in plasticity, humans would not have survived the climatic and geological upheavals faced—and not always survived—by all living organisms. But even plastic, when stressed too greatly, can weaken and begin to function below design. Unprecedented high-fat, high-sodium, and low-fiber diets, along with sedentary life, have done just that—stretched human plasticity beyond its limits. The "diseases of civilization" indicate how often this occurs.

The past resides within us; it must be acknowledged and accommodated. In making choices which affect our health, it should be a guide, but not an inviolate one—and certainly not our only one. We have the benefits of modern biological, medical, and behavioral research with which to enhance and modify the lessons of the past, just as our knowledge of the past can interpret and complement the results of modern scientific investigation.

For example, in the brief time since 1970 physicians have sequentially accepted serum cholesterol levels of 300, 240, 200, and now 180 mg/dl as upper limits for relative safety from atherosclerosis. However, the past suggests that this progression needs to proceed even further and that levels below 150 mg/dl will ultimately be recognized as being optimal. Yet, our health advice in other areas owes more to medical research than to paleontology. Our opposition to tobacco use, for example, is based not so much on the fact that few Paleolithic humans were exposed to it, as on the experience of physicians who consistently relate pulmonary emphysema, peripheral and coronary vascular disease, and many cancers (especially bronchogenic carcinoma) to its use. We suspect that naturally fermented alcoholic beverages were used by few preagricultural humans, but it is statistics on traffic fatalities, cirrhosis, breast cancer, and other alcohol-related diseases and injuries that make us argue against its use, except in the strictest moderation.

We need not—and ought not—attempt merely to recreate Late Paleolithic existence. An echo is hollow and weak, no matter how romantic. To be human is to make choices—intelligent choices. And we now have the insight upon which to base our choices—selections from both the past and the present—which, in concert, promise a future no prior humans have known.

NEW PROSPECTS: THE BEST OF BOTH WORLDS

The theme of this book is that our current lives are intricately tied to ancient experience, and that our task is to integrate contemporary science with the Paleolithic perspective. In most respects, the health of humans in today's affluent countries must surpass that of typical Stone Age people. Life expectancy now is over seventy years, double what it was in preindustrial times. Infant death rates are lower than ever before, and nearly 80 percent of all current newborns will survive to age sixty-five and beyond. The rate of endemic infectious disease (especially parasitism) and the prevalence of posttraumatic disability were both far higher 25,000 years ago than they are at present. These vital statistics certify that the health of current populations, at least in the affluent nations, is superior to that of any prior human group.

Furthermore, in countless ways the millennia since agriculture have expanded the dimensions of our world and unleashed the human spirit. The development of writing and mathematics, although late in human history, were contributions of ineffable importance. Our arts are the descendants of those that existed in the Stone Age, but over the centuries the range of creative traditions has expanded so that a vastly greater diversity of artistic expression has become possible. Our libraries, universities, museums, and laboratories afford possibilities far beyond the imagination of preagricultural humans, while computers and sophisticated communications systems seem to be the first stage in yet another unprecedented expansion of human accomplishment.

But the blessings of "civilization" are not unmixed. Our doubled life expectancy is both the crowning achievement of Western society and a telling comment on the ills of life in affluent nations. For many of us the second half of our lives is a time when we are unfit, unhealthy, and unattractive—unable to benefit maximally from, enjoy, or utilize the newly added years. Since our increased longevity is such a recent phenomenon, it is not surprising that its negative aspects—including chronic degenerative diseases—have been considered part of the natural consequences of aging. Only in the past generation have we begun to understand that these chronic conditions are actually "afflictions of affluence"—a result of the discordance between our contemporary lifestyle and our fundamental biochemistry and physiology.

As John Rowe, a noted gerontologist, and other authorities have observed, aging can either be "usual"—by our standards bad—or "successful"—the happy result of the right life-style choices against the background of good genes. "Usual" aging is not the inevitable expression of human biology.

This realization affords us an unprecedented opportunity and challenge. It is now within our reach to benefit from the positive aspects of modern life while at the same time reintroducing essential elements from the life-style of our Paleolithic ancestors. These features can minimize, delay, and in some respects prevent altogether the chronic degeneration that otherwise degrades the "extra" years made possible by modern accomplishments.

Increasing life span has also accentuated the marked divergence in patterns of aging. From a health standpoint, twenty-year-olds are generally quite similar, but there are fairly prominent differences between forty-year-olds, and the disparities become much greater among individuals in their seventh and eighth decades. Many of the original members of this cohort have died; others are sick to a greater or lesser extent; still others, while not clinically ill, are limited in their physical and mental capacities. A growing minority of the elderly, though, remain vigorous and alert: playing tennis, square dancing, and beating their grandchildren at chess while managing their business and social affairs with facility. Eighty-one-year-old Norman Vaughan, who in 1987 successfully completed his fifth 1,100-mile Iditarod Trail dog sled race, from Anchorage to Nome in Alaska, exemplifies the potential of older humans. Japan's sacred Mount Fuji, 12,388 feet in height, might be an appropriate symbol of this potential; in 1987 it was climbed by ninety-one-year-old Hulda Crooks and by one-hundred-year-old Teiichi Igarashi! At present such people are in the minority, but similarly impressive physical and mental capacities can and should become the rule.

Wide variation in health status is characteristic of older people in all societies, including ours. Yet, for us, the downside not only affects our personal lives, but also has great impact on the economy. High-cost users of medical care commonly suffer from one or more *preventable* chronic illnesses, and consume a major portion of medical resources. Faced with a limit as to how much of our gross national product can be allotted to health, we must either economize elsewhere, accept rationing of medical care, or somehow reduce our national need. We may not be able to extend our lives beyond biologically fixed limits, but we can reduce much premature mortality and compress the period of late-life impairment. And since the life-style required to prevent chronic disease involves increased physical and mental activity, it can prolong adult vigor beyond its previously accepted limits. As we delay or halt altogether the progression of many chronic diseases, it will become necessary to redefine "normal" human aging. Our current preconceptions are warped by habitual disuse of our faculties (we must "use it or lose it") together with the inexorable progression of degenerative illnesses promoted by our life-styles. But with proper vigilance, ever-increasing numbers of older adults will be able to retain mental and physical capacities now considered extraordinary.

To achieve these goals, we have the unprecedented challenge—and opportunity—to reinstate the essential elements of Paleolithic life into our modern existence, elements basic to the very core of our biology.

To realize full human potential for vigor and well-being, twentieth-century technology—including the diagnostic and therapeutic capabilities of modern medicine—must coexist with ancient formulas derived from the past. With this integration, we can restructure our lives so that we can enjoy our full potential for health—our legacy from the generations of ancestors whose genes we bear.

For Further Reading and Reference

The starred items are of particular importance and/or general interest.

Chapter 1: The Paleolithic Legacy

*Boyden, S. V., ed. *The Impact of Civilization on the Biology of Man*. Canberra: Australian National University Press, 1970.

Rousseau, J.-J. "Discourse on the Origin of Social Inequality." In J.-J. Rousseau, *The Social Contract and Discourses*. Paris, 1755.

Chapter 2: Our Ancestors, Ourselves

*Angel, J. L. "Health as a Crucial Factor in the Changes from Hunting to Developed Farming in the Eastern Mediterranean." In M. N. Cohen and G. J. Armelagos, eds., *Paleopathology at the Origins of Agriculture*. New York: Academic Press, 1984, pp. 51–73.

*Bicchieri, M. G., ed. *Hunters and Gatherers Today*. New York: Holt, Rinehart and Winston, 1972.

Brown, F., J. Harris, R. Leakey, and A. Walker. "Early Homo erectus Skeleton from West Lake Turkana, Kenya. *Nature* 316 (1985): 788–92.

Campbell, B. *Human Evolution*. 3d ed. New York: Aldine, 1985.

Cohen, M. N. *The Food Crisis in Prehistory: Overpopulation and Origins of Agriculture*. New Haven: Yale University Press, 1977.

Cronin, J. E., N. T. Boaz, C. B. Stringer, and Y. Rak. "Tempo and Mode in Hominid Evolution." *Nature* 292 (1981): 113–22.

Darwin, C. R. *On the Origin of Species by Means of Natural Selection*. London: Murray, 1859.

Eaton, S. B., M. J. Konner, and M. Shostak. "Stone Agers in the Fast Lane: Chronic Degenerative Diseases in Evolutionary Perspective." *American Journal of Medicine* 84 (1988): 739–49.

Gould, S. J., and N. Eldredge. "Punctuated Equilibria: The Tempo and Mode of Evolution Reconsidered." *Paleobiology* 3 (1977): 115–51.

Haddingham, E. *Secrets of the Ice Age*. London: Walker, 1979.

Johanson, D. C., and M. A. Edey. *Lucy: The Beginnings of Humankind.* New York: Simon & Schuster, 1981.

Johanson, D. C., F. T. Masao, G. G. Ech et al. "New Partial Skeleton of Homo habilis from Olduvai Gorge, Tanzania." *Nature* 327 (1987): 205–9.

Keene, H. J. "History of Dental Caries in Human Populations: The First Million Years." In J. M. Tanzer, ed., *Animal Models in Cariology.* Washington, DC: IRL Press, 1981.

Leakey, R. E. *The Making of Mankind.* New York: Dutton, 1981.

*Lee, R. B., and I. DeVore, eds. *Man the Hunter.* Chicago: Aldine, 1968.

*Lewin, R. *Human Evolution: An Illustrated Introduction.* New York: W. H. Freeman, 1984.

Nield, E. W., and V. C. T. Tucker. *Paleontology: An Introduction.* Oxford: Pergamon Press, 1985.

Pfeiffer, J. *The Emergence of Man.* New York: Harper & Row, 1978.

Reed, C. A., ed. *Origins of Agriculture.* The Hague: Mouton, 1977.

Smith, F., and F. Spencer, eds. *The Origins of Modern Humans.* New York: Liss, 1984.

Turner, C. G., II. "The Dental Search for Native American Origins." In R. Kirk and E. Szathmary, eds., *Out of Asia: Peopling the Americas and the Pacific.* Canberra: *Journal of Pacific History*, 1985, pp. 31–78.

Chapter 3: The Discordance Hypothesis

Blankenhorn, D. H. "Two New Diet-Heart Studies." *New England Journal of Medicine* 312 (1985): 851–53.

Blankenhorn, D. H., S. A. Nessim, R. L. Johnson, M. E. Sanmarco, S. P. Azen, and L. Cashin-Hemphill. "Beneficial Effects of Combined Colestipol-Niacin Therapy on Coronary Atherosclerosis and Coronary Venous Bypass Grafts." *Journal of the American Medical Association* 257 (1987): 3233–40.

*Cohen, M. N., and G. J. Armelagos, eds. *Paleopathology at the Origins of Agriculture.* New York: Academic Press, 1984.

*Doll, R., and R. Peto. "The Causes of Cancer: Quantitative Estimates of Avoidable Risks of Cancer in the United States Today." *Journal of the National Cancer Institute* 66 (1981): 1191–1308.

*Eaton, S. B., and M. J. Konner. "Paleolithic Nutrition: A Consideration of Its Nature and Current Implications." *New England Journal of Medicine* 312 (1985): 283–89.

Emerson, H., and L. D. Larimore. "Diabetes Mellitus: A Contribution to Its Epidemiology Based Chiefly on Mortality Statistics." *Archives of Internal Medicine* 34 (1924): 585–630.

Graham, S. "Alcohol and Breast Cancer." *New England Journal of Medicine* 316 (1987): 1211–13.

Jarvis, J. F., and H. G. Van Heerden. "The Acuity of Hearing in the Kalahari Bushmen: A Pilot Study." *Journal of Laryngology and Otology* 81 (1967): 63–68.

Kannel, W. B., P. A. Wolf, J. Verter et al. "Epidemiological Assessment of the Role of Blood Pressure in Stroke: The Framingham Study." *Journal of the American Medical Association* 214 (1970): 301–10.

Malinow, M. R., and V. Blanton. "Regression of Atherosclerotic Lesions." *Arteriosclerosis* 4 (1984): 292–95.

*Mann, J. I., K. Pyorala, and A. Teuscher, eds. *Diabetes in Epidemiological Perspective.* London: Churchill Livingstone, 1983.

*Manson, J. E., M. J. Stamapafer, C. H. Hennekens, and W. C. Willett. "Body Weight and Longevity: A Reassessment." *Journal of the American Medical Association* 257 (1987): 353–58.

Mizell, M., and P. Correa, eds. *Lung Cancer: Causes and Prevention.* Deerfield Beach: Verlag Chemie International, 1983.

Painter, N. S., and D. P. Burkitt. "Diverticular Disease of the Colon." In D. P. Burkitt and H. C. Trowell, eds., *Refined Carbohydrate Foods and Disease.* London: Academic Press, 1975.

Pilbeam, D. "The Origin of *Homo sapiens*: The Fossil Evidence." In B. Wood, L. Martin, and P. Andrews, eds., *Major Topics in Primate and Human Evolution.* Cambridge: Cambridge University Press, 1986.

Roberts, W. C. "Frequency of Systemic Hypertension in Various Cardiovascular Diseases." *American Journal of Cardiology* 60 (1987): 1E–8E.

Sibley, C. G., and J. E. Ahlquist. "The Phylogeny of the Hominoid Primates, as Indicated by DNA-DNA Hybridization." *Journal of Molecular Evolution* 20 (1984): 2–15.

Sims, E. A., R. F. Goldman, C. M. Gluck, et al. "Experimental Obesity in Man." *Transactions of the American Association of Physicians* 81 (1968): 153–70.

Tobian, L. "Salt and Hypertension." *American Journal of Clinical Nutrition* 32 (1979): 2739–48.

*Trowell, H. C., and D. P. Burkitt. *Western Diseases: Their Emergence and Prevention.* Cambridge, MA: Harvard University Press, 1981.

Zimmet, P. "Type 2 (Non-insulin Dependent) Diabetes: An Epidemiological Overview." *Diabetologia* 22 (1982): 399–411.

Chapter 4: The Stone Age Diet

*Angel, J. L. "Health as a Crucial Factor in the Changes from Hunting to Developed Farming in the Eastern Mediterranean." In M. N. Cohen and G. J. Armelagos, eds., *Paleopathology at the Origins of Agriculture.* New York: Academic Press, 1984, pp. 51–73.

*Crawford, M. A. "Fatty-Acid Ratios in Free-Living and Domestic Animals." *Lancet* I (1968): 1329–33.

*Eaton, S. B. "Fibre Intake in Prehistoric Times." In A. R. Leeds, ed., *Dietary Fibre Perspectives:* II. London: John Libbey, in press, 1988.

*Eaton, S. B., and M. J. Konner. "Paleolithic Nutrition: A Consideration of Its Nature and Current Implications." *New England Journal of Medicine* 312 (1985): 283–89.

Hughes, R. E., and E. Jones. "A Welsh Diet for Britain?" *British Medical Journal* I (1979): 1145.

*Ledger, H. P. "Body Composition as a Basis for a Comparative Study of Some East African Mammals." *Symposium of the Zoological Society of London* 21 (1968): 289–310.

McArthur, M. "Food Consumption and Dietary Levels of Groups of Aborigines Living on Naturally Occurring Foods." In C. P. Mountford, ed., *Records of the American-Australian Expedition to Arnhem Land.* Vol. 2. Melbourne: Melbourne University Press, 1960, pp. 90–135.

Morgan, K. J., and M. E. Zabik. "Amount and Food Sources of Total Sugar Intake by Children Ages 5 to 12 Years." *American Journal of Clinical Nutrition* 34 (1981): 404–13.

Nickens, P. R. "Stature Reduction as an Adaptive Response to Food Production in Mesoamerica." *Journal of Archaeological Science* 3 (1976): 31–41.

Schoeninger, M. J. "Diet and the Evolution of Modern Form in the Middle East." *American Journal of Physical Anthropology* 58 (1982): 37–52.

*Select Committee on Nutrition and Human Needs, United States Senate. *Dietary Goals for the United States*. Washington, DC: Government Printing Office, 1977.

Smith, G. C., and Z. L. Carpenter. "Eating Quality of Meat Animal Products and Their Fat Content." In National Research Council, *Fat Content and Composition of Animal Products*. Washington, DC: National Academy of Sciences, 1976, 147–82.

Chapter 5: Our Daily Bread

*Anderson, J. W., and C. A. Bryant. "Dietary Fiber: Diabetes and Obesity." *American Journal of Gastroenterology* 81 (1986): 898–906.

Anderson, J. W., and J. Tietyen-Clark. "Dietary Fiber: Hyperlipidemia, Hypertension, and Coronary Heart Disease." *American Journal of Gastroenterology* 81 (1986): 907–19.

Angel, J. L. "Health as a Crucial Factor in the Changes from Hunting to Developed Farming in the Eastern Mediterranean." In M. N. Cohen and G. J. Armelagos, eds., *Paleopathology at the Origins of Agriculture*. New York: Academic Press, 1984, pp. 51–73.

Brown, F., J. Harris, R. Leakey, and A. Walker. "Early Homo erectus Skeleton from West Lake Turkana, Kenya." *Nature* 316 (1985): 788–92.

Consolazio, C. F., H. L. Johnson, R. A. Nelson, et al. "Protein Metabolism During Intensive Physical Training in the Young Adult." *American Journal of Clinical Nutrition* 28 (1975): 29–35.

*Eaton, S. B., M. J. Konner, and M. Shostak. "Stone Agers in the Fast Lane: Chronic Degenerative Diseases in Evolutionary Perspective." *American Journal of Medicine* 84 (1988): 739–49.

Gey, K. F., G. B. Brubacher, and H. B. Stahelin. "Plasma Levels of Antioxidant Vitamins in Relation to Ischemic Heart Disease and Cancer." *American Journal of Clinical Nutrition* 45 (1987): 1368–77.

Grundy, S. M. "Monounsaturated Fatty Acids, Plasma Cholesterol, and Coronary Heart Disease." *American Journal of Clinical Nutrition* 45 (1987): 1168–75.

*Heaney, R. P. "Calcium, Bone Health, and Osteoporosis." *Bone and Mineral Research* 4 (1986): 255–301.

*Hegsted, D. M., R. B. McGandy, M. L. Myers, and F. J. Stare. "Quantitative Effects of Dietary Fat on Serum Cholesterol in Man." *American Journal of Clinical Nutrition* 17 (1965): 281–95.

Illingworth, D. R., W. S. Harris, and W. E. Conner. "Inhibition of Low Density Lipoprotein Synthesis by Dietary Omega-3 Fatty Acids in Humans." *Arteriosclerosis* 4 (1984): 270–75.

*Keys, A., ed. *Seven Countries: A Multivariate Analysis of Death and Coronary Disease*. Cambridge, MA: Harvard University Press, 1980.

*Leveille, G. A., M. E. Zabaik, and K. J. Morgan. *Nutrients in Foods*. Cambridge, MA: The Nutrition Guild, 1983.

*Meneely, G. R., and H. D. Batterbee. "High Sodium–Low Potassium Environment and Hypertension." *American Journal of Cardiology* 38 (1976): 768–85.

Miettinen, T. A. "Dietary Fiber and Lipids." *American Journal of Clinical Nutrition* 45 (1987): 1237–42.

Palgi, A. "Vitamin A and Lung Cancer: A Perspective." *Nutrition and Cancer* 6 (1984): 105–20.

Schonfield, G., W. Patsch, L. L. Rudel, C. Nelson, M. Epstein, and R. E. Olson. "Effects of Dietary Cholesterol and Fatty Acids on Plasma Lipoproteins." *Journal of Clinical Investigation* 69 (1982): 1072–80.

Select Committee on Nutrition and Human Needs, United States Senate. *Dietary Goals for the United States*. Washington, DC: Government Printing Office, 1977.

*Walker, A. R. P., and D. P. Burkitt. "Colonic Cancer: Hypotheses of Causation, Dietary Prophylaxis and Future Research." *American Journal of Digestive Diseases* 21 (1976): 910–17.

Walker, A., M. R. Zimmerman, and R. E. F. Leakey. "A Possible Case of Hyper-Vitaminosis A in Homo erectus." *Nature* 296 (1982): 248–50.

Watt, B. K., and A. L. Merrill. *Composition of Foods* (Agriculture Handbook No. 8). Washington, DC: United States Department of Agriculture, 1975.

Wilmore, J. H., and B. J. Freund. "Nutritional Enhancement of Athletic Performance." In M. Winick, ed., *Nutrition and Exercise*. New York: Wiley, 1986, pp. 67–97.

Chapter 6: Hunting and Gathering in the Supermarket

*American Cancer Society. "Nutrition and Cancer: Cause and Prevention." *Ca: A Cancer Journal for Clinicians* 34 (1984): 121–26.

Brenner, B. M., T. W. Meyer, and T. H. Hostetter. "Dietary Protein Intake and the Progressive Nature of Kidney Disease." *New England Journal of Medicine* 307 (1982): 652–59.

*Brown, P. J., and M. J. Konner. "An Anthropological Perspective on Obesity." *Annals of the New York Academy of Science* 499 (1987): 29–47.

Duncan, K. H., J. A. Bacon, and R. L. Weinsier. "The Effects of High and Low Energy Density Diets on Satiety, Energy Intake, and Eating Time of Obese and Non-obese Subjects." *American Journal of Clinical Nutrition* 37 (1983): 763–67.

*Eaton, S. B. "Fibre Intake in Prehistoric Times." In A. R. Leeds, ed., *Dietary Fibre Perspectives:* II. London: John Libbey, in press, 1988.

Eichner, E. R. "Alcohol Versus Exercise for Coronary Protection." *American Journal of Medicine* 79 (1985): 231–40.

Gamble, C. S. "Culture and Society in the Upper Paleolithic of Europe." In G. B. Bailey, ed., *Hunter-Gatherer Economy in Prehistory*. Cambridge: Cambridge University Press, 1983, pp. 201–11.

Graham, S. "Alcohol and Breast Cancer." *New England Journal of Medicine* 316 (1987): 1211–13.

Heaney, R. P. "Calcium, Bone Health, and Osteoporosis." *Bone and Mineral Research* 4 (1986): 225–301.

Klevay, L. M. "Hypercholesterolemia in Rats Produced by an Increase in the Ratio of Zinc to Copper Ingested." *American Journal of Clinical Nutrition* 26 (1973): 1060–68.

LaCroix, A. Z., L. A. Mead, K-Y. Liang, C. B. Thomas, and T. A. Pearson. "Coffee Consumption and the Incidence of Coronary Heart Disease." *New England Journal of Medicine* 315 (1986): 977–82.

*McArdle, W. D., F. I. Katch, and V. L. Katch. *Exercise Physiology: Energy, Nutrition, and Human Performance.* 2d ed. Philadelphia: Lea & Febiger, 1986.

Oscai, L. B., and J. O. Holoszy. "Effects of Weight Changes Produced by Exercise, Food Restriction, or Overeating on Body Consumption." *Journal of Clinical Investigation* 48 (1969): 2124–28.

Pavlou, K. N., W. P. Steffee, R. H. Lerman, and B. A. Burrows. "Effects of Dieting and Exercise on Lean Body Mass, Oxygen Uptake, and Strength." *Medical Science, Sports and Exercise* 17 (1985): 466–71.

Simoons, F. J. "Primary Adult Lactose Intolerance and the Milking Habit: A Problem in Biological and Cultural Interrelations." *American Journal of Digestive Diseases* 15 (1970): 695–710.

Stamford, B. "What's the Importance of Percent Body Fat?" *Physician and Sportsmedicine* 15 (1987): 216.

Von Schacky, C. "Prophylaxis of Atherosclerosis with Marine Omega-3 Fatty Acids." *Annals of Internal Medicine* 107 (1987): 890–99.

Wilmsen, E. N. "Seasonal Effects of Dietary Intake on Kalahari." San. *Federation Proc* 37 (1978): 65–72.

Zuti, W. B., and L. A. Golding. "Comparing Diet and Exercise as Weight Reduction Tools." *Physician and Sportsmedicine* 4 (1976): 49–58.

Chapter 7: The First Fitness Formula

Anderson, B., J. E. Beaulieu, W. L. Cornelius, R. H. Dominguez, W. E. Prentice, and L. Wallace. "Flexibility." *National Strength and Conditioning Association Journal* 6 (1984): 10–22, 71–73.

*Åstrand, P-O. "Exercise Physiology and Its Role in Disease Prevention and Rehabilitation." *Archives of Physical Medicine and Rehabilitation* 68 (1987): 305–9.

Ayalon, J., A. Simkin, I. Leichter, and S. Raifman. "Dynamic Bone Loading Exercises for Postmenopausal Women: Effect on the Density of the Distal Radius." *Archives of Physical Medicine and Rehabilitation* 68 (1987): 280–83.

*Balke, B., and C. Snow. "Anthropological and Physiological Observations on Tarahumara Endurance Runners." *American Journal of Physical Anthropology* 23 (1965): 293–98.

*Barnard, J. R. "The Heart Needs Warm-up Time." *Physician and Sportsmedicine* 4 (1976): 40–50.

Carter, J. E. L., and W. H. Phillips. "Structural Changes in Exercising Middle-Aged Males During a 2-Year Period." *Journal of Applied Physiology* 27 (1969): 787–94.

*Casperson, C. J. "Protective Effect of Physical Activity on Coronary Heart Disease." *MMWR* 36 (1987): 426–30.

Dimsdale, J. E., L. H. Hartley, T. Guiney, et al. "Post Exercise Peril: Plasma Catecholamines and Exercise." *Journal of the American Medical Association* 251 (1984): 630–32.

*Eaton, S. B., M. J. Konner, and M. Shostak. "Stone Agers in the Fast Lane: Chronic Degenerative Diseases in Evolutionary Perspective." *American Journal of Medicine* 84 (1988): 739–49.

*Fleck, S. J., and J. E. Falkel. "Value of Resistance Training for the Reduction of Sports Injuries." *Sports Medicine* 3 (1986): 61–68.

Franklin, B. A., E. R. Buskirk, J. Hodgson, et al. "Effects of Physical Conditioning on Cardiorespiratory Function, Body Composition and Serum Lipids in Relatively Normal Weight and Obese Middle-aged Women." *International Journal of Obesity* 3 (1979): 79–109.

Goldberg, L., D. L. Elliot, R. W. Schutz, and F. E. Kloster. "Changes in Lipid and Lipoprotein Levels After Weight Training." *Journal of the American Medical Association* 252 (1984): 504–6.

Jennings, G., L. Nelson, P. Nestel, M. Esler, P. Korner, D. Burton, and J. Bazelmans. "The Effects of Changes in Physical Activity on Major Cardiovascular Risk Factors, Hemodynamics, Sympathetic Function, and Glucose Utilization in Man: A Controlled Study of Four Levels of Activity." *Circulation* 73 (1986): 30–40.

Johnson, C. C., M. H. Stone, A. Lopez-S., J. A. Herbert, L. T. Kilgore, and R. J. Byrd. "Diet and Exercise in Middle-aged Men." *Journal of the American Dietetic Association* 81 (1982): 695–701.

Jurmain, R. D. "Paleoepidemiology of Degenerative Knee Disease." *Medical Anthropology* 1 (1977): 1–24.

*Krolner, B., B. Toft, S. P. Nielsen, and E. Tondevold. "Physical Exercise as Prophylaxis Against Involutional Bone Loss: A Controlled Trial." *Clinical Science* 64 (1983): 541–46.

Larsen, C. S. "Functional Implications of Post Cranial Size Reduction on the Prehistoric Georgia Coast, U.S.A." *Journal of Human Evolution* 10 (1981): 489–502.

Mann, G. V., R. D. Shaffer, and A. Rich. "Physical Fitness and Immunity to Heart Disease in Masai." *Lancet* 2 (1965): 1308–10.

Mazess, R. B. "Bone Mineral in Vilcabamba, Ecuador." *American Journal of Roentgenology* 130 (1978): 671–74.

Nabokov, P. *Indian Running.* Santa Barbara: Capra Press, 1981.

Nimuendaju, C. *The Eastern Timbira.* Berkeley, CA: University Publications in American Archaeology and Ethnology, 1946, pp. 136–43.

*Olson, J. R., and G. R. Hunter. "A Comparison of 1974 and 1984 Player Sizes, and Maximal Strength and Speed Efforts for Division I NCAA Universities." *National Strength and Conditioning Association Journal* 6 (1985): 26–28.

Paffenbarger, R. S., and R. T. Hyde. "Exercise as Protection Against Heart Attack." *New England Journal of Medicine* 302 (1980): 1026–27.

*Paffenbarger, R. S., R. T. Hyde, A. L. Wing, and C.-C. Hsieh. "Physical Activity, All-Cause Mortality, and Longevity of College Alumni." *New England Journal of Medicine* 314 (1986): 605–13.

Plum, P., and J. F. Rehfeld. "Muscular Training for Acute and Chronic Back Pain." *Lancet* 1 (1985): 453–54.

Prescott, W. H. *History of the Conquest of Mexico*. 1843.

Prives, M. G. "Influence of Labor and Sport upon Skeletal Structure in Man." *Anatomical Record* 136 (1960): 261.

Robertshaw, D. "Sweat and Heat Exchange in Man and Other Mammals." *Journal of Human Evolution* 14 (1985): 63–73.

Saltin, M. H., and P-O. Åstrand. "Maximal Oxygen Uptake in Athletes." *Journal of Applied Physiology* 23 (1967): 353–58.

Schneider, S. H., and H. Kanj. "Clinical Aspects of Exercise and Diabetes Mellitus." In M. Winick, ed., *Nutrition and Exercise*. New York: John Wiley, 1986, pp. 45–82.

Skyler, J. "Diabetes and Exercise: Clinical Implications." *Diabetes Care* 2 (1979): 307–11.

Stone, M. H., G. D. Wilson, D. Blessing, et al. "Cardiovascular Responses to Short-term Olympic Style Weight-Training in Young Men." *Journal of Applied Sports Science* 8 (1983): 134–39.

*Thompson, P. D., and J. H. Mitchell. "Exercise and Sudden Death: Protection or Provocation?" *New England Journal of Medicine* 311 (1984): 914–15.

Tipton, C. M., R. D. Matthew, J. A. Maynard, and R. A. Carey. "The Influence of Physical Activity on Ligaments and Tendons." *Medical Science and Sports* 7 (1975): 165–75.

Wathen, D., R. Borden, B. Dunn, et al. "Prevention of Athletic Injuries Through Strength Training and Conditioning." *National Strength and Conditioning Association Journal* 5 (1983): 14–19.

Wheeler, P. E. "The Loss of Functional Body Hair in Man: The Influence of Thermal Environment, Body Form, and Bipedality." *Journal of Human Evolution* 14 (1985): 23–28.

Wiktorsson-Moller, M., B. A. Oberg, J. Ekstrand, and J. Gillquist. "Effects of Warming-up, Massage, and Stretching on Range of Motion and Muscle Strength in the Lower Extremity." *American Journal of Sports Medicine* 2 (1983): 249–52.

Wood, P. D., and W. L. Haskell. "The Effect of Exercise on Plasma High Density Lipoprotein." *Lipids* 14 (1979): 417–27.

Chapter 8: The Natural Child

Arling, G. L., and H. F. Harlow. "Effects of Social Deprivation on Maternal Behavior of Rhesus Monkeys." *Journal of Comparative and Physiological Psychology* 64 (1967): 371–77.

Barry, H., III, and L. Paxson. "Infancy and Early Childhood: Cross-cultural Codes: 2." *Ethnology* 10 (1971).

*Bowlby, J. *Attachment and Loss*. 3 vols. London: Hogarth Press, 1969–77.

Goodall, J. *The Chimpanzees of Gombe: Patterns of Behavior*. Cambridge, MA: Harvard University Press, 1986.

Harlow, H. F. "Age-Mate or Peer Affectional System." In D. Lehrman, R. Hinde, and E. Shaw, eds., *Advances in the Study of Behavior*, vol. 2. New York: Academic Press, 1969.

Kagan, J. *The Nature of the Child*. New York: Basic Books, 1984.

Konner, M. J. "Aspects of the Developmental Ethology of a Foraging People." In N. G. Blurton Jones, ed., *Ethological Studies of Child Behavior*. Cambridge: Cambridge University Press, 1972.

*———. "Evolution of Human Behavior Development." In R. L. Munro, R. Munro, and B. Whiting, eds., *Handbook of Crosscultural Development*. New York: Garland Press, 1981.

———. "Infancy Among the Kalahari Desert San." In P. H. Leiderman, S. Tulkin, and A. Rosenfeld, eds., *Culture and Infancy*. New York: Academic Press, 1977.

*———. "Relations Among Infants and Juveniles in Comparative Perspective." In M. Lewis and L. Rosenblum, eds., *The Origins of Behavior*, vol. 3: *Friendship and Peer Relations*. New York: Wiley, 1975.

*Konner, M. J., and M. J. Shostak. "Adolescent Pregnancy and Childbearing: An Anthropological Perspective." In J. B. Lancaster and B. A. Hamburg, eds., *School-age Pregnancy and Childbearing: Biosocial Dimensions*. New York: Aldine, 1986.

*———. "Timing and Management of Birth Among the !Kung: Biocultural Interaction in Reproductive Adaptation." *Cultural Anthropology* 2 (1987): 11–28.

*Konner, M. J., and C. Worthman. "Nursing Frequency, Gonadal Function and Birth Spacing Among !Kung Hunter-Gatherers." *Science* 207 (1980): 788–91.

Leiderman, P. H., S. R. Tulkin, and A. Rosenfeld, eds. *Culture and Infancy*. New York: Academic Press, 1977.

*Munroe, R. H., R. L. Munroe, and B. B. Whiting. *Handbook of Cross-Cultural Human Development*. Chicago: Garland STPM Press, 1981.

West, M. M., and M. J. Konner. "The Role of the Father: An Anthropological Perspective." In M. Lamb, ed., *The Role of the Father in Child Development*. New York: Wiley, 1976. Revised second edition, 1981.

Whiting, B. B., and J. W. M. Whiting. *Children of Six Cultures: A Psychocultural Analysis*. Cambridge, MA: Harvard University Press, 1975.

Whiting, J. W. M., and I. L. Child. *Child Training and Personality: A Cross-Cultural Study*. New Haven: Yale University Press, 1953.

Chapter 9: Woman the Gatherer

Amoss, P. T., and S. Harrell. *Other Ways of Growing Old: Anthropological Perspectives*. Stanford, CA: Stanford University Press, 1981.

Berndt, C. "Interpretations and 'Facts' in Aboriginal Australia." In F. Dahlberg, ed., *Woman the Gatherer*. New Haven: Yale University Press, 1981.

*Dahlberg, F., ed. *Woman the Gatherer*. New Haven: Yale University Press, 1981.

*Friedl, E. *Women and Men: An Anthropologist's View*. New York: Holt, Rinehart, and Winston, 1975.

Griffin, P. B., and A. Estioko-Griffin, eds. *The Agta of Northeastern Luzon*. Cebu City, Philippines: San Carlos Publications, 1985.

Hausfater, G., and S. B. Hrdy, eds. *Infanticide*. New York: Aldine, 1984.

Holmberg, A. R. *Nomads of the Long Bow: The Siriono of Eastern Bolivia*. Garden City, NY: American Museum of Natural History, Natural History Press, 1969.

Howell, N. *The Demography of the Dobe Area !Kung*. New York: Academic Press, 1979.

*Hrdy, S. B. *The Woman That Never Evolved*. Cambridge, MA: Harvard University Press, 1981.

Hurtado, M., and K. Hill. "The Cuiva: Hunter-Gatherers of Western Venezuela." In *Anthroquest*, Leakey Foundation News, Winter 1986.

Hurtado, M., K. Hawkes, K. Hill, and H. Kaplan. "Female Subsistence Strategies Among Ache Hunter-Gatherers of Eastern Paraguay." *Human Ecology* 13 (1985).

Klein, L. "Tlingit Women and Town Politics." Ph.D. dissertation, New York University, 1975.

*Lee, R. *The !Kung San*. Cambridge: Cambridge University Press, 1979.

*Lee, R., and Irven DeVore. *Man the Hunter*. Chicago: Aldine, 1968.

*Martin, M. K., and B. Voorhies. *Female of the Species*. New York: Columbia University Press, 1975.

*Meltzer, D. *Birth: An Anthology of Ancient Texts, Songs, Prayers, and Stories*. San Francisco: North Point Press, 1981.

Quinn, N. "Anthropological Studies on Women's Status." In Bernard J. Siegel, ed., *Annual Review of Anthropology*. Palo Alto, CA: Annual Reviews, 1977, pp. 181–225.

Scrimshaw, S. "Infanticide in Human Populations: Societal and Individual Concerns." In G. Hausfater and S. B. Hrdy, eds., *Infanticide*. New York: Aldine, 1984.

Sharp, H. "The Null Case: The Chipewyan." In F. Dahlberg, ed., *Woman the Gatherer*. New Haven: Yale University Press, 1981.

*Shostak, M. *Nisa: The Life and Words of a !Kung Woman*. Cambridge, MA: Harvard University Press, 1981; New York: Vintage, 1983.

Turnbull, C. M. *Wayward Servants*. Garden City, NY: Natural History Press, 1965.

Zihlman, A. "Women as Shapers of the Human Adaptation." In F. Dahlberg, ed., *Woman the Gatherer*. New Haven: Yale University Press, 1981.

Chapter 10: The Paleolithic Prescription: Old Ways, New Prospects

Connor, W. E., M. T. Cerqueira, R. W. Connor, R. B. Wallace, M. R. Malinow, and H. R. Casdorph. "The Plasma Lipids, Lipoproteins, and Diet of the Tarahumara Indians of Mexico." *American Journal of Clinical Nutrition* 31 (1978): 1131–42.

*Cooper, K. H. *The Aerobics Way*. New York: Evans, 1977.

"Doctor Downplays Cholesterol as Main Cause of Atherosclerosis." *Atlanta Constitution* (from *New York Times*), April 9, 1987, p. 14A.

Gordon, T., W. P. Castaelli, M. C. Hjortland, et al. "High Density Lipoprotein as a Protective Factor Against Coronary Heart Disease: The Framingham Study." *American Journal of Medicine* 62 (1977): 707–14.

*"Lowering Blood Cholesterol to Prevent Heart Disease." Consensus Conference. *Journal of the American Medical Association* 253 (1985): 2080–86.

McManus, B. M., J. E. Wilson, and W. E. Miller. " 'Normal' Blood Cholesterol Levels." *New England Journal of Medicine* 312 (1985): 51–52.

Tanner, J. M. *Growth at Adolescence*. 2d ed. Oxford: Blackwell, 1962.

White, P. D. "The Historical Background of Angina Pectoris." *Modern Concepts of Cardiovascular Disease* 43 (1974): 109–12.

*Williams, R. R., S. J. Hasstedt, D. E. Wilson, K. O. Ash, F. F. Yanowitz, G. E. Reiber, and H. Kuida. "Evidence That Men with Familial Hypercholesterolemia Can Avoid Early Coronary Death." *Journal of the American Medical Association* 255 (1986): 219–24.

Index

300